DESTROYING SANCTUARY

Destroying Sanctuary

The Crisis in Human Service Delivery Systems

Sandra L. Bloom, MD
Brian Farragher, LCSW, MBA

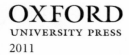

OXFORD
UNIVERSITY PRESS
2011

OXFORD
UNIVERSITY PRESS

Oxford University Press, Inc., publishes works that further
Oxford University's objective of excellence
in research, scholarship, and education.

Oxford New York
Auckland   Cape Town   Dar es Salaam   Hong Kong   Karachi
Kuala Lumpur   Madrid   Melbourne   Mexico City   Nairobi
New Delhi   Shanghai   Taipei   Toronto

With offices in
Argentina   Austria   Brazil   Chile   Czech Republic   France   Greece
Guatemala   Hungary   Italy   Japan   Poland   Portugal   Singapore
South Korea   Switzerland   Thailand   Turkey   Ukraine   Vietnam

Published by Oxford University Press, Inc.
198 Madison Avenue, New York, New York 10016
www.oup.com

Oxford is a registered trademark of Oxford University Press

Library of Congress Cataloging-in-Publication Data
Bloom, Sandra L., 1948–
Destroying sanctuary : the crisis in human service delivery systems / by Sandra L. Bloom,
Brain Farragher.
p. cm.
Includes bibliographical references and index.
ISBN 978-0-19-537480-3
1. Mental health services—United States. 2. Social services—
United States. I. Farragher, Brain J. II. Title.
RA790.6.B65 2011
362.1—dc22
2010012021

9 8 7 6 5 4 3

Printed in the United States of America
on acid-free paper

This book is dedicated to the administrators, managers, direct and indirect care staff in our healthcare, mental health, and social services who, every day, are willing to take on the emotional labor of doing whatever they can do to relieve the suffering of those in their care.

*The world is a daycare center and we are each given
some toys to play with.*

Roy Stern, M.D.

Contents

Preface

Looking back over the last 40 years, I can truthfully say that I know a great deal about the stresses and strains of starting, working in, managing, closing, then starting again and again and again, mental health programs. I began this work in the 1960s as a psychiatric department secretary and then a mental health technician. From the 1970s through 2001, I went to medical school, trained as a psychiatrist, ran five renditions of our inpatient psychiatric treatment program, managed an outpatient practice, maintained a large inpatient and outpatient private psychotherapy practice, chaired a department, owned a business, supervised professional and nonprofessional staff, and became a novice researcher. In this most recent decade I have become a writer, a teacher, and a consultant to almost every kind of social service delivery program for children, adolescents, and adults.

This book is a direct outcome of that varied experience and my passionate regard for the people who do the kind of work we do, trying as best we can, for as long as we can, to relieve the suffering of others. I know how difficult it is to provide social service work, and I know how frequently our services fail to measure up to the standards of critics or of ourselves. In 1997, my first book, *Creating Sanctuary: Toward the Evolution of Sane Societies*, was published. It described the intellectual and emotional journey of a team of mental health providers, colleagues, and friends, who happened upon the knowledge that most of the people they were treating as inpatients, and as outpatients, had been exposed to significant adversity usually beginning in childhood [1]. That adversity had changed them, had played a determining role in their cognitive, emotional, behavioral, social, and moral problems. As we wrestled with this new information, their exposure to adversity and all that went along with it changed us as well. We experienced a shift in our paradigm for viewing ourselves, other people, and the world around us. In the Introduction to that book, I said that my worldview had *"changed almost entirely as a result of what I have learned about what happens to human beings who are exposed to overwhelming stress"* (p. 13). That shift was best captured by one of my colleagues, Joe Foderaro, when he noted that we seemed to have changed the foundational question asked of troubled people, *"What's wrong with you?"* to the very different question, *"What happened to you?"* (p. 476) [2].

When I wrote that book I knew that our core values were radically diverging from the evolving values of the overarching U.S. health care system because what has become known as managed care was shifting the emphasis from what we considered quality care to profitable care. As this happened, patients stopped being the customer. Instead the customer became the largely for-profit managed care companies that became the middle managers between the service delivery programs and the insurance companies. Under these conditions, psychiatric beds were eliminated and the competition for filling the beds became more intense. The result was that specialty programs were no longer encouraged, and although we continued to be a profitable venture for the hospitals where we were located, it became possible to fill the hospital beds without having to hire specialists. I also think that the work we were doing, creating what has since been termed a "trauma-informed culture" was too disturbing, too challenging of existing mental models at a time of overwhelming adjustment and change for the systems we worked within. Thus, the program I described in that first book, moved to a new hospital in 1996, moved again in 1999 and divided into two separate programs, and we ultimately decided to close the program in 2001 rather than face the degradation and humiliation of slow and strangulating program demise.

Toward the end of that first book, I described work that still had to be done, as I saw it at that time. I noted that our program was struggling to survive under increasingly dismal conditions for the delivery of human services. I described a status quo of cutbacks in spending on programs and personnel in mental health, an almost exclusive focus on biological treatments, and significant decreases in the ability to provide psychotherapy and social therapy. As an organizational leader, I had also discovered that the greatest source of stress to leaders does not usually derive from internal problems—at least not at first—but from dealing with the world outside. *"We learned that the health of our system would always be limited by the health of the systems within which we were embedded"* (p. 182) [1] .

At that time, my main motivation for writing the book was memorializing an experience that I believed was drawing to a close. I believed that our work meant little if it remained the product of a unique group of personalities working in a specific place during a specific time. For me, writing that book was the beginning of a grieving process, a letting go of what had been the purpose of my life up to that point: treating adults as a psychiatrist on an inpatient unit and following many of those same people in long-term psychotherapy. But it was also a message in a bottle that I launched out into the ocean of information and hoped that someone, someday would pick up, read, and use.

To my surprise, the ocean of information was not as vast or impersonal as I had imagined. People did begin to respond to the message I had launched into the world even before the World Wide Web was much of a force. By that time, I had been winding down my clinical psychiatric practice and had begun consulting to and training a wide variety of mental health and other mental health, social service, and health care programs in what it means to help very traumatized people. I had the opportunity to interact with people working in inpatient and outpatient mental health programs for children and adults, domestic violence shelters, homeless shelters, emergency rooms, medical schools, health clinics, home visitation programs, HIV programs, child protection services, substance abuse facilities, and others. In traveling all around the country and internationally, I began to see the universal nature of the system problems that I had personally experienced in moving our program five times in 10 years.

Gradually I came to recognize that organizations are alive, and that as individuals, we can become very closely identified with the organizations that we join. I watched an organization come alive and learned what it meant to feed it, nurture it, revel in its successes, and suffer heartache when it failed. I learned what it is like to spring to the defense of a program when it is attacked, and to lose your own personal certainty and safety in the face of organizational demands. I discovered what it is like to face up to and face down a wide variety of leadership experiences that test one's inner strengths, fortitude, self-awareness, emotional intelligence, and beliefs. I witnessed the conflict over divided loyalties when sometimes people defended their organization instead of protecting the people in their care. And I had come to understand what it is like to mourn a system when it dies.

In the late 1990s, I had the opportunity to start a relationship with the Jewish Board of Children and Family Services (JBFCS) in New York to implement what we had started and I had written about—The Sanctuary® Model—in children's residential services. We obtained a grant from the National Institute of Mental Health to study the process of implementation, and this resulted in some significant positive changes that have led the Sanctuary Model to become an "evidence-supported" practice.

In 2000 I began consulting with the Julia Dyckman Andrus Memorial Center, or as it is more familiarly known, Andrus Children's Center. It was there that I met Brian Farragher and started a collaboration that has led to the development of the Sanctuary Institute, an outcome I never imagined in 1997 when the book about our experiences was published. Now I know what it looks like as organizations gradually, painfully, and sometimes traumatically transform themselves into something they were not born to be and as leaders within these organizations find themselves as excited, invigorated, and exhausted as any new mother. As of this writing, over 100 programs—residential and acute care mental health facilities for children and adults, substance abuse programs for adolescents and adults, homeless shelters, an urban child welfare program, an academic program, private hospitals and state hospitals, an insurance company, domestic violence shelters, and juvenile justice facilities, from coast to coast, across the Atlantic and the Pacific—have been through our Sanctuary Institute training and have become part of the Sanctuary Network.

This growing network of interconnected programs is setting new standards for what it truly means to have "trauma-informed" care for a wide variety of children and adults who have experienced repetitive exposure to adversity and trauma. Hundreds of administrators and thousands of clinicians and front-line workers are endeavoring to discover the keys to expanding democratic workplace practices, improving the quality of care, achieving better outcomes for the clients and better workplace environments for themselves, and transforming their systems to meet the needs of the twenty-first century.

I would like to express my gratitude to the Board of Trustees, the staff, and the administrators at Andrus Children's Center, and most of all to Nancy Ment, Brian Farragher, Sarah Yanosy, Lorelei Vargas and the entire faculty of the Sanctuary Institute for their unswavering support and commitment. None of us envisioned over ten years ago, that the Sanctuary Institute would be the good news of the beginning of this century. I am also very grateful to all of the state agencies, funding organizations, administrators, and staff members who are participating in the Sanctuary Network. They struggle with the issues we describe in these chapters, every day, often foregoing their own needs and desires to help the children and adults in their care. I also would like to thank Maggie Bennington-Davis and Tim Murphy as well as Kathy Wellbank and Cynthia Figueroa, and Judy Dogin who by their efforts helped me to believe that teaching this work to other programs was indeed possible.

In addition to my work with the Sanctuary Institute, I serve on the faculty of the Drexel University School of Public Health and am Co-Director with Dr. John Rich and Dr. Ted Corbin, of the Center for Nonviolence and Social Justice. Along with Linda Rich, Ann Wilson, Dionne Delgado, and our other staff members, we have the opportunity to explore what it means to view violence as a public health problem instead of simply an individual problem and put into practice some ideas about prevention. I am grateful to Dean Marla Gold, Dr. Arthur Evans, Director of Behavioral Health for the City of Philadelphia, and to Joe Pyle and the Scattergood Foundation for their continuing support of our work.

My mentor, who taught me all about how goofy systems can be a very long time ago, Dr. Roy Stern, says he doesn't remember saying what I wrote down as the epigraph of the book, but that may speak to how much we are both mis-remembering as we age—I know he said it! But I haven't misremembered the love and support from my parents, Dorothy and Charles Treen, and am grateful that I have been lucky enough to share most of my Dad's 95 years with him.

Whatever wisdom resides within these pages has been cultivated through interaction with many people over the years but most importantly, Joe Foderaro, RuthAnn Ryan, Beverly Haas, Lyndra Bills, Liz Kuh, Carol Tracy and. I am grateful for their continued laughter, friendship and support.

This book is about what happens to human service programs under the impact of unrelenting stress and multiple losses. At the urging of my colleague, Dr. Lyndra Bills, who has been "along for the ride" with me for the last 17 years, we have titled it *Destroying Sanctuary: The Crisis in Human Service Delivery Systems* because that is what has been happening for the last several decades. The important places of refuge—of sanctuary—for the most injured among us are in great jeopardy and are being destroyed. Never perfect places of safety in the first place, many mental health systems, health care systems, and social service programs of every size, shape, and variety are collapsing under over 30 years of system fragmentation even while public costs have escalated dramatically.

This book is the first of two volumes. In it we describe the problems we are facing and some causes for those problems. The next volume, *Restoring Sanctuary: A New Operating System for Trauma-Informed Organizations*, will describe what we have learned about the elements necessary for creating safe and healing organizational cultures in the world we live in today. Taken together, *Creating Sanctuary*, *Destroying Sanctuary*, and *Restoring Sanctuary* represent the cycle of life, at least mine so far. Throughout these past 40 years, although the rate of change in almost everything has become increasingly rapid, there is one thing that has not changed at all about the human race and that is the need for Sanctuary.

Sandra L. Bloom, MD

By 2000 the staff and administration at Andrus Children's Center had been intensively working on reducing the amount of restraints of children in our residential facility and exploring the outer dimensions of what it means to have a "trauma-informed system" for several years. When we at Andrus met Dr. Bloom and her team, we recognized our shared strengths and weaknesses and how we could complement each other. As a pioneer in applying a psychobiological understanding of traumatic experience to adults who had been abused as children, Dr. Sandy Bloom already had 20 years of experience in specially designed inpatient and outpatient treatment programs to treat psychological trauma and had consulted in a wide variety of other settings. I had extensive experience in the residential treatment of children and in management and had just become Chief Operating Officer at Andrus and had been the Campus Director at Andrus for approximately 6 years.

After many discussions, our Sanctuary process actually took off in the summer of 2001, so very early in the process we were confronted with the attacks of September 11th. The Andrus Children's Center is located in Yonkers, New York, just north of Manhattan so some people in the first Core Team lost close friends and family members. My brother Tom, is a New York City Firefighter as were many of the people I grew up with in Rockaway Beach. All of us were stunned and shocked by the images we saw nightly on the television, and we all had our sense of safety and security shaken in a major way. However, these events provided us with a powerful experiential learning opportunity about the nature of trauma and the impact it had on each of us. We talked about how it was hard to concentrate, to sleep, how irritable some of us were. These events were imprinted on our minds, and many of us will never look at a clear blue sky in the same way or hear a plane flying over head without thinking about that day. It became easier to imagine what life might be like for children who have had daily experiences of shock, betrayal, loss, or devastation. These events changed how we looked at the world, how we looked at each other, and how we looked at the kids.

Our collaboration has led to the development of the Sanctuary Institute, a training program for organizations who have the dedication and commitment (and some would say, the sheer madness) to engage in system change during difficult times. This book represents a snapshot of what we have learned to this point about the stresses and strains of trying our best to create healing environments for very injured children, adolescents, and their families.

Our hope in writing this book and in creating the Sanctuary Institute and the Sanctuary Network is that we can create a critical mass of people who can and will begin to push back. Let's face it: we know what is happening and why things are going in this wrong direction. It's not just about good and evil—it is about understanding how people and systems react under stress and being able to use this knowledge to think about how we can get better results in spite of the fact that we are under a great deal of pressure, stress, and strain ourselves. For most of the programs and systems we work with, this process is not like moving a sailboat, it's like moving the largest ship in the world and it takes time, practice, and getting a lot of people onboard. But if we can do it, we know other people can, too.

Meanwhile, I want to thank Nancy Ment, our C.E.O for being my partner in this venture all along the way and all of the people at Andrus: the staff, the management, the Board, and the kids and their families, who have taught me and inspired me for a very long time. Most of all I want to thank my very patient wife, Ann, and my kids, Brian and Katie, for their love and support. Without them, nothing works for me.

Brian Farragher, LCSW, MBA

Prologue: October 1996

Background

The narrative below is taken from material written by the management team of an adult inpatient, acute care mental health program in October 1996. The original Sanctuary® program, specializing in treating adults who had exposed to severe adversity as children in an acute care psychiatric setting, lasted for 10 years following the previous decade of development. This narrative was written at almost the precise halfway point in the life of that program. We had already treated several thousand trauma survivors and would treat several thousand more before we closed. I (Sandy) was in the middle of writing a book about the profound experiences that my colleagues and I had encountered along this journey of becoming "trauma-informed" and that book would be published the next year under the title, *Creating Sanctuary: Toward the Evolution of Sane Societies* [1].

All of our patients had very complex problems, co-occurring disorders, and comorbid physical conditions. They suffered from depression, various shades of psychosis, dissociative disorders, phobias, panic states, and other forms of anxiety. Their personalities had been skewed by the developmental impact of childhood adversity in a wide variety of ways. Many of them had experienced adult trauma as well as childhood adversity—everything from severe gunshot injuries, to domestic violence, to sexual assault, and even one truck driver who had the misfortune to be driving through Oklahoma City in 1995 at the time of the bombing. We treated people who were well-educated middle-class professionals, and we treated people who had grown up in extreme poverty who had very little education at all. We treated people with criminal histories, and we treated Philadelphia policemen who had been severely injured on the job and had posttraumatic stress disorder. We saw Vietnam veterans, Holocaust survivors, one alleged contract killer in his twilight years, and one madam of a "house of ill repute."

At the time when this report was made, we had just been forced to move the program from a for-profit hospital in the suburbs of Philadelphia, to a more urban, nonprofit hospital. Three members of this team, however, had been together for 16 years at this point, doing inpatient work that had evolved into The Sanctuary. The Sanctuary program itself would survive for 5 more years and would need to move again in 1999, split into two separate programs, and finally close in 2001. The situation we had left was ideal, during a very good era for the development of innovative services in private mental health settings. This account reflects our difficulties in adjusting to a new, and less welcoming, environment, in a not-for-profit hospital that was struggling to survive in an ever-more "managed" environment. On this particular day, the management team for *The Sanctuary* met from noon to five o'clock on Friday, October 25, 1996 to discuss the current situation on the unit and make recommendations for change. In attendance were all three Sanctuary psychiatrists, the Director of Social Work, the Clinical Coordinator, three creative therapists, two social workers, two primary therapists, the head nurse, and a social work student. The following is a summary of the retreat written immediately afterwards based on notes recording each person's comments. We believe these notes present a shared personal and collective background for this book.

Sanctuary Retreat, October 25, 1996

The most pervasive complaints voiced by everyone relate to problems with the pace of treatment and space constraints in our present physical setting. Last year we averaged 1.28 admissions a day. Since moving here the number of admissions has risen by 65%. At the same time the length of stay has decreased from an average length of stay of 14 days down to 9.8 days, a 30% drop that is predicted to continue to go lower [the length of stay did go down to 5 days].

The results of this dramatic and sudden increase in pace are manifold, dynamic, and interactive. We are accustomed to having frequent close communication between all members of the treatment team. We attribute much of our success to this level of communication, which has always provided a web of connection and support. Basically, we have always have had a "safety net" around our program that is invisible but very strong. It's really why we can contain people who are doing and saying dangerous things without locking anybody in, because that safety net keeps everyone safe. We stop dangerous things from happening before they happen because we know when something is wrong. It is unlikely that any patients will "fall through the cracks" and be ignored because every patient is connected to a number of people on the team and through those relationships connected to the entire team and the rest of the community—just like in a real web. Various members of the treatment team can get to know important aspects of each patient and then the information can be pooled in an efficient manner so that each patient's problems can be understood and explored in depth.

But our staffing pattern was designed to meet the treatment needs of a maximum of 22 patients, when our average occupancy was around 80%, meaning that periods of a full census would be interspersed with periods of a lower census. It's like having a weekend to do your laundry, change the sheets, clean the house, and go food shopping in the sense that during the down period the treatment team could catch up on all the things we don't get time to do when the myriad details of

running a good program—completing medical records, returning phone calls, pro-
gram development, program evaluation, quality assurance, training, and supervi-
sion. These periods also provided an opportunity for the staff to emotionally refuel,
reconnect with each other, debrief from the very high level of stress entailed
in intensively treating victims of trauma, share new learning, and intellectually
integrate the overall experience.

In our present situation we are operating 24 beds at 100%+ capacity (some-
times the administration puts extra beds in the hallway). In addition to this,
whenever an empty bed becomes available the hospital is using our unit to board
other patients who should not be—and don't want to be—on a specialty trauma
program. Not only does this increase the demands on us because their nursing
needs are no different than anyone else, but it creates unnecessary conflict on the
unit because neither they nor their doctors have to follow our program rules and it
interferes with the normal development of a sense of community. It would be like
having a classroom of fifth graders and suddenly you just plop in some kids from
another class who sit at unfilled desks but actually go somewhere else for all their
classes. It's a situation that breeds trouble because they never have the chance to
adopt the norms of the community. In addition, because of present admission pol-
icies in the managed care environment, the patients who are admitted tend to have
a much higher level of acuity. The increased rate of turnover means that it is more
difficult for a community to form and have the "older" patients help orient the
"newer" patients, formerly a powerful socialization tool. The physicians for these
patients, who don't know anything about how we approach treatment, are often
working at cross purposes to the goals of the program, and that requires more team
time as we debate what to do in trying to resolve what are actually deep philo-
sophical issues about treatment, like when the physician on the case believes that
the person's memories of abuse are just attempts at manipulation or when he has
administered so many drugs that the patient cannot even think or worse, becomes
disinhibited.

Since so much of our sense of safety is dependent on the maintenance of our
social safety net which depends on communication among all team members, there
is a constant state of stress and worry about the patients who do want to be there
and come specifically for treatment at The Sanctuary. We all feel a pervasive sense
of guilt and inadequacy over our ability to give the patients what they need in ever-
shortening lengths of time. There is no recognition that we deal with extremely
traumatized patients with very complex problems. Questions arise as to how decades
of mistrust can be overcome in a week, how years of trauma bonding and traumatic
reenactment behavior can be undone in 10 days time, how 5 days can provide
enough time for even the most elemental development of a contract for safety in
someone who is severely self-abusive. As the physicians and the hospital try desper-
ately to survive as viable entities in what feels like an impossible and abusive
system, punishment coming from some quarter seems to be increasingly common.

Such daily stresses raise important questions about meaning, purpose, priorities, and values that are unanswerable and often directly contradict our stated beliefs and values that are the core of our philosophical premises. Everyone is feeling increasingly helpless in the face of these changes that we have had no part in making and which undermine the recovery of our patients. Repeatedly questioning their own potential hypocrisy in preaching a philosophy of care and compassionate concern while being forced to practice in a seemingly cold-hearted and calculated fashion, the staff members are being confronted daily with complicated moral dilemmas that force them to choose only between evils, never the good.

In addition, since coming here we have lost our social workers to virtually all clinical involvement. Formerly, they were the bedrock of the program, providing the interconnecting "glue" for all aspects of the patients' care, including team meetings, regular meetings and groups with the patients, meetings with referral sources, and family therapy sessions. But at this facility the social workers have taken over the functions of case managers and quality assurance. At least 80% of their time is now consumed by inputting data into the computer, talking to insurance reviewers, spending vast amounts of time listening to "Musak" while on hold with these insurance companies, speaking to various other institutions, and supervising discharge plans. The institution is depending on these case managers to protect the hospital from what are becoming routine abuses of the managed care system. Any failure of protection is viewed as a personal failure of the social worker; the social worker gets blamed when patient days are refused so that the hospital will not get paid. These are jobs that the social workers are neither trained for nor ever wanted and are vastly different than the jobs they had come to love and for which they had developed a high level of skill. In a period of 3 months they have gone from being extremely capable, valued, connected, and fulfilled professionals to feeling like harried secretaries and isolated bureaucrats. Not only has this left the social workers unhappy and discouraged, but this has left a dramatic hole in our clinical programming and in our communication safety net because they just aren't available. This results in an increased workload on everyone else's part, less family contact, less communication with referral sources and with the patients.

This is compounded by the significant loss of the ability to obtain thorough psychological testing on any of our patients. We used to be able to include a deep assessment which often quickly surfaced critical problems such as underlying psychotic thinking, potential neurological dysfunction, and as yet unseen personality traits and vulnerabilities but insurers will no longer pay for psychological testing. As physicians, this is infuriating—it would be like not allowing radiologists to use their machines!

To make it even worse, we were not permitted to bring our trained nurses with us when we came here, so we have had to train the staff in the Sanctuary Model ourselves. This would be fine except for the fact that since arriving at this hospital we have had difficulty establishing a stable nursing pool, so people keep showing up who do not know us, do not know our patients, and do not know our program. The nurses themselves have been very supportive and cooperative but need more training in our treatment model for them to be effective, and yet there is no time for such training to occur. Every second is accounted for, even "double-booked," making teaching a luxury that we cannot afford and yet cannot afford to do without, producing yet another cycle of helpless frustration. In addition, the constant, uncontrollable, threatening, and often irrational interface with insurance companies is sometimes simply unbearable. It seems like there is a crisis everyday and the level of stress is growing exponentially, but not from the patients. They just want some help overcoming their problems. But they are definitely negatively affected by our frustration and stress: it's contagious.

As a result of all this, there is never a moment's respite for the treatment team. What we call secondary traumatic stress is increasing on the part of the staff. Free-floating anxiety, chronic feelings of anger, fear, depression, guilt, and loss are admitted to by everyone, and people are feeling the pressure not just at work but at home with increased marital, relational, and parenting discord. There has also been an increase in physical symptoms and actual episodes of physical and emotional illness on the part of staff members. Since our staff members universally pride themselves on their commitment to the patients and see this commitment not just in professional, but in moral and even spiritual terms, they so far have refused to compromise on the quality of care.

Since time cannot be manufactured, the result is a serious infringement on personal time, which further contributes to burnout. It is not unusual for both physicians to be still present on the unit until 11 p.m. after beginning work early in the morning. At our previous unit, some of the pressure on the physicians was relieved by a call schedule that included our primary therapists who were nurses. Until we arrived, we were unaware that the bylaws at this hospital were quite different and that the primary therapists would not be permitted to do the admission evaluations they had been doing for years because of the completely unrealistic regulations of managed care. As a result, our physicians are frequently required to work 7 days a week on alternate weeks, since they must be available on Saturdays for admissions. They must be present, even though the primary therapist is present on the unit, since only a physician can sign the history forms, not because there is any immediate medical necessity.

There is simply no time for the preventative and restorative activities that help make this work possible without damaging health. Most importantly, perhaps, there is no time for the mutual debriefing that formerly was the primary defense against compassion fatigue. We are doing trauma work. We are engaging with several dozen people every day who have the most disturbing histories imaginable, all of them leave and new people come in within days, and the process starts again. It's heartbreaking because we know we can help people recover, but we need time, *space, and emotional energy to do that. As one staff member put it, "There is not even any time for tears."*

Despite being overcrowded with people, there is a sense of complete alienation and disconnection from others, a sense of having no permanent sense of belonging and feelings of pervasive isolation and loneliness, all attributed to the extreme time constraints, multiple demands, and lack of control over external factors that bear directly on internal management. The staff is highly competent and yet the sheer volume of work is producing inefficiency and a general feeling of fear secondary to sensing that things are "falling through the cracks," that it is impossible to keep up, that disaster is always somehow imminent.

Rounds are held three times a week, but many times now we do not even know who the patients are if the Sanctuary doctors are not treating them, and other than the Sanctuary physicians, the attending doctors rarely come to the team meetings or participate in treatment. The time constraints mean that there is virtually no flexibility in the system. What each person does or doesn't do has an even larger impact on everyone else since the system is built to be tightly interconnected. When an unexpected medical problem arises, when the nurses are delayed in distributing medications, when patients arrive late from lunch, when the groups do not end immediately on time, then the entire schedule is disrupted, causing reverberating stress on every aspect of the system. Tempers shorten, frustration increases, stress soars, even from the slightest shift in timing, shifts that in real life and real time are inevitable.

Space is a chronic stressor. The unit we presently occupy is very poorly equipped for group functioning or for team treatment due to serious design flaws. One room was put together to provide for a staff room, but the number of phones ringing and beepers going off makes for a deafening level of inescapable noise. There is very little personal space and no place to gather in comfort or quiet. The nursing station is far away from the patient rooms. The main lounge that is used for group meetings is invariably oppressively hot. There is no boundary between the patient space and the nursing station, so confidentiality is constantly breached and there is no privacy in this critical area between staff and patients as a result of an extremely poor architectural design. Part of the unit is structured to be a locked intensive care unit, but when we are forced to utilize this space for this purpose, we are forced to further compromise our nursing staff since additional nursing staff are rarely, if ever, provided. We have always had unlocked doors and programmatically emphasize freedom from coercion as a basic treatment approach. But the hospital pressures us constantly to lock the doors of our program, which is in direct conflict with our professional and treatment philosophy and undermines the very goals of the program.

The fatigue is compounded by problems related to interfacing with a large, long-standing, stressed bureaucracy. Our treatment team is accustomed to a high degree of autonomous decision making, innovation, and problem solving that is not encouraged in the present system. There is a feeling among the team, that our work is undervalued, our philosophical principles poorly understood, and our boundaries not respected. The demands of the bureaucracy often appear to defy rational common sense and good care, but they are insisted upon even if time for patient care is sacrificed. There is little sense of being in control while having a continuing strong sense of being responsible for all that goes on, a situation that breeds helpless rage. Admissions appear on the unit regularly without any screening from the management team—an experience that was formerly unheard of and is extremely detrimental to good unit management. Any innovation requires a seemingly endless series of meetings and levels of permission before it can be implemented. There is redundancy built into the system that results in needless paperwork and more wasted time when there is no time to be wasted. In our conversations, over and over again, the issue of lack of control arose about every area of care from who gets admitted to the unit to the temperature of the front lounge, to who gets to interrupt any meeting by paging, to staff physicians who repeatedly refuse to cooperate with community norms...

Introduction: January 2010

Some months ago we were in a meeting in which a group of providers were talking about services to children in the child welfare system and the need to reduce or eliminate stays in residential treatment programs. It seemed that we were talking about the child welfare system as though it were a conveyor belt and its role was to deliver its kids, who sounded a lot like inventory, to the right place at the right time. The intention seemed to be to run the tightest ship in the shipping business. But what always seems to get lost in these conversations is that we are talking about *kids*—small people with flesh and blood, developing brains, and the potential to be almost anything, good or bad. Both of us were lucky; we had families, safe schools, stable neighborhoods, and an absence of violence in our lives. The kids we serve are coming to us after their fifth failed foster home placement, their sixth family, their sixth school, and their sixth community. They generally arrive with all of their worldly possessions in two or three large, black garbage bags. No family pictures, no trophies, no certificates of merit, and no real hope that things are going to be much better at this next placement. Many of them are children of color and their lives bear witness to the legacy of racism. The adults we serve have been beaten down by their experiences as children, often multigenerational experiences of poverty, abuse, neglect, discrimination, illness, and despair.

Regardless of what we do or where we work, we all need to begin by accepting the plain and repeatedly studied truth that the vast majority of the people we work with have been psychologically and socially injured. To help them it is crucial that we fully understand the nature of those injuries and the impact those injuries have had on their lives. But in the past, it has been very easy not to ask these questions or to ignore the responses, or over time just to forget the story. It is easy to forget just how much who we are today is shaped by where we come from and what we have experienced. It is hard to listen to the stories of profound injury day in and day out, whether they are being told with words or actions, while at the same time it is relatively easy over time to become hardened and calloused by these stories filled with sadness, trauma, and loss.

Because we all have our own stories, their stories sometimes come far too close to our own pain. We have found that the reason why we do not explore these stories more is not because it is too hard for our clients but because it is too hard for us.

Sanctuary

A sanctuary is a place of refuge from danger, threat, injury, and fear. It has been recognized since ancient times—and scientific research has validated—that for physical and emotional healing to occur, people need such a protected space in order to allow time, healers, and the natural powers of recovery to work their magic. In reviewing large numbers of studies that have looked at therapeutic outcomes, largely in mental health settings, what the client brings into a help-seeking environment accounts for about 40% of the outcome. But the other 60% of influence is determined by what helpers do and don't do within helping environments: the ability of a helper to be empathic, warm, and nonjudgmental accounts for a whopping 30% of influence, offering hope for about 15%, and providing people with an explanation for their difficulties and a method for resolving those difficulties accounts for about another 15% of outcome [3]. So a place that is a sanctuary for people who need help is one where the staff members are warm, caring, hopeful, have a clear theory and method for change, and are willing to deal with the problems that the clients bring into their doors.

This book is titled *Destroying Sanctuary* because it describes the multitude of ways that organizations and systems originally designed to afford injured people a healing refuge have instead become factories of neglect and abuse. One of the thoughtful people who reviewed this book before publication did not like the title we gave because the person did not believe that mental health programs—or presumably any of our social services—had ever actually been sanctuaries. Although never close to perfect, both of us—and many of our colleagues—remember a time when it was possible to provide more of a shelter than it is now, a time when well-intentioned, well-trained, and committed practitioners in every area of social service delivery and health care were able to feel that their work was valued and important, that they had control over the quality of service they provided, and that it was possible to "do no harm." Both of us have worked in helping environments where staff members of all educational backgrounds were well educated in theory, were able to use that theory to inform what they did, were hopeful about the capacity of their clients to heal, and were themselves warm, communicative, responsible, disciplined, nonjudgmental, and caring.

But for the reasons described in the Prologue—and detailed in this book— many people who work in health care, mental health, and social services do not feel that way today. Contradictory theories and methods abound with little time for integrating complex and conflicting ideas about human nature and human problems. Frustrated beyond measure, many who work in these settings have become inured to suffering, angry, punitive, avoidant, and despairing. Many function in their jobs day to day without really feeling much hope that their work is making a difference in anyone's life. They are challenged to create any sanctuary for their clients, and they do not feel they have any for themselves.

We do not believe that this outcome has ever been the intention of anyone managing or working in these systems. Rather, we believe it is the insidious result of an all-encompassing mental model and system of beliefs that promote a mechanistic view of care giving systems, the devaluation of those who choose to do emotional labor and who work with vulnerable populations of people in any and all of the social services, the dehumanization of anyone who cannot compete successfully in a cut-throat economic climate inappropriate for the delivery of quality human services, a culture that is more enamored of sex and violence than of love, and the universal impact of chronic stress and repetitive trauma that results. Our radical antidote to the moral deterioration that is the result of these insidious forces we call the Sanctuary Model. We will briefly describe what we mean by that at the end of this volume. A fuller description will be our next volume in which we explore *Restoring Sanctuary: A New Operating System for Trauma-Informed Organizations.*

"Aha" Experiences for Health and Human Services

One objective in writing this book is to offer our colleagues a different, expanded conceptual framework—a language, a way of thinking—about their clients, their organizations, their managers, and themselves. We hope that as you read this you have many "aha" moments that are at the heart of insight, epiphany, and creativity. Those moments occur when suddenly ideas come together, integrate and become a cohesive whole and you see into a problem in a way you never have before. Whether we are talking about individual trauma survivors or traumatized systems, these "aha" moments are the starting point for healing and recovery. They prepare us to move down entirely different pathways in our minds and in our actions and that means we stop ending up in exactly the places where we started and instead we begin to explore new possibilities.

We think this is vitally important for the simple reason that our care giving organizations are struggling and are suffering themselves. Over the last 30 years it has become increasingly difficult to deliver adequate services to the people most in need of them, and this has caused an untold amount of stress and moral distress that is felt at individual, organizational, and systemic levels. The end point of this disarray is that our services are, to a great extend, ineffective and this book explains the complex reasons behind the multiple ways in which good intentions go wildly astray.

Just an explanatory note: for those who have not worked in human services, the way we sometimes interchangeably use various words to describe components of the human service system may be confusing. We are aiming this book at the entire health and human service sector, but we often interchangeably discuss health care, mental health care, and social services or refer to them generically as human service delivery systems. Most of the concrete examples we use are from adult and child mental health care service delivery simply because that is the arena where most of our work has occurred. However, we draw additionally on our experience working with child welfare agencies; homeless shelters; medical hospitals; psychiatric hospitals for children and for adults; domestic violence shelters and programs; children's hospitals; substance abuse facilities; HIV prevention programs; faith-based support programs; juvenile and adult criminal justice systems; inpatient and outpatient services, community-based services, and virtually every component of the human service delivery network.

It is not a coincidence that beginning in 1980, the federal department in charge of everything from care of the physically and mentally ill, to substance abuse treatment, to child welfare and homeless services, to the Centers for Disease Control and the Public Health Service came under the jurisdiction of the Department of Health and Human Services (HHS). This structure designates an understanding that all human services dedicated to the HHS motto of "improving the health, safety and well-being of America" are interrelated and interdependent. That is our position in this book—that the problems that currently beset health care service delivery are mirrored in mental health care service delivery, substance abuse treatment, child welfare, services for the homeless and the poor, domestic violence services, and any other services devoted to improving the well-being of American citizens. And that this vast, interconnected network, so vital to the public health of the nation, represents both national success and national failure.

Systems in Crisis: The Impact of Biological Reductionism

A friend and change agent herself, lawyer Carol Tracy, once shared a quote about system change from a former Provost of the University of Pennsylvania, now the President of the Carnegie Corporation, Dr. Vartan Gregorian. She paraphrased a remark he made about system change, that *"In order to change a system you have to be either a loving critic or a critical lover."* In this book we have taken that admonition to heart and applied it to the human service delivery system. Over the last three decades we have watched a disturbing series of events unfold within the social service network that for us constitutes largely a disintegration of many components of this system. The result of this disintegration is what many officials now are calling "a crisis" in service delivery. Certainly widespread economic forces like managed care have been a major determining factor in creating this crisis, but predatory financial behavior can only occur in an environment that is already philosophically and morally weakened.

When we began working in the human services arena, we learned that there was an intimate relationship between the individual who showed dysfunctional behavior of some sort and the context within which the individual lived and breathed. This context extended in concentric, interactive, and permeable circles around the individual outward and included family, community, nation, and world. We were taught that to help someone, it was important to understand that person's unique position within those concentric circles and the multiplicity of interacting influences that could be determining his or her behavior. We learned that human beings are profoundly divided and that we all have a conscious *and* an unconscious life. We live partly in the light and partly in the shadows.

Throughout a period loosely running from the 1950s through the beginning of the 1990s, and frequently outside of state institutions, in private and non-profit clinical settings, as long as the customer was the client, there was an incentive to find methods that would deliver effective therapeutic services to the client. Innovations in mental health treatment have always been behind, and in many ways the stepchild of, general medicine. The technology that has advanced medicine has done relatively little to help us understand the complicated workings of the human psyche. But during this period, clinicians began experimenting with innovative methods for achieving significant gains in a time frame less onerous than that of the lengthy, expensive, and time-consuming methodology of psychoanalysis, while not losing the profound insights derived from a psychodynamic understanding of human systems. Innovation, spurred by the new knowledge about combat trauma, disaster trauma, child abuse and domestic violence, blossomed in what is still a young field of endeavor compared to other branches of medicine—traumatic stress studies [4].

Then, beginning about 30 years ago as the political climate became increasingly punitive, authoritarian, and "conservative" (perhaps less properly termed conservative than radically right wing), and a variety of pressures began to change the face of human service delivery so that in many ways it is unrecognizable today as the same system that existed two or three decades ago. The growing interest in the biological and genetic causes of mental disorder began to exclusively dominate the psychiatric field—what we refer to here as "biological reductionism." Various influences served to fuel deinstitutionalization resulting in the loss of many institutional settings for study and research and the shifting of 24/7 care to short-term, intensely "medical model," pharmaceutically driven psychiatric care. Innovation in many non-biological therapeutic methods within the mental health system virtually ceased when the customer ceased being the client and became instead the middle managers of insurance companies and the organizations they created or hired, a system known as "managed care."

System Degradation: Systems in Crisis

What we now find in health, mental health, and social service settings around the country is profoundly disturbing. In many different kinds of programs something is dreadfully wrong. The post-World War II spirit of extraordinary hope and belief in progress in all human affairs, even among the most disordered in our society, has given way to a passivity and pessimism. The belief in the "common good" and our individual responsibility to contribute to that common good has been eroded. The result is a cynicism and hopelessness about the clients our systems are supposed to serve. The clients haven't really changed very much, but the providers of care and entire systems of care have changed profoundly.

As a result, over the last few decades, serious problems within all of these systems have been accumulating and compounding insidiously. As historians have explored, the science of mind and body integration was in its infancy during the tumultuous 17th century when influential men like philosopher René Descartes turned over the body to physicians and the mind to the clergy and philosophers [5]. This remains the situation today, despite the fact that an enormous amount of mental health treatment is provided by primary care physicians and social services by religious organizations. Clients present at the doors of mental health and social service programs seeking remedy for their problems, but they often leave with few solutions and sometimes with even more difficulties than they brought with them. Staff in many treatment programs suffer physical and psychological injuries at alarming rates, become demoralized and hostile, and their counter-aggressive responses to the aggression in their clients create punitive environments. Leaders become variously perplexed, overwhelmed, ineffective, authoritarian, or avoidant as they struggle to satisfy the demands of their superiors, to control their subordinates, and to protect their clients. When professional staff and nonprofessionally trained staff gather together in an attempt to formulate an approach to complex problems, they are not on the same page because they lack a common theoretical framework that informs problem solving. Without a shared way of understanding the problem, what passes as treatment is little more than labeling, the prescription of medication, and behavioral "management." When troubled clients fail to respond to these measures, they are labeled again, given more diagnoses, and termed "resistant to treatment."

Meantime, the system grinds on, people go to work, and caregivers do the best they can. Caregivers frequently change jobs in search of a better place to work, while longtime workers become profoundly demoralized. Clients do not get the benefit they could and should be receiving. Managed care companies, recognizing the disarray, seek simple solutions by funding only "evidence-based practices" that selectively endorse only forms of interventions that meet medical standards of proof of efficacy. As important as it is to be able to show that what we do is effective, the present emphasis on a very narrow range of evidence-based practices allows people to ignore the long-established fact that most forms of psychotherapeutic interventions are effective as long as several key factors are present, most importantly, safe relationships and hope. At the same time, few programs actually hold themselves accountable for results that are based on whether or not the client has improved. Instead, they are often accountable only to productivity demands, budgetary requirements, and the completion of paperwork.

As is always the case when individual financial gain supersedes social welfare, the public system has been the most profoundly affected by these changes. It is still possible for wealthy and some upper middle class patients to seek out therapeutic interventions from knowledgeable and systems-informed therapists. But even for them, if they must be hospitalized, they are unlikely to have anything resembling the kinds of therapeutic experiences offered in years past, although the disassembling of the state hospital systems has also virtually guaranteed that no one will experience any form of inpatient care for more than a few days.

As a society, we have done a terrible job of taking care of our children, and we seem to have no sense that our failure to care for our kids has really long legs. As a result of a series of decisions, many of which have been made because of increasing financial pressures, we may have lost a whole generation of children and families. Our justice system is exploding because we have not done a good job with these men and women from the very beginning. There is no sense of foresight that each dollar we cut out of education, children's mental health, child welfare, housing, Head Start, and other programs that support the vulnerable, young, and oppressed will likely cost us thousands of dollars down the road. Politically-based decisions are made with very short-term goals in mind but the problems that are left unaddressed have very long legs that reach far out into the future. Our failure to address our front end has left us crushed under the back-end results.

From what we have seen, it has become evident that there is no quick fix. We need an entirely different way of thinking about, planning, and addressing our current problems. We need new "mental models" and a multitude of "aha" moments.

New Mental Models

Mental models are deeply held assumptions. They are so deeply held and operating outside of our individual awareness that we don't even realize the role these assumptions are playing in determining what we think, feel, and do. Our mental models are activated when we observe the exact same event as someone else but describe it—or experience it—in entirely different ways. As you read this book, we challenge you to think about your own mental models.

At least two different mental models, each of which has a number of component parts, presently exist in our organizational world. We describe these as *Organizations as Machines* vs. *Organizations as Living Beings*. These two categories are themselves misleading because, as you will see in our description, no person, organization, or society falls neatly into our idealized category; rather, each exists somewhere along a continuum. We believe that over the last few decades, the human service delivery system can be described more like a machine than as a living organism delivering complex services to living individuals and families.

Organization as Machine

The mental model that has dominated group life—and therefore individual existence—for the last several hundred years views organizations as machines that operate more or less like clocks with interchangeable parts, lacking feelings, able to perform their function without conflict—regular, predictable, ordered, and controlled [6]. In the model of system as machine, individuals are cogs in the organizational machine, functioning independently and competing with other individuals for survival. And each organization is itself a machine that is embedded within a larger mechanistic view of society that includes local, county, state, and federal component parts. Organizations can become dysfunctional and fixing them requires external expertise and some form of top-down social engineering.

Organization as Living Being

It was not until the 1940s that mechanistic thinking began to broadly change, and this overly simplistic view of how organizations work became much more complex. The hallmark of all living systems is interratedness and interdependence and an understanding of these characteristics became known as "general systems theory" [7]. A system can be defined as a set of interrelated elements that respond predictably and interact with each other consistently over time. As a result, change at any one point will eventually have an impact on the total system and its component parts [8]. Another characteristic of living systems is "emergence," which occurs when the whole is greater than the sum of the parts. For example, in your body, organs emerge from combinations of cells, and an organization's collective identity emerges out of the combined individual identities of everyone within the organization.

Living beings have both conscious and unconscious processes. For a living organism to be consciously aware, all the time, of everything that is going on to sustain life would require brain power not available to individuals or organizations. So over time, and in the course of development, much activity that may have at one point been conscious, deliberate, and strategic, takes on a kind of life of its own, outside of conscious awareness. The longer an organization has been in operation the more likely it is that much of what occurs in the organizational culture is happening at the level of unconscious norms and basic assumptions, built on mental models that are completely out of view. Any challenges to these basic assumptions—which provide our individual and shared organizational minds with stability and security—are likely to give rise to anxiety and to "social defense mechanisms" that we will discuss in Chapter 4.

In this book, we make the case that instead of being seen as living systems, chronic and unrelenting stress has had and continues to have extremely detrimental effects on the overall functioning of the health and human services. Toxic stress—the strong, unrelieved activation of the body's stress management system—has destructive impacts on the social body just as it does the individual body. As a consequence of this toxic stress, individual workers within the organizations, as well as managers and leaders of organizations and of systems, are likely to become more primitive, inflexible, aggressive, authoritarian, and punitive and therefore unable to grapple with the level of complexity that characterizes every organization. *Destroying Sanctuary* describes the long-term, toxic effects of treating living systems as if they were emotionless machines. The next volume, *Restoring Sanctuary,* now in preparation will describe the ways in which living systems—families, groups, organizations, systems, and societies—can begin restoring themselves to health.

Thinking About Operating Systems: A Useful Metaphor

We believe these two categories—machines versus living beings—represent two very different ways of viewing ourselves, other people, our organizations, and the world around us. We will use an everyday analogy to mediate between the two conceptual frameworks: the computer.

Computers are machines, yet scientists are on the verge of integrating the components of these machines into human bodies and are using living systems as models to improve machines, a field known as *bionics*. Until recently *androids,* synthetic organisms designed to look and act like human beings, and *cyborgs,* beings that are partly organic and partly mechanical, have been relegated to the world of science fiction. But there is now global competition to produce robots that are increasingly like living beings, modeled on the way living systems work.

Hardware, Software, and Operating Systems

Computers and people have hardware and software. Hardware in a computer includes microchips, hard drives, input devices, and a "motherboard." People have hardware that includes our DNA, genes, cells, and all of our organs, including our brains. But neither computers nor people really can do anything without software programming. There are basically two kinds of software: foundation software and application software.

In a computer, the foundation software is called an "operating system," a master program that controls a computer's basic functions and allows other programs to run on a computer *if* they are compatible with that operating system. Examples of operating systems include Microsoft Corporation's various versions of "Windows," Apple's Mac OS, and the –open source operating system Linux. All the things that a computer can do such as word processing, photography programs, and spreadsheets are all "application software." In order to function properly the application software must be compatible with the operating system.

Like people, computers can get "sick." A computer virus is a small piece of software that piggybacks onto real programs. Each time the program runs, the virus has a chance to spread and to wreak havoc on the entire computer. Computer viruses masquerade as other things and are transmitted through personal contact. They are hard to diagnosis, difficult to treat, malevolent, and contagious. They may lie dormant for years and then attack the system. As anyone knows whose life space has been violated by a computer virus, they represent a form of violence since they are created with the intention of doing harm to others. Now let's use these basic concepts and apply them to human beings.

The Human Operating System and the Virus That Disrupts It

Over the last few decades, research on the nature of attachment relationships has made clear that for human beings, healthy attachment is a fundamental requirement for physical, emotional, social, and moral development. We understand attachment as the basic "operating system" for individuals. Without an attachment relationship in early development, people cannot become fully human. As the grandfather of attachment studies, John Bowlby pointed out, we remain attached to others from cradle to grave.

During this same period there has also been the emergence of a different way of viewing the impact of traumatic experience and prolonged exposure to adversity, particularly in childhood. Trauma theory brings context back to human services without denying the importance of the biological discoveries of the last several decades; instead, it integrates those discoveries into a more comprehensive understanding of human beings.

Exposure to trauma, toxic stress, and severe adversity disrupts the human attachment system in a wide variety of ways. Such disruption can wreck havoc on the "applications" we use to adapt to the world, such as learning, emotional management, and memory. Trauma and sustained adversity do to the human operating system what a computer virus does to a computer. The problems that result are complex and interrelated, which is why people with a history of exposure to trauma and adversity often are carrying around three, four, or five different diagnoses and are taking at least that many medications.

If people are to heal from sustained exposure to adversity and traumatic experience, then we need to shift the usual level of focus on treatment approaches or the "applications," to a deeper level. We need to figure out how to promote change in their "operating system," what we commonly call their "personality."

Over the last few decades the growth in knowledge of two interrelated fields of study—disrupted attachment and trauma—when combined, offer us a different paradigm for defining what we mean by "treatment". For people who have suffered complex exposure to trauma and adversity, deep, structural personality shifts have occurred—trauma-organized shifts in the individual's "operating system"[9]. People with these very complex disorders are the same people who populate our mental health, substance abuse, child welfare, and criminal justice systems. If they are to heal, they must experience a new trajectory of experience that shifts their personalities, changes their operating system, and changes their brains.

This change can begin when clinicians start exploring new possibilities and in doing so come to believe that significant alteration in deep structure is achievable. This internal shift may keep them from resorting to the more routine explanations that afford little hope of reasonably rapid alteration in personality structure. The second major change is in implementing the complex, holistic, integrated, trauma-informed, attachment-based, organizational approaches that are necessary for such alterations to occur and proving that they can. The third major change is in convincing policy makers that funding such intervention and treatment approaches is worth it and the earlier in a person's life that intervention occurs, the bigger "bang for the buck" the society will achieve. The secondary or collateral costs of failing to address these individual and family problems early in their development is socially and economically staggering and rather than minimizing treatment, we should be radically increasing effective approaches, including primary prevention efforts directed at young children and their families in an effort to forestall the inevitably greater need for increasingly expensive secondary and tertiary forms of prevention and intervention.

Organizational Culture: The Organizational Operating System

Like computers and people, organizations also have operating systems. The operating system for the organization is embedded within the organizational culture. Organizational culture arises spontaneously whenever groups of people come together for any length of time and focus on tasks long enough to create common traditions, rites, and history. It is binding in that it determines how people enter the organization, survive within it, and learn to solve problems.

As we will learn in future chapters, there are close and interactive relationships between individual identity and organizational identity. The organizational culture has both conscious and unconscious components and both elements get transmitted to new organizational members. Their ability to translate these elements—to read and respond to the "visible and the invisible group"—determines whether they are able to survive in the organization [8; 10].

We believe that the current operating system for the human service delivery system is outdated, mechanistic, and inappropriate to human health and well-being. This helps to explain why there are so many chronic clashes between our organizations and the living individuals who entirely comprise them. In order to adequately address the needs of the traumatized clients who fill the ranks of our trauma-organized human service delivery system, we need a new operating system—what is being referred to now as a "trauma-informed" operating system—for human service delivery organizations. Just as attachment is the basis of the individual operating system, social relationships are the basis of organizational functioning as well. We believe that in a parallel way, traumatic experience and adversity can profoundly disrupt the operating systems of organizations. We believe that the current mechanistic model of organizational functioning is a result of destructive and potentially lethal *parallel processes* secondary to chronic stress that have created a seriously flawed operating system for human service organizations and entire systems.

Organizational Stress, Parallel Process, and Trauma-Organized Systems

The issue of organizational stress turns out to be particularly salient for anyone involved in delivering human services. It is possible to imagine that car batteries, vacuum cleaner parts, and cushion covers could still be produced, even if everyone in each factory is under considerable stress. But there is no easy way to define the "product" that comes out of human service delivery organizations. People come to social service programs seeking "help" and when they get what they came for, that goal has been achieved through human relationships, not a factory production line.

Organizations, like individuals, can be traumatized, and the result of traumatic experience can be as devastating for organizations as it is for individuals. The outcome of a traumatic experience will be in part determined by the pre-traumatic level of organizational health and integrity. We believe that at this point, our social service network is functioning as a *trauma-organized system* still largely unaware of the multiple ways in which its adaptation to chronic stress has created a state of dysfunction that in some cases virtually prohibits the recovery of the individual clients who are the source of its underlying and original mission, and damages many of the people who work within it.

Just as the encroachment of trauma into the life of an individual client is an insidious process that turns the past into a nightmare, the present into a repetitive cycle of reenactment, and the future into a terminal illness, the impact of chronic strain on an organization is insidious. As seemingly logical reactions to difficult situations pile upon each other, no one is able to truly perceive the fundamentally skewed and post-traumatic basic assumptions upon which that logic is built. As an earthquake can cause the foundations of a building to become unstable, even while the building still stands, apparently intact, so too does chronic repetitive stress or sudden traumatic stress destabilize the cognitive and affective foundations of shared meaning that is necessary for a group to function and stay whole.

Our emphasis on changing organizational operating systems so that they become trauma-informed systems is so important because we now recognize that most of the clients who require services in the human service delivery system are survivors of overwhelming life experiences and multiple kinds of adversity. Decades of clinical experience and previous research have demonstrated that creating a *trauma-informed culture* in and of itself could help staff and clients make better recoveries than has previously been possible. It also provides the necessary context for implementing *trauma-specific treatment* approaches.

A Word About Vocabulary

Now is a good point to clarify the terminology we use so frequently in the upcoming chapters. In this book we refer to "chronic stress," "toxic stress" "adversity," "trauma," "dissociation," "disrupted attachment," "acute stress disorder (ASD)," "posttraumatic stress disorder (PTSD)" and "complex PTSD" (also sometimes called "developmental trauma disorder"). But are these words interchangeable? No, they are not interchangeable, but they are related.

Stress as we use it in this book refers to the pressure that life exerts on us and to the way this pressure affects us. Thus, stress is both external and internal, and the effects of stress on our minds, bodies, and behavior can be positive or negative—or both [11]. The stress response is built in to our mammalian makeup and is a basic survival response, just like eating, sleeping, and reproducing are basic to survival. By chronic stress we refer to the fact that there are many situations in modern life that stimulate the physiological survival response, even when survival—in the moment—is not at stake. As mammals, our bodies and minds are adapted to experience a survival threat, respond with the stress response, take survival-based action, and then either recover or be killed. We are not designed to live with the chronic arousal of these basic survival responses.

Toxic stress is another word for chronic stress, generally applied to the prolonged experiences of exposure to adverse conditions that occur in childhood when the body's stress management resources are overused and overtaxed. It is now well established that such experiences can be damaging to children's brains and bodies, rather like a toxic chemical [12].

Adversity can be defined as a state, condition, or instance of serious or continued difficulty or adverse fortune that implies that the person who experiences adversity is under conditions of chronic stress, but it is also true that individuals vary greatly in their response to adversity. Children often experience adverse experiences, sometimes for many years of their childhood, and as we will see later, there are indicators that this exposure can have very detrimental effects on the body, mind, and spirit. However, it is also true that the capacity to "bounce back" from adversity, also known as "resilience," may be a response to adverse childhood experiences. For many survivors, resilient strategies and maladaptive coping skills are interlaced and occur simultaneously.

A *traumatic event* has been defined in many ways, but our favorite definition is one that explains that a traumatic event is one that overwhelms the person's internal and external resources that enable him or her to cope with an external threat [13]. Traumatic events that are experienced directly include, but are not limited to, military combat, violent personal assault (sexual assault, physical attack, robbery, mugging), being kidnapped, being taken hostage, terrorist attack, torture, incarceration as a prisoner of war or in a concentration camp, natural or human made disasters, severe automobile accidents, or being diagnosed with a life-threatening illness. For children, sexually traumatic events may include developmentally inappropriate sexual experiences without threatened or actual violence or injury. Many people believe that there are also events like threats to one's safety or the safety of others, sexual harassment, and various manifestations of psychological abuse that can also be defined as traumatic.

Witnessed events include, but are not limited to, observing the serious injury or unnatural death of another person due to violent assault, accident, war, or disaster or unexpectedly witnessing a dead body or body parts. Events experienced by others that are learned about include, but are not limited to, violent personal assault, serious accident, or serious injury experienced by a family member or a close friend; learning about the sudden, unexpected death of a family member or a close friend; or learning that one's child has a life-threatening disease.

Dissociation is an automatic mental response that involves a failure to integrate or associate information and experience in the way our minds usually are able to do. Dissociation appears to be a central part of many traumatic experiences and is viewed by some as a "state"—a special type of consciousness that we all have access to under normal and traumatic conditions—and by others as a "trait," that is, a characteristic quality or property of an individual that may be heritable. There is still debate in the field about exactly what dissociation is and how important it is in understanding PTSD, but for now, a useful way of thinking about these differences is as "normal dissociation," meaning dissociation that is not associated with maladaptive response, and "pathological dissociation" that is maladaptive [14–16].

After a traumatic event, most people experience "*acute stress*" and if they come to medical attention may be diagnosed with "*acute stress disorder*," which by definition must occur within 4 weeks of the traumatic event and be resolved within that 4-week period. Calling this a "disorder" may be a bit of a stretch, since so many people experience this after an overwhelming event, but not everyone.

According to *The Diagnostic and Statistical Manual* (*DSM-IV-TR*), published by the American Psychiatric Association and regarded as the standard for diagnoses, if acute stress-related symptoms persist for longer than a month, then a person is suffering from *post-traumatic stress disorder* or *PTSD*. If so, the person has experienced or witnessed a traumatic event, is suffering from intrusive reexperiences, such as nightmares and flashbacks, actively avoids encountering reminders of the traumatic event, and experiences symptoms of increased physiological arousal [17].

Because of the vital importance of attachment behavior for human survival, traumatic experience is associated with *disrupted attachment*—a disruption in the ability to trust and feel safe with other people. The experience of disrupted attachment can occur at any age, but it is well established that disrupted attachment in childhood is a major source of *toxic stress* and a wide variety of long-lasting negative consequences for the developing child and the adult he or she becomes [18–21].

Complex PTSD or *developmental trauma disorder* as of this writing are not yet officially considered diagnoses as defined by the American Psychiatric Association. Nonetheless, people working in this field believe it is necessary to understand the very complex changes in a person's body, mind, identity, personality, relationships with others, ability to differentiate right from wrong, and meaning-making that may be the result of exposure to toxic stress and disrupted attachment beginning in childhood, or to chronic, severe interpersonal violence that occurs at any age [22–25].

This book focuses on the crisis in the human service delivery system. The most difficult clients, with the greatest degree of complexity and who are the most challenging to all health and human service delivery environments, are those who have a history of exposure to adversity, toxic stress, and trauma. At the same time, the people who work in these organizations may have experienced traumatic events themselves and many will have experienced adversity as children. And the organization as a whole often has in its history some terrible events that have occurred. But for the most part, it is not the traumatic events themselves that cause the systematic dysfunction that we will describe in the upcoming chapters. It is instead caused by chronic stress that is the context within which many traumatic events occur and that is the result of the attempts to address a traumatic event unsuccessfully. When we are talking about the conditions of the workers and the workplace in this book, and referring to whole organizations, an actual traumatic event is likely to be only one of the causes of the problems we describe here. It may have been the incident that triggered a response after years of tolerating toxic organizational environments.

Chapter Summaries

The goal of this book is a practical one: to provide the beginnings of a coherent framework for organizational staff and leaders to more effectively provide trauma-informed care for their clients by becoming *trauma-sensitive* themselves. This means becoming sensitive to the ways in which managers, staff, groups, and systems are impacted by individual and collective exposure to overwhelming stress. But most research about organizational dynamics and the process of change is not to be found in the mental health literature or in most health and social service training programs. For that, we must look to the worlds of business, management, organizational development, and communication, and little of this knowledge seems to have found its way into clinical or social service settings in the last few decades.

Our task has been to integrate a wide survey of existing knowledge of organizational dynamics with our understanding and experience in human service delivery environments. We hope that this expansion in knowledge will ultimately improve clinical outcomes, increase staff satisfaction and health, increase leadership competence, and enable human service delivery systems to develop an advanced technology for creating and sustaining healthier systems. We believe that a shift in mental models is a critical first step in enabling the mental health system and its "sister" social service systems to make a more effective contribution to the healing of traumatized children, adults, and families and therefore contribute in a positive way to the overall health of the nation.

The book is divided into 12 chapters. In *Chapter 1: Human Service Organizations: Dead or Alive?* we expand on the idea of organizations as living beings, not machines. Treating a living system as a machine may be useful in the short term but creates significant long-term, sometimes disastrous problems as we are seeing today throughout the human service field as each service sector decries the current, imminent, or future crisis in workforce development, in service delivery, in mission fulfillment, and in funding. Applying an economic mental model that applies to making "things" and believing the same principles will apply to delivering services to human beings can cause insurmountable obstacles to good care. We do not need to empathize with machines, but human beings require empathic regard in order to heal. To address these crises, we need to look at some basic mental model conflicts that exist between our economic system and human service delivery systems. To do this, we will briefly look at our current health care insurance system (pre-health care reform)and use the mental health system as an example of one component of human service delivery that represents a "system under siege."

Most people may not recognize that stress has become a major risk for a wide variety of health and mental health problems, although when surveyed most people talk passionately about the stress they confront at work. Nowhere is that more true than in human services. *Chapter 2: Workplace Stress as a Threat to Public Health* focuses on workplace stress in general and specifically around the kinds of stressors and the sources of the stress that most impact human service delivery workers, including the collective risks of working in social services.

The backbone and scientific underpinning of our work as applied to individuals, families, organizations, and communities is trauma theory—all that has been gathered in the last 30 or so years about the complex biopsychosocial impact of toxic stress on people and systems. The purpose of *Chapter 3: When Terror Becomes a Way of Life* is to summarize what trauma theory means for the way we understand each other and the groups we create.

In *Chapter 4: Parallel Processes and Trauma-Organized Systems*, we discuss what we mean by "sanctuary trauma" and the ways in which organizations are designed to help us achieve tasks that are both conscious and unconscious, giving rise to powerful and largely unconscious social defense systems that become problematic under conditions of chronic stress. As a result, parallel processes emerge in which organizational problems can mirror the problems in the clients, and continue to unfold as our organizations begin to buckle under the influence of toxic stress. This chapter outlines these parallel processes that are individually covered in subsequent chapters, so readers that need the short-hand version of what is to come should focus on this chapter.

In *Chapter 5: Lack of Safety: Recurrent Stress and Organizational Hyperarousal*, we describe how acute crisis often leads to chronic states of organizational crisis and organizational hyperarousal. We look at the impact of workplace violence and the loss of social immunity that occurs when unrelenting stress occurs in system of care.

Emotional intelligence is finally recognized as an important component of any workplace environment that hopes to be productive and healthy. *Chapter 6: Loss of Emotional Management* explores what happens when emotional intelligence is slow to develop because of fear, recurrent crisis, and the group contagion of distress. We also explore the notion of "emotional labor" as an undervalued but vital component of caring work, the fears that accompany change and the role that conflict and conflict management plays in organizational health and dysfunction.

The next chapter, *Chapter 7: Organizational Learning Disabilities and Organizational Amnesia* has a wide focus, covering many of the cognitive problems that are secondary to chronic organizational stress, including problems with organizational learning, organizational memory, and decision-making abilities. Stressed groups are frequently unwilling to perceive and discuss problems that the group denies and are more likely to actively and dangerously silence dissent.

Chapter 8: Miscommunication, Conflict, and Organizational Alexithymia discusses the multiple communication problems that arise normally among groups of people and that are exacerbated under the impact of recurrent stress. Here we review the notion of "undiscussability" and how that leads to alexithymia at an organizational level—the inability of groups of people to talk about the feelings that are destructively influencing organizational function. Without the ability to discuss vital subjects, the organizational grapevine becomes poisoned, conflict compounds, and without adequate communication, collective disturbances emerge that, if not stopped, will lead to violence.

Rarely does the subject of power—who has it, who doesn't, and how it is used and abused—come up for open discussion in social service environments and yet it is a critical component of any organizational setting. In *Chapter 9: Authoritarianism, Disempowerment, and Learned Helplessness*, we discuss research findings on learned helplessness, authoritarianism, and risk avoidance and how likely these are to increase under stress and crisis, but how detrimental these approaches are in solving complex dilemmas. Increases in authoritarianism among leaders produce increases in helplessness and decreases in performance in staff. Although this has long been recognized, true efforts to implement workplace democracy have often become forms of bogus empowerment and bullies are given license to intimidate other people.

The notion that "punishment works" is simply taken for granted as true, as part of our existing mental model for dealing with other people. Here we ask whether punishment actually is effective and under what conditions. In *Chapter 10: Punishment, Revenge, and Organizational Injustice*, we recognize that human beings who believe they have been treated unfairly quite naturally seek revenge, and we tie that to manifestations of organizational injustice and how employees deal with perceived injustice. We also look at the powerful influences that people exert on each other to do good or to do harm.

Because the existing mental model for organizations is based on notions of rationality, control, and social engineering, the human reactions to loss of attachments is given little recognition. Nonetheless, loss, grief, and traumatic loss have become commonplace components of human service environments. All change involves loss, but without an ability to acknowledge, honor, and work through repetitive loss, organizations are likely to develop ever-increasing problems and a powerful tendency to repeat ineffective strategies. This reenactment behavior can ultimately lead to decline and even organizational death. *Chapter 11: Unresolved Grief, Reenactment, and Decline* deals with these issues at length, including the disturbing idea that the broader society may have unconsciously set up the social service sectors to actually be successful failures.

The final chapter, *Chapter 12: Restoring Sanctuary: Organizations as Living, Complex Adaptive Social Systems*, offers a brief introduction to what we consider a parallel process of recovery: The Sanctuary Model. The Sanctuary Model offers an evidence-supported trauma-informed theory and methodology for changing organizational cultures. We will only touch on the main components of the model here and explore the subject in more depth in the next volume of this work.

A Cautionary Note

Please do not be surprised if you find the content of this book disturbing. Another of our reviewers suggested that we provide the reader with a "disclaimer warning" because the content is "blunt, provocative, and requires courage on the part of the reader." We have both lived with and in the situations we describe for so long that what we describe in this book no longer seems remarkable. This book is meant to disturb the state of perplexed, helpless bewilderment that most people who work in the human service delivery professions are currently in. As you read this, it is easy to get hopeless, it is easy to feel helpless, and it is easy to retreat and just protect what little you have from what sometimes feels like "the hordes" at the door. It is also possible to just rail against "those people" however we define "them," who we believe are doing us in. It is quite another thing to be thoughtful and rational, considerate and civil. We believe that this is easier to do when you know you are not alone—that the problems you perceive in your workplace are happening everywhere. As of the beginning of 2010, we have trained over a hundred programs across the United States and in several other countries in the Sanctuary Model and we can assure you that you are definitely not alone. We believe it is easier to be thoughtful and rational, considerate and civil in groups and in communities. We believe in Benjamin Franklin's advice to his colleagues of the Continental Congress of 1776, when those enlightened revolutionaries were daring to speak Truth to Power and were about to sign the Declaration of Independence, "*We must, indeed, all hang together, or most assuredly we shall all hang separately.*"

The ultimate goal of our work is to individually make the changes in our own lives and together, to make the changes in our systems in order to create the energy and power to take action on a larger scale. We know that it is possible to *Create Sanctuary* if a group of people have the shared will, commitment, drive, and vision to do so. It isn't rocket science, but it is hard work. We know because we have been doing that work for decades.

We hope this book helps others to transform their own organizational cultures so that what emerges is a critical mass of people to create a tipping point to a new culture more supportive of life, growth, development, and peace. We feel an urgency about this. As a species, we don't have much time left if we keep going down the path we are on. The Earth is getting smaller and its people grow hungrier every day. This is the only Earth we have, and we are in great danger of losing our true Sanctuary forever. It is time for creation and restoration. It's time for us to recognize that our organizations, our systems, our governments, and our societies are living beings, comprised of living beings. We need to begin figuring out what that means and creating some new structures and some new rules for helping living systems to stay alive, grow, thrive, and be self-sustaining. We will be fulfilled if this work makes even a small contribution to that larger effort.

Chapter 1

Human Service Organizations: Dead or Alive?

SUMMARY: *Mental models are the largely unconscious ideas and beliefs that structure what we think about—and what we do not consider. Mental models represent mental shortcuts and limitations. In this chapter we look at the mental models that shape our organizations, especially health care and human service delivery environments. Looking through the lens of mental models enables us to see the ethical conflicts that lie at the heart of many caring environments today. We then focus the lens on the mental health system and discuss the ways in which the chronic and disabling conditions that affect the mental health system represent a "system under siege."*

The Case of the Separated Garbage

If you have ever worked in, lived in, or needed help from an organization, then you know that organizations have a "mind of their own" and can be as contrary as any individual human being. This is because organizations, like individuals, are alive. The Julia Dyckman Andrus Memorial Center was founded by John Andrus as a memorial to his wife, Julia, in the early part of the twentieth century. Julia had herself been an orphan and creating a beautiful place in the country where orphaned children could grow up, be educated, and thrive was the founding dream [26]. In those days, Andrus was a working farm with apple orchards, cornfields, cows, pigs, and sheep. When Brian Farragher arrived in 1986 as a cottage supervisor, all that was left of the farm were the apple and peach trees.

Children lived in the original cottages that had been built for them and staff served them meals in a family dining room. At that time, the practice of the cottage staff was to use two separate garbage pails in the kitchen. The larger of the two containers was used for trash. Things like wrappers, napkins, empty containers, and such were thrown in this receptacle (this is long before recycling started). The smaller of the two containers was used for food scraps that were not eaten by the children and staff. Everyone would scrape his or her plate into the smaller pail under the sink and throw other items into the larger pail.

23

All the staff who worked in the cottage were adamant about the importance of maintaining this process correctly, and children were chided and disciplined when they put paper in with the food or food in with the paper. There was a significant commitment to this entire procedure.

Each day the maintenance staff would come to each cottage and pick up the refuse from both pails, grabbing the bags from each one, tying them off, and carrying them out. In his role of cottage supervisor, Brian had an explanation for the two garbage pails in his own mind that for awhile went unquestioned. At the time, there was a large cooler in the maintenance barn where apples from the orchard were stored through the winter months. He just assumed that the maintenance staff were keeping the garbage in the cooler during the summer months to reduce the smell. He was completely off base about that, but his own rationalization kept him from questioning the process earlier. This was the way it was when he arrived, and he simply assumed there was some logical rationale. It took about 2 years on the job, but then circumstances of supply and demand got Brian to question the entrenched policy—and his own assumptions.

For those of you who have not worked in a residential program, it may not be common knowledge that there are certain supplies that are provided to cottages in great abundance and others that are always scarce. At Andrus, bread and condiments are never in short supply. It is not unusual to end a week with four or five loaves of unused bread. Nor is it uncommon to end a month with 20 jars of hot sauce. But plastic garbage bags are always in short supply. Garbage bags then as now were like gold. There were never enough and it was impossible to pry more out of the food service staff. It was this garbage bag shortage that led to cracking the mystery of the separated garbage.

In an effort to see if the garbage bag ration could be stretched, Brian began to pay closer attention to the management of garbage. He watched as the maintenance men would pick up the two bags of garbage each day, throw both bags into the waiting truck, and move on to the next cottage, seemingly without any attempt to keep the now unidentifiable food garbage separate from the other trash.

Finally, one day Brian grabbed the maintenance foreman and asked him about the whole separate garbage bag story. The maintenance foremen, Bob Peters, had grown up on the campus, spent time in the military, and had come back to work at Andrus as a young adult. In all, he had spent almost 40 years on the grounds and Brian figured he would be his best key informant. As it turned out, Mr. Peters was the person to ask.

He told Brian that in the days when Andrus was still a working farm, the food scraps were segregated because the scraps were used to slop the hogs. Well, the hogs had left the campus in the mid-seventies and no one had seen a pig or anything resembling a pig since. It was now 1989, 12 to 15 years since anyone had seen a scrap-eater on the campus and people were still putting a plate aside for them.

The next day Brian announced that garbage segregation was over. Seemingly, this would solve the problem. But this was not the case; staff and children continued to do what they had always done—separating trash from scraps—and in doing so they were wasting precious garbage bags. After about 4 weeks of repeatedly telling everyone to use only one garbage pail, Brian finally took action and removed the small scrap pail from the kitchen and threw it out (a pail that was older than Brian). This seemed to be the first real signal for the staff that they could now comingle the garbage and would not get into any trouble for doing so! Brian remembers being struck by the oddity in how organizations deal with memory. The memory of the pigs on the farm was lost, but the behavior involved in caring for the pigs was still present in the system. Until those two pieces of memory could be brought back together, resistance to change was inevitable.

Mental Models Shape Our World

This story illustrates the ways in which working in organizations can be amazingly frustrating. The seeming irrationality of systems can drive any employee to the point of distraction. Systems don't work the way we want them to and, in fact, they often seem to move in exactly the opposite direction. We think we know a little bit about why this is so frequently the case. System change is usually embraced with methods more appropriately applied to our cars and washing machines. And therein lies a fundamental problem. A central position of this book is that all human service delivery organizations are alive. They function as living, complex adaptive systems, not at all like machines.

Mental models help our brains to organize important information without us having to do much conscious mental work. But the result is that we tend to pay attention to and remember only the information that reinforces our existing mental models, determining what we screen out and what we allow in, and what choices are available to us [27]. In this way, our mental models inhibit change—automatically, apparently thoughtlessly, and outside of our awareness.

Mental models are assumptions that are so deeply held that we usually don't even know that what we think, feel, and do are determined by these assumptions outside of our individual consciousness. Your mental models are activated when you and someone else observe the exact same event but describe it— or experience it—in entirely different ways. Our mental models are being challenged when we respond automatically and defensively (often with what in retrospect seems an irrational amount of anger) to an idea that is different. At least two different mental models exist in the organizational world: Organizations as machines versus organizations as living beings [28–29]. As you read this book, we challenge you to think about your own mental models.

Organizations as Machines

In a mechanistic model of organizational life, the goals and directions for the way the organization functions are imposed from outside or above. Authority and power are centralized, and authoritarian leadership is generally viewed as good leadership. Decisions are made above and communicated as instructions to those lower in the hierarchy—or as it is usually referred to, the chain of command. Control is the primary job of managers, and there are clear lines of authority with everyone lower in the hierarchy expected to be obedient to those higher and to expect obedience from those below. Tasks are clearly divided, work is broken down into its smallest part, and each person specializes in those individual tasks that are controlled through detailed rules and regulations and a hierarchical system of supervision. When something needs to be fixed, somebody has to fix it.

Machines do not have emotions, so in a machine model engendering trust is not essential but control and order are. It is not necessary to feel for a machine, to be concerned about the machine's welfare, or to empathize with either the machine's joy or suffering. Machines do not feel. To the extent there is a recognition that these are people, not machines, emotions are not so much to be respected as to be manipulated. Fear is seen as vital to maintain control and order. Other emotions are a bothersome complication of dealing with human beings and thus are largely ignored. Stress is seen as inevitable and any parts of the organization that cannot handle the stresses of operation should be replaced. Knowledge, information, and the power that accompanies it are held at the top of the hierarchy that exists. Dissent is unwelcome and information is distributed on a "need to know" basis. Decision making is bureaucratic, inflexible, rule bound, and hierarchically determined. Communication is seen as a source of power and is highly controlled. Secrets abound. Conflict is suppressed to the extent that it interferes with the proper function of the individual or the organization. Justice is retributive and punishment is designed to inflict pain and arouse fear, thereby setting an example to others that obedience to authority is necessary. Violence is used as necessary to obtain and maintain power and control. Social injustice is tolerated and even encouraged or simply ignored. Since human attachment is only marginally important, loss of those attachments is not recognized or honored. Since traditional solutions to problems are preferred, the compulsive reenactment of previous failed strategies is both compulsive and unrecognized. There is a focus on past success, entrenchment and a tendency to only respond—not prepare—for crises. Over time, the system wears out, degrades, declines and sometimes fails.

In a machine, there is no concept of awareness, consciousness, or the unconscious. There is no part that is not known. If a part breaks, replace it. If you have a part that is no longer needed, eliminate it, ignore it, work around it, or even promote it. In a mechanistic model of organizational life, the goals and directions for the way the organization is to function are imposed from outside or above.

People are not expected to learn; whatever they need to know will be told to them, and if they follow the rule book all will be well. Supervision is strictly hierarchical, with every lower level reporting and responsible to someone in the hierarchy above them. There are detailed rules and regulations to direct everyone's behavior, and work is broken down into the smallest parts. When you hear people talking, you are likely to hear command and control language with mechanistic metaphors: slot to fill, reengineering, insubordination, precision, speed, efficiency, and productivity. People are hired to operate the "machine" and everyone is expected to behave in a predetermined way. The machine is owned by someone and machines do not learn [6]. People who spend the most time with the clients are frequently called "line workers" referring originally to workers on assembly lines.

There are some conditions that make this kind of mechanistic model the ideal approach: when tasks are very simple and require a high level of precision and efficiency, when the exact same outcome is desired every time, when human "machine parts" can be expected to be compliant and obedient (rare, but possible). This mechanistic mental model is the one that dominated the entire organizational landscape in the nineteenth and early twentieth centuries, creating the Industrial Revolution. Although many areas of industry have had to change their operating style in order to survive, this mental model still dominates the educational, health care, and social service environments today.

The problem is that when an organization must constantly adapt to a changing environment, when learning and creativity are essential components of achieving organizational goals, and when the tasks are complicated, interactive, and complex, then applying a mechanistic way of working can be devastating to organizational function. To understand some of the dimensions of the current crisis in human service delivery, we have to take a brief summary look at the health care system in the United States as the backdrop for not just physical health care, but mental health care and all of the social services.

Health Care as Commodity: The Failed Balancing Act of U.S. Health Care

The greatest art is to attain a balance, a balance between all opposites, a balance between all polarities. Imbalance is the disease and balance is health. Imbalance is neurosis, and balance is well-being.

Osho, twentieth-century Indian mystic

In the Buddhist understanding of the world, the Fourth Noble Truth is that of the Middle Path, the life path that avoids extremes but rather maintains a balance between opposites. As a wise ancient Egyptian carved into stone at the Temple at Luxor, "one foot isn't enough to walk with." It is a basic life truism that anything taken to extremes becomes a hazard rather than an asset or as we colloquially say, "too much of a good thing is poison." Rarely, however, is this commonplace wisdom applied to our economic system and nowhere is this observation more accurate than in the evolution of the present health care system. It's not at all clear who originally noted that "the road to Hell is paved with good intentions," but it might have been a health care provider.

The care of the ill, the disabled, the destitute, and the mentally ill has too long a history to fully explore here, but since it is at the root of what we focus on in this book, we feel a need to provide a selective background on the issue of service delivery. Although health care—and its poorer stepsister, mental health care—has become a valuable commodity, it wasn't always looked at through the lens of capitalism, and today in many other parts of the developed and developing world, health care is not seen as a privilege, but as a fundamental right. The United States, however, has not yet decided that health care is a basic human right. The 2009–2010 health care debate has epitomized the conflict between those who see health care coverage as an individual responsibility and those who see it as an issue related to the common good. But even in the United States it was not until the late 1940s that commercial insurance companies became interested in the health care market and not until the 1980s was it possible for people to accumulate fantastic wealth by building health care insurance empires.

Mental Models of the Healing Professions

As we mentioned earlier, mental models are the unspoken foundational assumptions for any enterprise. These fundamental ideas are generally embodied within the ethical structure of every human service delivery organization. Provider organizations each have their own mission statements and guiding values or statement of beliefs. Professional organizations have codes of ethics that practitioners are expected to follow and for which they can be professionally and/or legally punished if they violate these principles. Whether we look at physicians, nurses, psychologists, social workers, or counselors, there is a consistency about ethical principles that are the keystones for practice.

For physicians, this is embodied in the Hippocratic Oath—or some version of it—that most graduates of U.S. medical schools recite at their graduation ceremony. Even earlier, they have been taught the ancient standard for all medical practice, "Primum non nocere" or "First, do no harm." According to the American Medical Association Code of Ethics, *"The medical profession has long subscribed to a body of ethical statements developed primarily for the benefit of the patient. As a member of this profession, a physician must recognize responsibility to patients first and foremost, as well as to society, to other health professionals, and to self*" [30]. Nursing professionals follow ethical codes embodied in the American Nursing Association that address human dignity and the primary commitment to the patient [31].

According to the Code of Ethics of the American Psychological Association, psychologists strive to benefit those with whom they work and take care to do no harm; to establish relationships of trust with those with whom they work; to seek to promote accuracy, honesty, and truthfulness in the science, teaching, and practice of psychology; to recognize that fairness and justice entitle all persons to access to and benefit from the contributions of psychology and to equal quality in the processes, procedures, and services being conducted by psychologists; and to respect the dignity and worth of all people, and the rights of individuals to privacy, confidentiality, and self-determination [32].

According to the National Association of Social Workers, "*the primary mission of the social work profession is to enhance human well-being and help meet the basic human needs of all people, with particular attention to the needs and empowerment of people who are vulnerable, oppressed, and living in poverty*" and the core values of the profession include service, social justice, valuing the dignity and worth of the person, the importance of human relationships, integrity, and competence [33].

According to the American Counseling Association, the primary responsibility of counselors is to respect the dignity and to promote the welfare of clients [34]. Similarly, the American Mental Health Counselors Association asserts that "*mental health counselors believe in the dignity and worth of the individual. They are committed to increasing knowledge of human behavior and understanding of themselves and others. While pursuing these endeavors, they make every reasonable effort to protect the welfare of those who seek their services, or of any subject that may be the object of study. They use their skills only for purposes consistent with these values and do not knowingly permit their misuse by others*" [35].

Aesculapian Authority

At an ethical level, even while practice differs, all of the helping professions are complexly interrelated as is visible in the similarity and overlap in the ethical codes. They are also very frequently interrelated on a practical level, especially in the cases of people who have multiple and/or complex problems. All derive some sense of authority from the ancient positions of practitioners of the healing arts: physicians and their predecessors, all those shamans and "witch doctors," witches and medicine men who were singled out as healers in earlier times. In 1957, T. T. Paterson was investigating types of authority in management and realized that his theory of types of authority did not accurately describe medical authority. He defined this other type of authority as

"Aesculapian authority" after Aesculapias, the Greek god of healing whose symbol of a snake, twined around a staff, has long been recognized as the symbol of medical authority.

Aesculapian authority consists of three of the types of authority Paterson was describing at the time: sapiential, moral, and charismatic. By "sapiential" he meant the right of someone to be heard by right of their knowledge or expertise. The second type, "moral authority," refers to the right to control and direct others by reason of the rightness and goodness according to the ethos of the work, as expressed in the Hippocratic Oath. The third ingredient of Aesculapian authority is what he characterized as "charismatic authority" or the right to control and direct by reason of God-given grace, reflecting the original unity of medicine and religion, the arbitrary nature of life and death, the mystery and the art of healing [36–37]. To become a health care, mental health, social work, or counseling professional means partaking both of this authority in some measure *and* of bearing the responsibility and commitment that goes along with that authority.

Community Responsibility

For many centuries, the care for those impacted by any kind of illness was viewed as primarily a family responsibility set within the context of community responsibility. The relationship between doctor and patient was sacrosanct, and deep moral commitments were involved in that relationship. Physicians were honored members of the community, expected to care for the old, the sick, and the needy. In the nineteenth century local lodges and fraternal orders provided assistance to their members through sickness funds when their families were absent or overwhelmed. As health care analyst Dr. David Barton Smith has written, "*The idea behind these sickness funds was that 'we' whoever that was (a church congregation, fraternal order, new immigrant group or recently emancipated slaves) are all in this together and we will take care of each other, just the way we would for a sick family member. It was a moral obligation, not a product one could choose to purchase* (p. 68)" [38]. Hospitals began creating voluntary community hospital insurance plans during the Great Depression, and these evolved into local Blue Cross plans, not initially considered a business but just a way of taking care of those who fell ill. In order to attract a scarcity of workers during World War II, employers used health care benefits as an incentive for recruitment, but as costs continued to rise over the ensuing decades, "*health-care insurance moved from its position of great employer gift to the burden of the worker*" (p. 2) as it remains today [39].

Health Care and the Threat of Communist Enslavement

In other countries, earlier community efforts to fund health care evolved into national health plans assuring universal health insurance coverage, but not in the United States. Since President Truman in 1948, every national health insurance proposal has gone down to defeat largely because, *"to be against choice and market competition seemed un-American. Indeed, medical associations had waged a successful campaign against the Truman National Health Insurance plan, arguing that 'compulsory' health insurance was the first step towards communist enslavement"* (p. 89) [38]. As we were writing this manuscript, the same arguments against a national health care agenda filled the airwaves. President Obama was finally able to wring some kind of health care reform out of Congress, but it is still not universal health insurance coverage. Virtually all European countries, even moderately poor countries and formerly Communist countries in central and eastern Europe, guarantee all of their citizens health care and at a lower cost than here. And despite the cost of our health care, we are ranked 37th for overall health care system performance [40]. Here the recent extreme and irrational nature of the concern that somehow providing health care for the uninsured will topple the nation is an indicator that a threat to mental models is activated and it has happened for many years whenever the need for a different health care system is raised.

In the 1940s and 50s, employers began buying health care benefits for their employees, and commercial insurance companies began developing instruments to buy into this market. In this way a fundamental philosophical shift, not fully recognized at the time, began to evolve. The costs of illness are not like other products or services because at any time—other than during epidemics—only a small part of any population accounts for a large proportion of its health expenditures. For example, in any given year in the United States, 1% of the population accounts for 25%–29% of all health expenditures (p. 67) [38]. In the previous nonprofit environment, the 50% who accounted for 3% of the costs paid the same as the 1% that accounted for as much as 29% of the cost, a philosophical cornerstone known as "community rating," spreading the costs of everyone's health care across the entire community.

But for profit-making companies, this made no sense. They believed that the amount each person paid should be based on individual experience and risk so that an employer with a young and healthy workforce should pay less than one with older and sicker employees. The result was what has been termed "cream skimming" by commercial insurance companies. As these for-profit companies catered exclusively to the less ill, less disabled, younger, and healthier, the nonprofits had to use the same measures in order to survive. Ultimately, so did physicians and hospitals. As Dr. Smith has pointed out, *"As a result, those that needed it the most were left to the government to insure or became uninsured. The United States has been struggling to address the social and economic consequences of this ever since"* (p. 69) [38].

Privatization Rules

Between 1960 and 1980, the federal government passed a series of health-planning legislation designed to shape a system of care and contain costs.

Costs, however, continued to rise, driven by a variety of causes, including significant advances in technology. This resulted in the promotion of health maintenance organizations (HMOs) in the 1970s and the HMO Act of 1973 that provided grants and loans for planning and developing nonprofit HMOs and required employers to provide an HMO option. As a prime example of the result, former pharmacist Len Abramson created HMO/PA and in doing so created a structure that would be copied by similar companies throughout the nation. He had a model that weeded out physicians who used more services than others and selected those who had practices comprised mainly of younger and healthier patients—yet another version of "cream skimming." To support competitive practices between providers—a model that spread rapidly—care had to be highly "managed" and an entire bureaucracy was created and/or funded in every insurance company to reduce costs.

In the 1980s under the Reagan administration, the federal grant program for the development of nonprofit HMOs was ended and the promotion of HMOs as an opportunity for private investment took off. Supported by changes in Medicare regulations, hospitals began to be paid in an entirely different way, shifting hospital reimbursement to a flat rate regardless of how long a patient was hospitalized. In order to survive, hospitals had to take steps to reduce hospital stays, reduce physician involvement, reduce staff, and more aggressively manage budgets. Meanwhile, nonprofit HMOs were able to become profit-making engines, the end result of which was that someone like Mr. Abramson, who originally built his business on a federal loan, ended up walking away 25 years later with $8.3 billion [38].

And what has happened over the last 30 years to health care, mental health care, and social service delivery? We have been and still are in a health care crisis, a social service workforce crisis, a crisis in the delivery of service to children, adults, and families, an institutional crisis, and a financial crisis. As a nation, we spend almost $2 trillion annually on health care alone, and costs continue to escalate, while more and more people have lost access to health care insurance, producing an unheard-of level of personal and family bankruptcy due to medical costs [41].

We will detail the impact of these changes on mental health and other social services later. For now it is enough to know that mental health and substance abuse treatment has been devastated by the shifts in costs, as mental health and drug treatment benefits were "carved out" of health care plans in a wide variety of ways. Reliable estimates for the economic burden of serious mental illness indicate that mental illness is associated with an annual loss of earnings totaling $193.2 billion [42] and that the total estimated economic burden is $317 billion, which excludes costs associated with comorbid conditions, incarceration, homelessness, and early mortality, yet this sum is equivalent to more than $1000/year for every man, woman, and child in the United States [43].

Studies have shown the annual cost of substance abuse to be $510.8 billion in 1999 dollars. More specifically, alcohol abuse costs $191.6 billion; tobacco use costs $167.8 billion; and drug abuse costs $151.4 billion [44]. Based on data drawn from a variety of sources, the estimated annual cost of child abuse and neglect is $103.8 billion in 2007 value and this is a very conservative estimate [45].

Despite these costs, significant components of the mental health system have been systematically deconstructed over the last 30 years, and as a result care of the severely mentally ill has often shifted to families and to prisons, while prison growth has increased exponentially with enormous rolling, multi-generational implications for the entire human service delivery system. The United States now incarcerates 1 in every 100 citizens and spends an estimated $60 billion each year on corrections—more than any country in the world [46–47]. But this figure excludes the costs of lost earnings, costs to child welfare to take care of the children of prisoners, the welfare and homelessness service costs that often follow incarceration, or the comorbidity associated with mental illness, lack of substance abuse treatment, or inadequate medical care.

The bottom line is that efforts to contain costs, prevent crime, reduce mental illness, and reduce health care costs over the last 30 years, based on sound principles of practice in a typical capitalist enterprise, do not seem to have been effective. If anything, these efforts have made things far worse.

Managed Care and Ethical Conflicts

There is quite a low status attached to 'management' in the medical field, and business is almost a dirty word. The literature on strategy for health care organizations is virtually nonexistent. Finally, in health care, many practitioners consider the whole idea of competition to be suspect. Physicians are taught that competition is wasteful, that it promotes self-interested behavior, and that it undermines patient care. Many equate competition with price cutting. (p. xiii) [41]

Porter and Teisberg (2006), *Redefining Health Care: Creating Value-Based Competition on Results*

The resistance among health care and social service providers to the introduction of cost-saving business practices into their environments is generally not because of a nonspecific distaste for business. Although it may not have been well articulated, this reluctance is based on both an intuitive and practical perception that the two just don't mix well for reasons that have more to do with basic philosophy and mental models than individual inclination. Years ago, clinicians were warning that "*the managed care approach to provision of human services will dominate professional work for the near future and possibly beyond. This approach raises serious concerns about the capacity of professionals to work within the structure of managed care without encountering serious ethical and clinical conflicts*" (p. 47) [48]. In other social services, welfare reform for example, has been demonstrated to have caused a significant increase in ethical conflicts for social workers responding to the demands of welfare-to-work requirements, regulations, and demands [49].

Question any health care, social service, or mental health professional who has been working in his or her field for any length of time and you will hear testimony to the near-universal nature of the ethical dilemmas facing providers. Dr. Ivan Miller, writing for the National Coalition of Mental Health Professionals and Consumers, has pointed out the 11 most unethical managed care practices that have plagued the delivery of health care, mental health care, and social service delivery. These include the following: *(1)* disregarding personal and medical privacy; *(2)* using false advertising; *(3)* using deceptive language—calling cost cutting "quality improvement" or gatekeepers "patient advocates"; *(4)* violating traditional scientific ethics; *(5)* practicing outside of a professional's area of competence as when utilization reviewers do not have the credentials or training necessary to confirm that they are competent to overrule and change the decisions of the treating professional; *(6)* creating and intensifying conflicts of interest; *(7)* keeping secrets about financial conflicts of interest; *(8)* violating informed consent procedures; *(9)* using "kickbacks" to keep patients away from specialists; *(10)* squandering money entrusted to their care; and *(11)* disregarding information about harm to patients [50].

It is not that there was an absence of unethical behavior prior to managed care. But providers did feel that they had a *choice* about whether to engage in shady practices and often looked askance at, and sometimes reported, those colleagues who did make that choice. The takeover of managed care, particularly those that are for-profit companies, not only deprived practitioners of that same level of choice, but instead has frequently placed them in untenable positions. In the highly managed mental health environments, some of the greatest sources of stress are the conflicts of interest that are intrinsic to many aspects of the system [51–52]. Should the clinician promote the interests of individual patients over all other interests, as is consistent with professional codes of ethics? Or should the clinician promote what is considered the "general social good" by rationing care? If a reviewer with at most a college degree tries to push you toward a different form of treatment, will you, as the patient's physician or provider, be punished in some way for refusing? Should the clinician promote his or her own financial well-being, which may be at the expense of the other interests [53]? If a representative of managed care requires information that a clinician believes is private and definitely not relevant to the current treatment decisions, must the clinician reveal that information rather than have the sessions denied? If the clinician disagrees with the treatment recommendations that the reviewer decides on, will the hospitalization be denied? Should clinicians advocate for their clients with managed care companies even if there will be potential acts of retribution [54]? Is it unethical to give a client a wrong diagnosis if that is the only way to get the client necessary services because of the diagnoses that managed care companies will and will not cover [55]?

These kinds of dilemmas have been the daily experience of many people providing care. If clinicians do not comply with the demands their organizations are forced to make by the dictates of managed care, they risk losing their jobs and their incomes. If they do comply, they may have to make decisions and engage in behavior that they inwardly believe compromises the level of care they offer to their clients. And all of these ethical dilemmas occur within the context of an extremely divided theoretical base. Insurance company reviewers have relatively clear guidelines in health care. In other areas of medicine, organs and organ problems can be isolated—or someday will be—and both clinical presentation and laboratory tests will demonstrate—often with a high degree of precision—whether an intervention strategy has worked. It is not the same in mental health or the human services. Here we are dealing with the enormous and often overwhelming complexity of human nature. There are dozens, perhaps hundreds, of theories about various components of human existence: thoughts, feelings, beliefs, behaviors, intentions, attitudes, and motivations. Many of these theories have led to various intervention strategies for a wide variety of problems. But no single theory, no unified field theory, explains everything about human beings—and probably never will. And even when we have evidence that one theory, and the intervention it is based upon, is supported, that does not mean that other theories are invalidated. So improvement is often very much in the "eye of the beholder" and open to interpretation of what exactly improvement means.

Today, significant problems remain and the effects of these last 30 years will be with us for some time to come, even if we were to create a very different health care delivery system immediately. For many providers of a wide variety of services, the term "managed care" has become synonymous with "mangled care." This is not entirely fair. As is usually the case, egregious behavior is what is noted and remembered, not the thousands of positive interactions with agents of managed care companies that occur every day. Given the contending and countervailing forces of providers; insurers; county, state, and federal governments; lawyers and consumers, the delivery of services does have to be managed if access to care, the quality of care, and fiscal prudence are all to be considered. But the never-ending search for ever-increasing profits that is the cornerstone of our financial system encourages practices that systematically delete compassionate care and sometimes reinforce inadequate care. Because nonprofit companies have slightly less accountability for the bottom line, they are often justifiably regarded in a more favorable light than for-profit companies.

But the reality is that everyone—insurers, providers, and clients—must function within the confines of a broken system.

What has happened? Under other circumstances, management control measures appear to make things better, not worse. Why then is the health care system—and all its related social service delivery systems—in such crisis? Let's look for a moment at the underlying and fundamental assumptions of a capitalist economic system.

Mental Models for U.S. Capitalism

The standard Merriam-Webster definition of capitalism is: "*an economic system characterized by private or corporate ownership of capital goods, by investments that are determined by private decision, and by prices, production, and the distribution of goods that are determined mainly by competition in a free market*" [56].

In reviewing the present health care system, Professors Porter and Teisberg struggle to understand why the typical practices of the corporate world have met with such abysmal overall results in the world of health care. As they investigated, "*It became increasingly clear that the nature of health care delivery needed to be transformed. We also began to believe that to reform health care, one had to reform competition itself. And to reform competition, one had to transform the strategies, organizational structures, pricing approaches, and measurement practices of the various actors in the system. We came to see that the problem was less a technology problem or a regulatory problem than a management and organizational problem. The overall result was that many talented and well-intended individuals working the system were often working at cross purposes to patient value and were increasingly aware of, and disheartened by, this conflict*" (p. xv) [41].

They went on to point out some of the basic discrepancies between normal markets and health care:

> *In a normal market, competition drives relentless improvements in quality and cost. Rapid innovation leads to rapid diffusion of new technologies and better ways of doing things. Excellent competitors prosper and grow, while weaker rivals are restructured or go out of business. Quality-adjusted prices fall, value improves, and the market expands to meet the needs of more consumers. This is the trajectory of all well-functioning industries...health care competition could not be more different .... The reason is not a lack of competition, but the wrong kind of competition. Competition has taken place at the wrong levels and on the wrong things. It has gravitated to a zero-sum competition, in which the gains of one system participant come at the expense of others. Participants compete to shift costs to one another, accumulate bargaining power, and limit services. This kind of competition does not create value for patients, but erodes quality, fosters*

inefficiency, creates excess capacity, and drives up administrative costs, among other nefarious effects. (pp. 3–4) [41]

Sandy can give a good example of this out of her own experience:

During the 1990s we became part of a large health care organization. We thought that allying ourselves with this national company would give our program a longer life because managed care was taking over the mental health environment with ever-increasing demands for more paperwork, fewer resources, less income without any concern for what we considered meaningful performance: helping our very traumatized patients to get in and out of the hospital quickly and with significant improvement in their mental state. We believed a larger organization would have more clout and be able to more adequately protect our small program. In fact, that was true. Our program lasted years longer than it otherwise would have because of this fundamental change.

Around the same time, however, this large organization brought into their organizational fold four other national experts in treating the complex problems associated with trauma. Our practices were widely spread out across the entire country, each program addressed different clients, and each of us had developed our own innovations. We had expected to collaborate and create a national network of superior programs, decades before "trauma-informed" treatment became any kind of standard. Unfortunately, all of our joint efforts to create this kind of creative collaboration failed due to the unforeseen clash between the corporate business culture and our own professional aspirations. We were not permitted to meet, plan, or collaborate within the corporate context and in fact were expected to compete with each other for clients. Competition, however, was actually impossible given our wide geographic dispersal, varied treatment objectives, referral sources, and referral patterns. From our point of view, we were indeed competing, but competing with all of the other programs that were not trauma-informed and that it was self-defeating to be competing with each other. But because the concept of competition was accepted as an almost religious tenet, there was no way any of us were able to surmount this obstacle and a very valuable opportunity for the company, ourselves, our patients, and the mental health field as a whole, was lost.

Profitability is another fundamental mental model issue at the bedrock of our economic system. But profitability in terms of health care and social service cannot be addressed in the same way as making and selling cars or chairs. Quarterly reports and yearly distribution of profits to stockholders may make sense in most other industries, but when it comes to any kind of human services, the focus on short-term gain can spell disaster. *"At the most basic level, competition in health care must take place where value is actually created. Herein lies a big part of the problem. Value in health care is determined in addressing the patient's particular medical conditions over the full cycle of care, from monitoring and prevention to treatment to ongoing disease management ... The problem is that competition does not take place at the medical condition level, nor over the full care cycle"* (p. 5) [41].

As we will see from research like the seminal Adverse Childhood Experiences Study in the upcoming chapters, many childhood experiences play a formative role in later adult physical, emotional, and social problems. Trying to assess "profitability" at only one point along that lifespan course becomes a futile— and potentially dangerous and destructive—exercise. If treatment of relatively minimal symptoms at age 5 stands a reasonable likelihood of preventing signifi- cant and costly problems at age 30, 40, 50, or 60, isn't that a sound social invest- ment? But to make those kinds of decisions, we require notions of profitability that are anything but short term. If we do intensive family therapy with an abused child (cost to the mental health sector and maybe child welfare) and as a result that child does not go to jail as a teenager (cost to the criminal justice sector), or does not end up a victim of domestic violence as an adult (cost to the domestic violence, judicial, child welfare and health care sector), or does not end up with diabetes (health care costs), and does become a good parent (costs distributed throughout society), how do we determine what exactly is profitability?

Lessons Learned?

This story of human social service delivery in the United States is, of course, incomplete, but some lessons can be drawn from the last few decades. The first is that our public policy is rarely based on the notion of a healthy balance. As a society we are frequently drawn to extremes, and the health care debacle of recent years is no exception. Public policy cannot be divorced from social con- text and since the 1980s there has been a fundamental shift in social norms with greed radically shifted from its previous ranking as one of the Seven Deadly Sins to one of the highest virtues.

A second conclusion is that we are notably unable to self-protect, to ade- quately insure "social immunity" as a society, against selfishness bereft of the balancing notion of social responsibility and the common good. In this way our current notion of "self-interest" cannot be considered enlightened self- interest at all. When the social and political frenzy to achieve ever-increasing levels of wealth became widespread in the professional world, physicians and other health care providers who had developed their careers as a social mission became enticed by the promise of profitability, falling like dominos to the lures and threats of managers schooled in the nuances of corporate warfare. The result has been a loss of innovation and profound demoralization among many of our most valuable health care, mental health, and social service providers and a decrease in the general social welfare.

Thirdly, as a society we are very short sighted, always looking for the fast solution and the quickest buck and as a result creating inconceivable long-term loss. As a result, we do not have well-established mechanisms for taking intergenerational, preventive approaches that could save us vast amounts of unnecessary physical, emotional, social, and financial suffering in the future.

A fourth conclusion is that when the same standards used to assess the success of a factory that builds widgets are applied to health care and social welfare, we all lose. But those who are the youngest or the oldest, the most ill, the most fragile, the most disenfranchised, and those with the least resources will lose the most. If we treat living systems as if they were machines, they will become increasingly dysfunctional. Providers of any kind of human service should be accountable for what they do and how well they perform but that performance cannot contradict their basic ethical principles. In order to bring about any true reforms in health care, mental health care, or social service delivery, the system will need to change based on *results*, and these results have to be results that the consumer and the providers mutually struggle to achieve in the most efficient, cost-effective way. *"Competition on results means that those providers, health plans, and suppliers that achieve excellence are rewarded with more business, while those that fail to demonstrate good results decline or cease to provide that service"* (p. 6) [41].

But this leads to a fifth conclusion: that as an entire society we are not yet capable of addressing complex problems. Currently, there actually is very little emphasis on this key concept of results or "does it work?" in part because there is often little agreement as to what "works" means, at least in mental health and social services. Much of this lack of agreement is due to the complexity of human problems that end up interactively affecting so many different parts of a person as well as the people in that person's social network. So immediate relief of depressed mood with an antidepressant may be judged as effective treatment. But what if the underlying causes of the depression are ongoing, as in situations of domestic violence? What if a parent is now less depressed but still goes on secretly abusing his child? Is this effective treatment? A child is taken into the custody of child welfare because the mother is incarcerated on a nonviolent drug offense and the mother's sentence is longer than the permanency requirements of the state, so the child is adopted out to another family and never sees his mother again. Is this a successful result? Successful for whom? If a child is being abused and witnessing family violence, is unable to concentrate, acts out in the classroom, and is diagnosed with attention-deficit/hyperactivity disorder and prescribed medication as the only intervention, can we view this as success if he grows up to abuse his own children?

In the next part of this chapter, we are going to use the mental health system as an example of the issues we have been raising so far and to set the stage for the rest of the book. Keep in mind, however, that whatever affects a component of the mental health system will reverberate throughout the rest of the human service delivery system because of the interrelated nature of human problems and efforts to resolve those problems.

Mental Health: An Example of a System Under Siege

If we look at the human service system as a whole living system and we look at the characteristics of unhealthy organizations, what do we see? A dictionary describes a "siege mentality" as a shared feeling of helplessness, victimization, and defensiveness that evolved from real sieges when an army attempted to capture a city, town, or fortress by surrounding and blockading it. Today it is a phenomenon that is particularly common in business as a result of competition, economic downturns, or downsizing [57]. We contend that the entire human service system designed to serve the most desperate members of our culture is "under siege" after decades of system degradation, mission erosion, chronically unrelenting toxic stress, and repetitive crises. Here we use the mental health system as an example.

System as Machine

Society's charge to the mental health system is to take care of the "problem" of the mentally ill. Depending on the historical era, sometimes the emphasis shifts to rehabilitating, curing, or at least treating the mentally ill, and at other times the emphasis has been on preventing the mentally ill from interfering with the smooth running of society. Whatever the case, historically the mentally ill have been seen as jamming the gears of industrial progress and putting a drain on the system [58]. They have largely been considered society's waste. One of the results of this devaluation is that those who labor in the industry designed to take the mentally ill off society's hands are doing work that has sometimes been considered noble and infrequently heroic, but remains work that is largely undervalued, relatively low paid, low-status employment.

The issue of control is a primary component of the mental health system since the system is hired by the public to restrict and restrain behavior on the part of the mentally ill who are by definition "out of control." The definition of what constitutes out-of-control behavior is itself strictly controlled by the intricate diagnostic labeling system of the *Diagnostic and Statistic Manual* that allows entry into the mental health system and from which it is virtually impossible to extricate oneself once drawn into it, particularly if you are also poor, young, inadequately educated, and poorly resourced. Brian discusses a very tangible example of a treatment program acting as if the children they were treating were little machines who could be brought into line—as would the staff—if the administration said so:

We have had a long history of autocratic, top-down management. In fairness this style was not abusive; it was a kind of benevolent dictatorship. It was, however, grounded in a belief that those of us with fancier titles, more experience, more investment, more of something were better equipped to make decisions about kids, families, purchasing, admissions, discharges, planning, and any number of other issues. Years ago when a child committed a serious behavioral infraction (going AWOL, doing serious property damage, hurting another child, stealing, and so on), the child was brought up to the administration building at the beginning of the day. The child would sit in the breezeway with a milieu staff and wait for a senior administrator to call him or her in. The administrator would read the child the riot act, make some effort to chop the child down to size, and then present the child with his or her "consequences." The consequences usually consisted of some combination of room restriction, activity restriction, allowance reduction, level reduction, trip restrictions, work details, house restriction, loss of recreation, or loss of some other privilege like a TV in the child's room. The consequences would then be typed up and sent to the cottage. Generally the consequences would fit on a 8 ½ by 11" sheet of paper, but occasionally a second sheet of paper was required for the really bad stuff.

The cottage staff would then be expected to enforce the consequences they had no hand in constructing. More often than not the cottage staff viewed these consequences as either far too harsh or way too lenient. When they were too harsh they would be ignored after a day or two, sometimes immediately. When consequences were ignored, administrators would get very upset with the staff—after all, they took the time to meet with the child, ponder the perfect punishment, and type up the directives, a considerable investment of one's work time. When consequences were deemed too soft by the cottage staff, the punishment would be carried out as directed, but not without considerable complaining about what a bunch of dopes were running this place.

Mental health organizations and virtually all social service agencies are strictly hierarchical in structure. Top-down control is exerted over the employees whose job it is to control the patients/clients in their care. In an era of dominance by biopsychiatry, the patients are expected to take medications that will control their symptoms. Charles Barber, in his critique *Comfortably Numb: How Psychiatry Is Medicating a Nation*, writes about his experience working in a homeless shelter in New York City beginning in the 1980s and watching changes in social services unfold as if patients were cars that could be brought in for a tune-up:

In some ways, things were actually worse by 2000. The emergence of managed care—the handmaiden of the medication revolution—had severely shortened hospital stays. Under managed care, psychiatric hospitalization came to be viewed not as an opportunity to work on treatment issues or to arrive at a thoughtful discharge plan, but primarily as a place to tinker with medications. Once a medication regimen was arrived at, and patients were no longer considered unsafe, they were out, sometimes on the streets. My clients were routinely hospitalized and rehospitalized, and discharged and redischarged, always before they were ready. This caused incalculable confusion and pain. (p. xix) [59]

When the management hierarchy fails to adequately control its charges, some form of external authority must come in to "fix" the program machine. If it is the patient that needs to be fixed, a new medication will be prescribed. If it is the employee that needs fixing, the process will begin with the employee's immediate supervisor. If it is the organization itself that is broken, then some regulatory body will step in to impose some sort of action intended to correct the problem. Andrus Children's Center is located in New York State, and Brian describes the regulatory situation:

> *Our agency must comply with regulations set forth by the New York State Office of Children and Family Services, New York State Department of Education, New York State Department of Health, State and Federal Medicaid, Occupational Health and Safety Administration, Westchester Department of Social Services, Westchester Department of Community Mental Health, No Child Left Behind, Health Insurance Portability and Accountability Act, Equal Employment Opportunity Commission, Department of Labor, Employee Retirement Income Security Act, and Sarbanes-Oxley Act, to name just a few. As an organization we are expected to monitor literally tens of thousands of pages of regulation and standards, some of which change daily. An organization with annual revenue of $1 million is as accountable as an organization with $100 million in revenue. Although ignorance of the law is no excuse for breaking the law, few nonprofits have the resources to monitor this landscape effectively. Most are forced to close what they believe to be their highest areas of risk and monitor those most closely.*

Social Engineering Cannot Address Adaptive Problems

Most efforts to change an organization or an entire system have been tried through a methodology known as "social engineering"—a perfect mechanistic term—which bears a striking resemblance to the whole "behavior management" approach to traumatized children. In social engineering, the main premise is that cascading intention is supposed to flow from the top of the chain of command and then be communicated downward so that everyone lower in the hierarchy rolls out the changes, which are carefully planned, predictable, and controllable.

The problem is that according to well-informed estimates around the world, 70% of change efforts using this method in companies have failed. Is it then likely that anyone is going to be able to successfully socially engineer system change in the social service system? To put it succinctly, "*Social engineering as a context is obsolete—Period*" (p. 13) [60].

Machines change only if someone changes them and mighty efforts have been and still are expended in trying to make the mental health system change. If you replace the headlamps in your car, you do not expect your car to complain about missing its familiar companions. Machines do not generally react to imposed change, except perhaps to operate more smoothly when repairs are made. Machines do not lead change and machines do not resist change. Machines challenge managers with mostly fixable technical problems, but technical problems are relatively rare in human services. As Brian notes,

> In our line of work—residential treatment of children—we are not dealing with technical problems; rather, the problems we are dealing with are generally adaptive problems. Technical problems generally lend themselves to cookbook kinds of solutions: "How do you put this backyard grill together?" "How do you process this piece of paper?" But most of the problems we face in our work lives are adaptive problems: They have never been solved before and there is no rulebook. We may have solved a problem "like" this before but not this one. This is a different client. This is a different day, a different year. The people involved in delivering the new response are different. If we do the same thing we did before, the outcome could be entirely different. There are always different variables that make this problem different from the last one. In our work we yearn for technical problems and as result we often treat adaptive problems as if they are technical problems. This is why we love to invest a great deal of time in "behavior management systems" or earlier, "token systems." The rage now is for "manualized treatment." Point systems, cookbook therapies, and Standard Operating Procedures on how to handle this or that crisis might help us feel better, but they cannot replace a good discussion between a group of caring and committed people who are constantly adapting—their approaches and themselves—to changing conditions.

Interlocking Crises

The latest spate of changes in the mental health system have revolved around "cost savings" and "fiscal discipline" and "managed care" and "increased productivity." The mental health system-as-machine should logically respond no differently than your car to the significant infrastructure changes that accompany this change in focus. But that is not what has happened. The fundamental changes in structure necessitated by radical changes in funding have precipitated multiple, interlocking crises throughout the human services field, including mental health treatment delivery systems. The onset of this fundamental change occurred sometime in the late 1970s when the fashionable terminology changed from the dominant usage of the words "mental health" (mental referring to the complex biopsychosocial processes, unconscious and conscious, that affect human behavior) to the different currently dominant terminology of "behavioral health" (need to focus exclusively on changing behavior).

Human beings in an organization-as-machine are simply parts of the machine and the machine is there to make profit for the owner. If the part wears out or breaks, it is to be replaced by a similar part to keep the machine operating in the most cost-effective way possible. In this model, occurrences like layoffs, dramatic changes in trained professional staff-to-patient ratios, or therapist turnover should really have relatively little effect since other people-as-machines have been designated to fill in the holes left by others. And besides, the job of the staff is to just "change behavior." Isn't that a lot like giving a car a lube job—almost anyone can do it? And if the key to "behavioral health" is actually changing neurotransmitters because all of this is genetic anyway, then all you really need to do is get them on the right medication and you will achieve the best result you can get.

Again an observation from Charles Barber:

> *Between 1987 and 1997, while the rate of pharmacological treatment for depression doubled, the number of psychotherapy visits for depression decreased. These days, only about 3% of the population receives therapy from a psychiatrist, psychologist, or social worker. What has happened is that in the last twenty years, as insurers have paid for psychotropic medications, they have compensated for the extra costs by "carving out" the rest of mental health care— inpatient stays, intensive outpatient, residential services, and psychotherapy— from their general benefits package. Those "specialty services" are managed by subcontractors, "managed behavioral health care" groups. Which in my experience have a reputation for watching expenses and denying services with even more vigilance and ruthlessness than general managed care. Talk to almost any social worker or psychologist, and they will tell you, probably for longer than you want to hear, how brutal managed care has been to their practice.* (p. 104) [59]

Of course, the whole machine can break down and if that happens, it is the job of management to rebuild it. In some cases, the society comes to view the machine as obsolete and simply throws it away, as has largely happened to our large state hospital systems. In other cases, the society strips them down to such an extent that they are no longer very useful, as in acute care inpatient psychiatric programs and many other psychiatric settings. It is logically acceptable then, that if the machinery is obsolete and thrown away, you can also throw away the instruction manuals. So the mental health field periodically cleans out its cupboards and throws out whole realms of knowledge like social psychiatry, psychoanalytic theory, transactional analysis, systems theory, group dynamics, therapeutic community development, and the connections between recovery and expressive arts. All you need to do is stop teaching a skill set to one generation of professionals and the knowledge is lost. The result is that many of the therapeutic approaches informed by this knowledge are also thrown out. As Barber points out:

> In the last two decades there has been a tremendous bias in academic psychiatry against psychological and social forms of inquiry... In this era, one could hardly get an article published in an academic journal of psychiatry that was purely qualitative (i.e., didn't include statistics) or that told the story of an individual patient, or that included any personal thoughts or feelings on the part of the authors about the people or the work they were engaged with. All that would be deemed not appropriately robust for the new standards of the profession. In our particularly American zeal for simple explanations, quick fixes, and overwhelming the enemy with technology, we've too quickly lost sight of the centrality of social and environmental factors. And despite undeniable progress in the pharmacological realm, the enduring truth is that the human factor, and the human approach, remains crucial to healing (p. xviii) [59].

It does not matter what the context of their actions are because machines will work in the dark, in the heat, in the cold, crowded together, often twenty-four hours a day without rest. Machines do not learn; they can do no more than their individual parts allow them to do, and experience has no effect other than to wear them out. Ultimately, when the machine model no longer allows the organization to adapt to changing circumstances, what unfolds is "a crisis" and according to the Substance Abuse and Mental Health Services Administration (SAMHSA) we are definitely in one:

> It is difficult to overstate the magnitude of the workforce crisis in behavioral health... The improvement of care and the transformation of systems of care depend entirely on a workforce that is adequate in size and effectively trained and supported. Urgent attention to this crisis is essential. (p. 2) [61]

Let's look at a little of the background on how this devolution of the mental health service delivery system has unrolled.

What Happened to the Social Psychiatry?

Rarely referred to today, "social psychiatry" was the dominant discourse in psychiatry in the 1950s and 1960s. It rode in on the back of World War II, the Holocaust, and the atomic bomb. But by the 1970s the United States was going through a fundamentally disruptive but profoundly creative period. Involved in an unpopular and arguably illegal war, conflict was apparent everywhere. Authority in all of its forms—civil, military, religious, educational, artistic— was being challenged. In 1973, thanks in part to the activism of many members of the organization and the emerging Gay Rights movement, the American Psychiatric Association removed homosexuality from the *Diagnostic and*

Statistic Manual thus ending the diagnosis as a category of mental illness. Women were meeting in consciousness raising groups, rapidly developing an awareness of gender-related discrimination and violence that had been used for millennia to keep half of the species oppressed. Race riots sparked by centuries of discrimination and segregation broke out in major cities. Protests erupted on virtually every college campus as young people and many of their teachers— raised on the idealistic patriotism of Mickey Mouse and John Wayne— encountered Richard Nixon, Vietnam, the segregated South, Watergate, the slaying of students at Kent State, and the triple assassinations of John F. Kennedy, Robert Kennedy, and Martin Luther King, Jr. All these events, though almost forgotten by many people today, were traumatic for the country as a whole [62].

The Personal Is Political

In the decade of 1970–1980, individual suffering, collective experience, and clinical observation about the impact of traumatic experience started to converge and began to develop into a field of study. In the subsequent years, the field of traumatic stress studies has come to present a significant challenge to the existing psychiatric paradigm. Immersed in the political connections between the problems of patients they were seeing in their offices and the social disparities around race, class, sexual orientation, and gender that were ever more evident, many psychiatrists joined in civil rights and anti-war protests, writing letters that allowed women to get what were then dangerous illegal abortions and allowed men to avoid being sent to Vietnam.

The convergence of so many forms of study represents a significant historical moment. In 1972, psychiatrist Chaim Shatan described "post-Vietnam syndrome" that ultimately led to the inclusion of post-traumatic stress disorder as a legitimate problem for combat veterans [63]. By this time, William Niederland, Henry Krystal and others who had already devoted twenty-five years to working with concentration camp survivors who were experiencing "survivor syndrome", noted that the same delay preceded their "survivor syndrome" as was being recognized in the work with Vietnam veterans [64–65]. In 1974, Ann Burgess and Linda Holstrom at Boston City Hospital described the "rape trauma syndrome" noting that the terrifying flashbacks and nightmares seen in these women resembled the traumatic neuroses of war [66]. Similarly, Lenore Walker published her landmark study on victims of domestic violence in 1979, giving birth to the "battered woman syndrome", while Gelles and Straus released the results of major studies on the enormous problem of family violence [67–68].

During the same era, other investigators were beginning to describe the impact of natural and man-made disasters and a rising crime rate. K. Erikson wrote a book about the survivors of the Buffalo Creek disaster of 1972 and other researchers started to explore the impact of disasters on the community [69–70]. In 1975, the National Organization of Victim Assistance (NOVA) was founded and other victim-centered groups emerged, such as Mothers Against Drunk Driving and Parents of Murdered Children [71]. At this point in time, arguably the beginning of what is now "trauma-informed" approaches, both Robert Rich and Susan Salasin became involved in developing mental health programs and social policies to meet the needs of victims [72]. Events such as the 1974 robbery of a bank in Stockholm, Sweden and the kidnapping, capture and sentencing of heiress Patty Hearst led to the notion of the odd form of bonding in captivity situations known as the "Stockholm Syndrome" [73].

In 1962, physical child abuse was identified as such for the first time when pediatricians in Colorado identified the battered baby syndrome [74], but by the 1970's, Susan Sgroi (1975), David Finkelhor (1979) and others had begun to document the widespread incidence of the sexual abuse of children and the harm it caused [75–76]. Around the same time, Judith Herman and her colleagues in Boston began to document the effects in adult women of having been sexually abused as children [77]. In 1979, Lenore Terr published the first of her series of papers and a book on the children of the Chowchilla, California kidnapping which introduced a developmental focus on the effects of trauma [78].

During this period, the context of individual and social existence were seen as relevant and extremely important in understanding and responding to a wide variety of problems. Many psychiatrists and other mental health practitioners were in the forefront of practicing a different kind of psychiatry—therapy that involved the family, therapy that listened to the meaning behind the schizophrenic's unique language, group therapies of all sorts from psychodrama to Tavistock groups, therapy that was socially and politically engaged under the rubric of "community mental health." Many of them believed that, as Ullman wrote in 1969, *"the mentally ill person is seen as a member of an oppressed group, a group deprived of adequate social solutions to the problem of individual growth and development"* (p. 263) [79]. They tried to place the patient and his or her symptoms within a total sociopolitical context, viewing each patient's symptoms as an adaptive response to dysfunctional systems, most importantly the patient's family. The French philosopher Foucault had written about mental illness as a social construct leading to the possibility that social forms of intervention could significantly change the outcome for those labeled as "mentally ill" [80]. Recognition grew that deviant behavior was not just irrational, insane, animalistic, and inexplicable, but could be understood in a relational context. "Deviant behavior can be seen as a form of communication, but to elicit and understand what lies behind such behavior is a difficult and painful process" (p. 61) [81].

Change was in the air and alongside the anxiety associated with seemingly chaotic and sometimes violent change, there was a surge of hope and vision that was captured in a number of ways: in communal settings where people of all stripes experimented with alternative living environments, and even in a mental health treatment climate that implied that mental illness—along with poverty, racism, sexism, and economic inequality—could be abolished. The human rights movement became a true international movement, people of color began to overcome 200 years of oppression, gay men and women started to openly express their own individuality and rights, while women surged into almost every occupational and educational setting and liberated themselves by taking control of their own capacity for reproduction. The long climb toward children's rights even gained momentum with the "discovery" of child abuse and child sexual abuse, and new efforts directed at child protection and an understanding of child development took off [4].

A Biopsychosocial Model and General Systems Theory

In 1977, Dr. George Engel wrote an article published in *Science*, and expanded on in 1980 in the *American Journal of Psychiatry*, in which he attacked reductionism of the traditional biomedical model and discussed how general systems theory provided a link between all levels of organization, important because the course of the illness and the care of the patient could be importantly influenced by processes at all system levels interactively [82–83]. He recognized that *"all medicine is in crisis"* (and this was almost 35 years ago) and that the crisis derives from a basic fault, namely *"adherence to a model of disease no longer adequate for the scientific tasks and social responsibilities of either medicine or psychiatry"* (p. 129) [83]. He saw that psychiatry was dividing into two separate camps: one which would exclude psychiatry from the field of medicine and the other that would limit psychiatry to behavioral disorders that were a consequence of brain dysfunction—what we here call "biological reductionism." He wrote that the result was that psychiatry was forgetting that it is now *"the only clinical discipline within medicine concerned primarily with the study of man and the human condition"* (p. 134) [83].

But the rebellions of the 60s and 70s with all the talk of equality—of races, classes, genders—were a direct challenge to the status quo that included several hundred years of racial segregation, the oppression of women and children over thousands of years, a growing separation of socioeconomic classes, and white male supremacy. The cultural changes that followed pushed more conservative elements in the society into disequilibrium. By the end of the 1970s, the social and economic systems of the United States responded strongly to the perturbations of the previous two decades by invoking the powerful equilibrium-seeking devices of large systems, in this case American right-wing, authoritarian, religious conservatism. The Presidency of Ronald Reagan beginning in 1980 marked a change in the climate of the United States that swung progressively and radically away from the liberal agenda of prior centuries.

The System Bites Back

The human services version of this extreme rightward swing resulted in the criminalization of the mentally ill and the profound reductionism of biological psychiatry and behaviorism. Starting in the late 1970s, biological psychiatry was inexorably displacing psychodynamic forms of training in virtually all residency programs across the country. Biological psychiatry depends upon the expertise of—and several layers of—established authority: physicians, pharmaceutical manufacturers, and the Food and Drug Administration. In contrast, psychodynamic forms of treatment, at their best, insist upon multiple layers of complexity and creativity. The individual is the expert about herself—even if she doesn't know it yet. And social forms of treatment look at the interactive social determinants of health and illness. Those inclining toward biological fundamentalism have always been in conflict with those who place a stronger emphasis on social and environmental factors as the sources of psychiatric dysfunction. In the world of psychiatry in particular and in the mental health field generally, there has long been a tension between those who favor doing whatever it takes to simply stabilize a patient—drugs, restraint, punishment —and those who see strategic and creative possibilities within the chaos created by the onset of acute emotional problems.

Reductionistic Behaviorism

Particularly in programs directed at children, behaviorism came to dominate programs during this era. Teaching behaviorist techniques to well-trained and supervised professionals who knew other ways of understanding children and their families was one thing. Teaching behaviorist techniques to people who had no other experience with treatment was quite another. Behaviorist techniques started to be practiced with religious fervor and in many places other beliefs and practices were ushered out the door. Under this regime it was no longer necessary to understand what had happened to the children in care, or to understand what they were trying to say with their symptoms. It was simply necessary to change their behavior through a rigid set of what consequences and if that didn't work, then it was because the consequences were not severe and punitive enough. As the executive director of one of our residential children's programs declared at a training while discussing the history of his very large organization, "... and then in the 1970s we all became behaviorists and that has been an unqualified disaster."

Many psychodynamic psychotherapists would agree that the proper role for therapy is to be a safe container for the chaos of the patient's experience. The therapist's role is to validate the importance of letting change occur, despite the disruptions that may attend the process. A seasoned therapist knows how to alternate between provoking enough anxiety to propel the person, family, or group into the vortex of change while sufficiently soothing anxiety that may be threatening to overwhelm the system thereby forcing it into regressive solutions. But such a system of care is fundamentally anti-authoritarian when the patient, not the professional, becomes the expert and ultimate decision maker. Such an approach can be perceived as dangerous because in a destabilized system, deviants must remain deviants. Deviance must be suppressed or at least held in check, and it is the socially assigned task of institutionalized psychiatry to assist in this process.

Deinstitutionalization and Deregulation

As all these changes were gradually unfolding, inpatient treatment in mental health settings was taking on a new face. The public system had deteriorated to such an extent that a movement called "deinstitutionalization" had already begun to close down most of the state facilities and put the patients out into the community. A good idea on its face, it was evident even as this was happening that the "community" was not about to provide the kinds of services that these chronically impaired patients needed, and they began showing up as the ubiquitous "street people" in all of the major urban areas while representing a substantial portion of the inmates in jails and prisons. On the other hand, general hospital psychiatry was expanding as a countermeasure to deinstitutionalization so that patients could be treated acutely in their own communities and because the hospitals saw opportunities for new sources of income.

The dominance of the market economy, the value of profit above all else, was a movement that was well under way by the mid-1980s and dramatic transformation via the psychiatric health care system occurred. Corporate America discovered that there was a great deal of money to be made by treating the mentally ill in private facilities under the notion that "the market rules"; and that meant that wherever money was available to be made, there was an obligation to make it. Insurance companies of the day still provided coverage for inpatient treatment and often long-term coverage for severe mental health problems. As a result the private for-profit and not-for-profit sectors mushroomed and as it grew, intense competition for patients developed between the various hospitals and hospital chains.

At first, this competition produced innovation, and it was possible to provide high-quality care without ethical compromise. But it was a system that bred corruption, particularly in the mental health sector, largely because there were insufficient checks and balances, promoted by a philosophy of deregulation. Unchecked growth is what happens in cancerous conditions when the body's normal regulatory feedback mechanisms cease to function properly. Without any regulation the same thing can happen in formerly healthy organizations. In order to keep the flow of patients coming in under the influence of rapidly expanding competition, and therefore keep their stockholders happy, health care corporations began engaging in corrupt practices that included bribery, paying referral sources for patients, intense and not always truthful marketing practices, and the practice of keeping patients in hospitals much longer than they needed to be there. Because recovery from an emotional disturbance is often more difficult to define than recovery from a medical illness, the psychiatric field was particularly prone to these kinds of abuses.

Little meaningful thought or action went into anticipating the results of turning professionals into entrepreneurs and money managers, of having them switch their ancient loyalties to patient care to loyalty to the financial stability of their institutions. Little consideration was given to the implications of having our health—individual and national—determined purely by the morality of the "free market."

And That Brings Us to Today

We have used the metaphor of a "system under siege" purposefully to express the notion that the mental health system has been systematically blocked and strangulated, while many of its component parts are weakened, starving for resources, and profoundly demoralized. Managed care for mental health is a system that has reduced mental health benefits that never had achieved parity with physical health care, reduced inpatient stays to only a few days, reduced the number of hospital beds, virtually eliminated specialty programs, reduced coverage for outpatient treatment to a minimum, while placing physicians and other health care providers into what can be described as a constant state of ethical conflict. Only in October 2008 was legislation finally passed requiring insurers to provide coverage for mental illness commensurate with coverage for physical illnesses, but there are many loopholes in that legislation. At its worst, unless a bureaucrat on the other end of the phone—who may or may not have credentials similar to your own—agrees with your treatment plan, you cannot give your patient the treatment you believe is the right thing to do. You may be told what medications you should start or change and if you do not comply, the patient's stay or treatment regimen is likely to be disallowed. And all of these judgments are made by someone who has never even spoken to the patient. If you administer treatment against the will of the managed care company, you may plunge your patient into overwhelming debt, it may become impossible for you to make a living, or you may compromise the survival of the organization that hires you.

As summarized in an article for the *Journal of the American Medical Association*, "*The current trend toward the invasion of commerce into medical care, an arena formerly under the exclusive purview of physicians, is seen ... as an epic clash of cultures between commercial and professional traditions in the United States. Both have contributed to US society for centuries; both have much to offer in strengthening medical care and reducing costs. At the same time, this invasion by commercialism of an arena formerly governed by professionalism poses severe hazards to the care of the sick and the welfare of communities: the health of the public and the public health"* [65].

The result of these seismic changes has been the radical expansion of the number of human service delivery systems that are ailing or in crisis. Even as the extent of mental illness in the population of children and adults was reported as increasing, expenditures on mental health care were plummeting while profits for managed care companies were soaring. As one consumer group has pointed out: *"In mental health, managed care creates administration and profit expenses that consume over 50% of the money that was previously available for treatment"* [50]. In a system where the only meaningful shared value is financial gain, this is entirely acceptable.

A starving body can live for a prolonged period consuming ever-decreasing levels of food. Most people—at least in America—have stores of fat to depend on that provide the energy necessary for survival. But beyond a certain point, fat stores are gone and as starvation continues, overall health begins to be negatively affected. By the mid-90s, human service organizations began to literally starve. Just as the human body consumes resources to stay alive and to grow, organizations consume resources for the same purposes, and as those resources are withdrawn the organization adapts by doing what it can to eliminate "fat." But if the resources continue to diminish, starvation and organizational dysfunction ensue.

The Economic and Human Burden on the System

As we noted earlier, recent cost analyses inform us that we are spending $1000/year for every man, woman, and child in the United States just for the burden of mental illness, and this excludes the costs of incarceration, homelessness, comorbid conditions, and early mortality [43]. Mental illness, more prevalent than cancer or diabetes, ranks first among illnesses causing disability in the United States. According to the former Surgeon General of the United States, about one in five Americans experiences a mental disorder in the course of a year, or 44 million people per year. Approximately 15% of all adults who have a mental disorder in one year also experience a co-occurring substance (alcohol or other drug) use disorder, which complicates treatment [84]. About 10% of the U.S. adult population uses mental health services in the health sector in any year, with another 5% seeking such services from social service agencies, schools, or religious or self-help groups. Approximately one in five children and adolescents experiences the signs and symptoms of a *DSM-IV* disorder during the course of a year [84].

Critical gaps exist between those who need service and those who receive service. Given that 28% of the population has a diagnosable mental or substance abuse disorder and only 8% of adults both have a diagnosable disorder *and* use mental health services, one can conclude that less than one-third of adults with a diagnosable mental disorder receive treatment in one year. In short, a substantial *majority* of those with specific mental disorders do not receive treatment [84]. In the United States, mental disorders collectively account for more than 15% of the overall burden of disease from *all* causes and slightly more than the burden associated with all forms of cancer [85]. Racial and ethnic minorities are even less likely to obtain care; when they do, it is often of poorer quality [86]. There are indications that the newly enacted reforms will change the discriminatory practices that for so long have determined mental health care practice but it will take years to undo the systemic damage already done.

Unlike the for-profit world that is investing in new product development and innovation all the time, we do not have adequate research and development funds. In the social service sector, change is promoted through resource reduction and punishment, which doesn't really make sense, not through investment in development. On other domains, research and development dollars often are funneled through nonprofit foundations. Through the 1990s although foundation grants substantially increased, behavioral health—meaning mental health and substance abuse—became a smaller proportion of all foundation giving (dropping from 2.2% in 1991 to 1.5% in 2000) as well as a smaller proportion of foundation health giving (dropping from 13% in 1991 to 7% in 2000). For the decade 1991–2000, funding for behavioral health averaged just under 2% of all foundation giving and 11.5% of health giving [87]. Foundation giving for mental health was $20.4 million in 2004—approximately 6% of total health giving. From 2003 to 2004, funding for mental health dropped 11.2%. Foundations making grants included the few funders that focus solely on mental health and a broader number that also fund in other areas [86].

According to the National Alliance on Mental Illness, state budget cuts are impacting mental health systems at a level never faced before. Across the country, demand for public mental health care is increasing while budget cuts are reducing coverage for and access to treatment for children and adults with mental illness. According to the Bazelon Center for Mental Health Law, federal block grant appropriations which support services to the states had not increased for decades (as of 2005) [88]. The states' major source of support from SAMHSA is the mental health block grant. This program has received level funding for many years, losing ground due to inflation. When expressed in constant dollars to reflect purchasing power, 2005 block grant spending was barely over half the 1983 total of $230 million [89]. Mental health spending by the states in 2006 was less than 12% of what was spent in 1955 when adjusted for medical inflation and population. A recent review of state mental health funding found that in the years 1981–2005, similarly adjusted spending declined by 0.2% each year, dropping from 2.09% of all state spending to 1.98%.

Given states' budget cutting in the current dismal economy, it is thought that this trend may well worsen [89].

Managed Care and Inadequate Payment

To understand what has happened to mental health organizations and the workforce, a little more information about the economic changes over the last two decades and the results of these changes may be useful. As the former American Psychiatric Association president pointed out, the genesis of the current crisis in the mental health care system is inadequate payment for care [90]. Between 1987 and 1997, the current insurance system had cut mental health and substance abuse benefits by more than 50% [91]. In reviewing claims from large employers responsible for 1.7 million covered lives, researchers have found that behavioral health spending dropped from 7.2% of total private health insurance spending in 1992 to 5.1% of total spending in 1999 (primarily because of a dramatic decrease in hospital treatment due to shorter lengths of stay and reduced probability of admission). In fact, as overall health spending *increased* by 15.7%, mental health and substance abuse spending *decreased* by 17.4% during this period [92].

In part these decreases reflect major shifts in inpatient spending which was 48% of total behavioral health spending in 1992 but by 1999 it was only 18%. From 1992 to 2000, the number of state mental hospitals declined by 29%, private psychiatric hospitals declined by 38%, and general hospital units declined by 14% [92]. This reduction in facilities and beds has had widespread reverberations, including substantial increases in admissions to the remaining hospitals. According to a survey of members of the National Association of Psychiatric Health Systems (NAPHS), admissions per facility on average have increased 11% (from 2113 in 2000 to 2354 in 2001). Occupancy rates have also substantially increased over the past few years. Based on the NAPHS survey, occupancy rose from 69.2% in 2000 to 74.1% in 2001—a 7% increase in occupancy rates in one year. In 1996 occupancy rates were 55.6%, compared to 74.1% in 2001. In addition, 25% of the respondents to the survey had occupancy rates greater than 88% in 2001 and even with these high occupancy rates the programs can barely scrape by financially [92].

Transinstitutionalization and Inappropriate Care

In 1970, state hospital beds represented 80% of all psychiatric hospital beds. By 1998 this had dropped to 24% of all psychiatric hospital beds. One of the results of this precipitous drop in state mental hospital beds, as every urban dweller can attest, is the rise in the number of mentally ill homeless people frequenting shelters and simply living on the streets, subject to repeated victimization and exposure to violence and subjected to "revolving door" brief psychiatric hospitalizations. It also helps explain the increase in mentally ill people who are incarcerated [93–95]. As E. Fuller Torrey wrote 15 years ago, "*Quietly but steadily, jails and prisons are replacing public mental hospitals as the primary purveyors of public psychiatric services for individuals with serious mental illnesses in the United States*" (p. 1611) [96]. This phenomenon has been called "transinstitutionalization" as people are moved between institutions [97].

Approximately half of people experiencing homelessness suffer from mental health issues. At a given point in time, 45% of homeless report indicators of mental health problems during the past year, and 57% report having had a mental health problem during their lifetime. About 25% of homeless people have serious mental illness, including such diagnoses as chronic depression, bipolar disorder, schizophrenia, schizoaffective disorders, and severe personality disorders [98]. Although benefits of deinstitutionalization have been described, "*most of the mental health field has seen it as a failed policy, or as a failure to implement policy*" (p. 161) [97]. As a result, injured people are being continuously reinjured on the street or in poorly staffed facilities. They often become inadequate parents who fail to adequately provide for the physical and emotional needs of their children and the pattern continues. The systemic focus is and has been on maintenance not recovery.

Rarely is it the bureaucrats or legislators who have made the structural decisions that have led to the crisis in care who actually must face the human consequences of their decisions. Instead it is emergency room mental health crisis worker (or the emergency room doctor where, as is frequently the case, there are no mental health staff in the emergency room), the staff in inpatient settings who must refuse admission or force these destitute and deranged souls back onto the streets, or law enforcement personnel who must arrest them. By mid-year 2005 more than half of all prison and jail inmates had a mental health problem, including 705,600 inmates in state prisons, 78,800 in federal prisons, and 479,900 in local jails. These estimates represented 56% of state prisoners, 45% of federal prisoners, and 64% of jail inmates [99].

This failure to implement policy can be witnessed in the outpatient sectors. The shift away from inpatient treatment was not compensated for by partial hospital or intensive outpatient/alternative programs. Many have closed or limited the number of patients they can accept. While 82.5% of respondents to the National Association of Psychiatric Health Systems' *Annual Survey* offered partial hospitalization services in 2000, in 2001 only 66.7% of respondents offered this level of care. Fewer partial hospital slots exist as facilities have struggled with administrative costs due to Medicare regulations, fewer payors for partial hospital services, and managed care organizations' pressure to look to lower cost alternatives. While the number of facilities offering partial hospitalization programs has shrunk, those that remain have seen substantial increases in their admissions and visits [92]. Nor have outpatient programs been able to meet the needs. As a report from the Bazelon Center for Mental Health Law pointed out, *"the squeeze on state mental health systems is resulting in fewer and fewer services in the community ... most communities in nearly all states lack the necessary continuum of appropriate care"* (p. 5) [100].

And as multiple investigators have pointed out, the services for children are in even worse disarray than those for adults, with children stuck for days and even months in emergency rooms waiting residential programs [100]. According to a report requested by Senators Waxman and Collins, about 15,000 children with mental illnesses were improperly incarcerated in detention centers in 2003 because of a lack of access to treatment, and 7% of all children in detention centers remain incarcerated because of a lack of access to treatment. In addition, the report found that 117 detention centers incarcerated children with mental illnesses younger than age 11. The report also found that 66% of detention centers said they incarcerated children with mental illnesses "because there was no place else for them to go." Some witnesses who testified at the hearing said that children with mental illnesses often are incarcerated in detention centers because their parents do not have access to treatment in schools or lack health coverage for such treatment [101].

Managed behavioral health care has now impacted the public sector as well as the private with mixed results thus far. But as one author put it:

> The empirical and anecdotal evidence of the negative effects of public sector managed care is as compelling as the evidence for its benefits.... The populations most vulnerable to serious and persistent mental disorders are often at risk due to failure to recognize their special circumstances or failure to treat them soon enough or at the appropriate level of care with specialty services. Economic incentives to provide less-intensive services and for shorter periods place those who need long-term services at risk of missed diagnoses, more complications, longer hospital stays, and poor recovery.... In attempts to reduce pharmacy costs, some publicly financed managed care programs have constrained formularies, excluding the newer, more costly psychopharmaceuticals and promoting generic substitutes and lower-cost alternatives. With little evidence of clinical substitutability or effectiveness, this approach limits treatment alternatives. (pp. 163–64) [97]

Under these pressures, inpatient psychiatric programs become little more than "holding tanks" for the most severely ill patients while medication is rapidly and frequently injudiciously adjusted. Outpatient providers are then left to fend for themselves when the patients are sent back to them in little better condition than when they were admitted, having received little information from the overextended inpatient staff as to what to expect or how to proceed.

Shorter lengths of stay, increased occupancy, and increased admissions per year means greater savings and profitability for the companies managing the benefits, but for the staff working in these settings it is a prescription for a wide variety of individual and organizational dysfunctions. The impact of this dysfunction spreads throughout the system and does not just affect the inpatient care programs. For example, inpatient teams do not have time to gather a client's history or even establish a relationship of sufficient length to gain the level of trust necessary for someone to reveal the kinds of intimate information that are required in order to make an accurate assessment. The impressions of one mental health program administrator are shared by thousands of others:

> As things have changed over the years it has rarely, if ever, been for the better. The rules become increasingly more punitive and the changes lauded as innovative are thinly disguised cost-cutting measures. There is generally just enough money invested in the system to keep it running, but never enough to really make it work. While the mental health system is gutted, the prison system thrives, but few people seem to make the connection. Apparently we have solved our mental health issues by criminalizing mental illness.

Just Don't Ask About Trauma

At the same time as all of these changes have been instituted, four significant fields of endeavor have emerged with revolutionary implications for the treatment of all forms of physical, psychological, and social injury: the biopsychosocial study of attachment, traumatic stress studies, research on the social determinants of health and disease, and the consumer recovery movement defined as "*an ongoing, dynamic, interactional process that occurs between a person's strengths, vulnerabilities, resources, and the environment. It involves a personal journey of actively self-managing psychiatric disorder while reclaiming, gaining, and maintaining a positive sense of self, roles, and life beyond the mental health system, in spite of the challenges of psychiatric disability*" (p. 10) [102].

Unfortunately, the emergence of radical new knowledge requires a capacity for innovative change and high-level integrative practices that are not available to significantly stressed systems. Instead, staff members in mental health organizations frequently react to the increased demands and the stress of rapid turnover by a "just don't ask" policy. As a result, important information such as an accurate trauma history is not obtained. A study in 1996 showed that trauma histories were poorly documented on patients' charts. In 1996, trauma knowledge was just percolating into the system and this finding reflected that only 15% of the reviewed histories had a trauma history documented on the charts. Sadly, when the study was replicated 10 years later, things had not gotten that much better. Although at this point 56% of charts had a description of trauma severity, only 14% compared to 9% in the original study had a documentation of diagnostic formulations or treatment plans for patients with a trauma history [103]. If this were a medical issue instead of a mental health issue, it would be comparable to finding an underlying cause for heart disease, diabetes, or cancer and 10 years later having clinicians still not ask about that cause or take advantage of advances in treatment. In fact, as we will explore in the next chapter, the past history of trauma may even be related to these very kinds of medical problems.

Systems in Crisis

The result of all these conflicts, clashes, and confusion is that our systems of service delivery are in crisis. In their Interim Report for the President's New Freedom Commission on Mental Health, the Commission concluded that:

> *Our review for this interim report leads us to the united belief that America's mental health service delivery system is in shambles. We have found that the system needs dramatic reform because it is incapable of efficiently delivering and financing effective treatments—such as medications, psychotherapies, and other services—that have taken decades to develop. Responsibility for these services is scattered among agencies, programs, and levels of government. There are so many programs operating under such different rules that it is often impossible for families and consumers to find the care that they urgently need. The efforts of countless skilled and caring professionals are frustrated by the system's fragmentation. As a result, too many Americans suffer needless disability, and millions of dollars are spent unproductively in a dysfunctional service system that cannot deliver the treatments that work so well.* [104]

This represents a description of a very broken system. This is not the first time organizational dysfunction has been described. Because a system is alive, it can become unhealthy just as our individual bodies can become ill. The illnesses that systems manifest can be acute and short term, or chronic and long term. Living systems can become self-destructive and suicidal and they can even die. Unhealthy organizations have a great deal in common and have been variously referred to as "the declining organization" [105], the "neurotic organization" [106], the "snakepit organization" [107], the "addictive organization" [108], or the "high fear organization" [109]. Whatever the term used, there is a general air of degradation and a sense that everything is always falling apart and one must be very careful to make sure that it does not fall on you. There is a general lack of energy, low motivation, and low morale among the people in the organization. Organizational goals and standards are not generally agreed upon by the employees, and frequently the stated goals are not consistent with what actually occurs, although this discrepancy is never directly confronted.

Little attention has been given to the impact on the workforce of downsizing, increased workload, increases in job complexity, loss of role definition, frustrated career development, increased levels of risk, toxic organizational cultures, and severe ethical conflicts in the workforce. And funding to provide the ingredients known to be major contributors to sustaining a satisfied workforce has been increasingly elusive: team management; opportunities for professional development; learning opportunities; shared decision making; a substantial rewards system; recognition for innovation and creativity; a high tolerance for different styles of thinking and ambiguity; respect for tensions between work and family demands; job sharing; parental leave; child care; a specific corporate social agenda; job safety awareness; and change management. And yet all of these factors affect the ability of professionals to create and sustain relationships that provide the fundamental building blocks of healing, the very factors known to make the largest contribution to positive therapeutic outcome: relationships, hope, and therapeutic healing rituals [3].

And yet despite the recognition that there are enormous problems *and* a workforce crisis, the factors that contribute to a healthy organization receive little attention in most of the recent national reports on health, mental health, and social service delivery systems, which are notably silent about the people who actually do the work in those systems. It is as if the worker is invisible except when he or she is actually invisible—when there are noticeable shortages of human beings adequately trained to do the work. Although a report from the National Mental Health Association addresses the lack of cultural diversity among mental health clinicians and notes the workforce crisis in mental health because "faced with high stress and low paying jobs, many potential clinicians have turned away from the mental health service sector," little else is mentioned about what it truly takes to create and sustain health within an organization [110].

This lack of attention to the people who actually deliver the service that is the centrally stated mission of the mental health system and the entire human service delivery system is not surprising if we consider the working model of mental-health-system-as-machine. In such a model, the workers are simply pieces of the machinery, and being such, their feelings, beliefs, and thoughts do not need to be considered, any more than you would consider the feelings, beliefs, or thoughts of your refrigerator. All that matters is the behavior, and if the behavior fails to meet the needs of the system, you replace the people and get new ones, just as you replace your old refrigerator. It is ironic that factories that make widgets and companies that do financial planning pay more attention to the well-being of their employees than systems designed to deliver vital health, social welfare, and mental health care services to human beings.

Don't be surprised if, when you read this book, it sounds like we are describing the places where you work. Wherever we speak about these issues, people immediately recognize the place where they work now or the place where they used to work. Students in classes we offer, when asked to write papers about the impact of stress on organizations, poignantly describe their personal experience working in very dysfunctional health and human service delivery systems of all sizes, shapes, and variety. The lack of anything resembling a healthy organization in the health care and human services field at this moment is so endemic that when someone comes up to us after a talk and asks, "How do you know so precisely the place where I work?" we respond, "It's not where *you* work—it's where *everyone* works." Sure, misery does love company, but it is also oddly empowering to know that the problems are not unique and that there are explanations that go beyond one's own individual situation that may provide some alternative means to change those situations.

From his position as the C.O.O. of a residential treatment setting for children, Brian has had a close-up and personal view of the results of all this:

> *The workload of staff is complicated enough just dealing with clients, but without a doubt the largest source of frustration for our staff in the Mental Health Division is the mounds of paperwork and the draconian rules related to documentation and authorizations. Clearly staff have their hands full managing very difficult issues with children, but the needs of insurance companies take far more of their time and attention some days than the clients do. I would venture to guess that most folks don't get into the field of social work or psychology because they yearn to complete outpatient treatment reviews or sit on the phone for an hour trying to get through to the managed care company. They want to spend time with the kids, but more and more of their time is committed to pushing papers around and demonstrating that this kid—who has been suspended three times, is failing all his courses, and fights constantly with his mother and siblings—needs therapeutic intervention.*

Conclusion

Unhealthy organizations are likely to be those that have been subjected to chronic and unrelenting stress and create environments that promote workplace stress for everyone that works within them. In Chapter 2 we will turn to exploring the public health nightmare that is workplace stress—what it looks like, its sources, and the impact it is having on service delivery systems.

Chapter 2

"I Gotta Get Out of This Place": Workplace Stress as a Threat to Public Health

SUMMARY: *It is impossible to understand the full impact of the last 30 years of changes in human service delivery without understanding the impact of acute and chronic stress on workers at every level of the system. In this chapter, we review what we know so far about the magnitude of stress impacting daily existence with a specific focus on workplace stressors. The issue of workplace stress is a public health problem of enormous proportion, not dissimilar to what existed 200 years ago before we understood that microbes cause disease—only now the infectious agent is violence in all of its forms.*

It's All about Stress

There's stress in all of our lives, and then there is stress. We experience stress—the internal or external influences that disrupt an individual's normal state of well-being (p. 3) [111]—throughout our lives even before we are born. Without it, we would not be able to grow and develop normally. The science of stress provides the integrating conceptual bridge between physical, emotional, social, and moral health. The physiological effects of stress are profound because every major organ system in our body becomes mobilized under conditions of stress to enable us to adapt to change and to overcome whatever threat to survival the stressor is posing. Because our bodies and minds evolved within an intensely social context, much of our adaptation and ability to survive is dependent on others of our kind. As a result, the physiological effects of stress are contagious. The effects of social contagion can be profoundly important and a door that "swings both ways." A certain amount of stress is vital for growth and development of the individual and social systems. But too much stress or the wrong kind of stress and people get sick and so do social systems.

Kinds of Stress

All stress is not alike. According to researchers at The National Scientific Council on the Developing Child, brain research is demonstrating the many ways in which biological events that occur during fetal and postnatal life predispose the child to an elevated risk of subsequent problems in physical and mental health [112–113]. The impact of stressors depends on the kind of stress a child—and later the adult he or she becomes—is subjected to, and investigators have described four major types of stress—positive, tolerable, toxic, and traumatic—that lead to very different outcomes.

Positive Stress

Positive stress promotes growth and development and is necessary for a healthy mind and body. When children experience positive stress, they have short-lived physiological responses, including changes in heart rate, blood pressure, and some neurohormones. In the context of supportive relationships from the adults around them, the normally stressful experiences of childhood help a child develop mastery, self-esteem, confidence, self-discipline, and self-control [112–113].

Tolerable Stress

Tolerable stress events are experiences that are intense but relatively short-lived such as death of a loved one, parental divorce, or a natural disaster. Tolerable stress may trigger enough physiological response to disrupt brain architecture, but when relieved by the support of caring relationships the brain has sufficient buffering to provide adequate protection for a child's vulnerable central nervous system [112–113]. Most children and adults will recover and suffer no long-term difficulties.

Toxic Stress

Toxic stress is associated with prolonged and intense activation of the body's stress response systems when a developing child lacks the buffering necessary from socially supportive people in his or her environment for the brain to be adequately protected. Recurrent child abuse or neglect, severe maternal depression, parental substance abuse, community violence, and family violence all increase the likelihood that a child will be repeatedly exposed to toxic stress.

Because of technological advances in the last few decades, we know now that the child's brain architecture—the very way the brain is structured—is determined by the interaction of the brain with the environment. When the child is exposed to frightening environments, his or her brain is persistently bathed in elevated stress hormones. These altered levels of key brain chemicals produce an internal physiological state that disrupts the architecture and chemistry of the developing brain. Although individuals differ in how they respond and adapt, the result can be long-term difficulties in learning and memory as well as health-damaging behaviors of many different kinds. Continuous activation of the stress response system also can produce disruptions of the immune system and metabolic regulatory functions [112–113].

Traumatic Stress

Traumatic stress occurs when a person experiences an event that is overwhelming, usually life-threatening, terrifying or horrifying and they are helpless to adequately protect themselves. In situations of traumatic stress, the individual's coping skills are overwhelmed and they are insufficiently buffered by resources that exist in their social environment. Much of what we describe in this book is a result of exposure to toxic stress or traumatic stress—and the impact of such exposure on clients, staff, and entire organizations. In Chapter 3 we will explore these effects in greater detail.

Allostatic Load

In understanding the impact of stress on body, brain, mind, and social context, it is important to recognize that the interactions between the individual, the social environment and the stressors themselves are interactive and complex. Two concepts are helpful in registering this complexity: allostasis and allostatic load. (1) *Allostasis*, defined as a dynamic regulatory process in which balance is maintained by an active process of adaptation during exposure to physical and behavioral stressors, and (2) *Allostatic load*, is defined as the consequence of allodynamic regulatory wear-and-tear on the body and brain promoting ill health, involving not only the consequences of stressful experiences themselves, but also the alterations in lifestyle that result from a state of chronic stress [114]. Using these bridging concepts, researchers are becoming able to calculate the various kinds and components of stress and its impact on the individual including the impact of socioeconomic factors and the kinds of exposure to childhood adversity that we describe next.

Adverse Childhood Experiences: A Public Health Nightmare

One sobering illustration of the enormity of the public health problem posed by exposure to toxic stress comes from the Adverse Childhood Experiences Study done by Kaiser Permanente in San Diego and the Centers for Disease Control and Prevention in Atlanta, Georgia [115–121]. The purpose of the study was to examine the impact of exposure to toxic levels of stress across the life span. So far, this is the largest study of its kind to examine the long-term health and social effects of adverse childhood experiences and included almost 18,000 participants. The researchers asked these willing participants—all members of the Kaiser HMO in San Diego—if they would take a survey. The majority of those who participated were Caucasian, 50 years of age or older, and were well educated, representing a solidly white, middle-class population.

An adversity score or "ACE" score was calculated by simply adding up the number of categories of exposure to a variety of childhood adversities that the person had experienced before the age of 18. These categories included severe physical or emotional abuse; contact sexual abuse; severe emotional or physical neglect; living as a child with a household member who was mentally ill, imprisoned, or a substance abuser; living with a mother who was being victimized by domestic violence; or parental separation/divorce. So, for example, a client comes for treatment or for some kind of help, and you find out that she was sexually abused by an uncle as a child, her parents were divorced, her mother was hospitalized for depression, and her father drank heavily and used drugs. Her ACE score would be at least "4"—one each for sexual abuse, parental divorce, mental illness in her mother, and substance abuse in her father. Or a client tells you that his father spent time in prison when he was growing up, his mother was a drug addict who neglected his psychological and physical needs, and his stepfather beat him. His ACE score would be five—score 1 for living with someone as a child who was in prison, another for his mother's drug addiction, one each for emotional and physical neglect, and one for physical abuse.

Of this largely white, middle-class, older population, almost two-thirds of the participants had an ACE score of one or more, one in six individuals had an ACE Score of 4 or more, and one in nine had an ACE Score of 5 or more. Women were 50% more likely than men to have experienced five or more categories of adverse childhood experiences [122]. Once they had gathered this data, the researchers compared the ACE score to each person's medical, mental health, and social health data. What they found was startling and very disturbing. The higher the ACE score, the more likely a person was to suffer from one of the following: smoking, chronic obstructive pulmonary disease, hepatitis, heart disease, fractures, diabetes, obesity, alcoholism, intravenous drug use, depression and attempted suicide, teen pregnancy, sexually transmitted diseases, poor occupational health, and poor job performance [123].Worse yet, the higher the ACE score, the more likely people were to have a number of these conditions interacting with each other. In other words, the higher the ACE score, the greater the impact on a person's physical, emotional, and social health.

According to the study findings, if you are a woman and have adverse childhood experiences your likelihood of being a victim of domestic violence and rape steadily increases as the ACE score rises and if you are a man, your risk of being a domestic violence perpetrator also rises. The study showed that adverse childhood experiences are surprisingly common, although typically concealed and unrecognized and that ACEs still have a profound effect 50 years later, although now transformed from psychosocial experience into organic disease, social malfunction, and mental illness. The authors of the study concluded, *"We found a strong graded relationship between the breadth of exposure to abuse or household dysfunction during childhood and multiple risk factors for several of the leading causes of death in adults"* (p. 245) [123].

A replication of the Adverse Childhood Experiences Study—one that would take into account, for example, the other kinds of exposure that inner-city children have, in addition to the existing categories of adversity —has not yet been attempted. We do know, however, that many children who live in conditions of urban poverty are exposed to dreadful experiences. Surveys done in Detroit, Chicago, Los Angeles, and New Orleans suggest that about a quarter of youth surveyed had witnessed someone shot and/or killed during their lifetime [124–127]. Among children at a pediatric clinic in Boston, 1 out of every 10 children witnessed a shooting or stabbing before the age of 6 [128]. Another group of researchers showed in a 1998 study of 349 low-income black urban children (ages 9–15), that those who witnessed or were victims of violence showed symptoms of posttraumatic stress disorder similar to those of soldiers coming back from war [129]. The Justice Department recently completed the most comprehensive nationwide survey of the incidence and prevalence of children's exposure to violence to date [130]. The findings are extremely disturbing confirming that most of our society's children are exposed to violence in their daily lives, over 60% in the past year. Nearly half of the children and adolescents had been assaulted at least once in the past year. We have not even begun to reckon with the long-term public health effects of this kind of violence exposure, nor have we addressed that in less than 20 years, the number of children with incarcerated parents has increased by 80% [131]. It is also disturbingly true that one in six black men, as of 2001, had been incarcerated and that if current trends continue, one in three black males born today can expect to spend time in prison during his lifetime [132].

So how fit is our human service delivery system to respond to the overwhelming needs facing it? Not very fit at all. But it gets even more complicated. Remember, the people studied in the Adverse Childhood Experiences Study were 50 years old or older when the study was done in the 1990s. They are now reaching retirement age, so the exposure of children to adversity is not new and cannot be blamed on recent cultural changes. These are people who are in the workforce, who are making the policies, and directing organizations. These are the judges, the police officers, the hospital administrators, the social workers, the Congressmen and women. Many people who are drawn to a social service environment have experienced overwhelming adversity themselves, so let's look at that for a moment.

Adverse Childhood Experiences and the Workforce Crisis

Given the rate of exposure to adverse childhood experiences in the general population, many of us who work in health care, mental health, child welfare, housing, and other human services are consumers of those services from time to time. And even if we haven't sought formal assistance, people who work in the social service field are, if anything, more likely to have suffered from childhood adversity. Many people go into this work as a helping professional because of their own struggles with loss and injury.

Several years ago we did a very simple survey of the residential staff at Andrus Children's Center and found that over 80% of the staff had suffered some form of childhood adversity. In our various training experiences, several of our faculty have asked the participants of the Sanctuary Institute trainings (anonymously of course) about their own experiences of childhood adversity as defined in the ACE Study. Out of 350 human service workers with a wide variety of experience, training, and professional education, 37% said they had been psychologically abused by their parents and 29% said they had been physically abused. When asked about neglect, 35% of them said they had been emotionally neglected, while 12% said they had been physically neglected. A quarter of those surveyed said they had been sexually molested while they were still children. An astonishing 40% said that as children they had lived with someone who was a substance abuser while 41% of them came from broken homes. Over a fifth of them had witnessed domestic violence as children, while 10% of them grew up in households where someone was in prison.

This does not suggest that these social service workers are ill equipped to do their jobs, but it might suggest that they could be prone to having reactions to stress not unlike the clients that they serve. Add to this the reality that the work in residential care and virtually all social service settings is routinely stressful, and it is not always clear who is triggering whom when we unpack incidents. Making the assumption that the clients are the most volatile ingredient in these situations is often wishful thinking.

The issue of childhood adversity is tied to the workforce crisis in social services. There is serious concern for the future in terms of social policy and the impact of exposure to adversity on a significant number of the workforce. As discussed in an article published in the *Proceedings of the National Academy of Science:*

> *A growing proportion of the U.S. workforce will have been raised in disadvantaged environments that are associated with relatively high proportions of individuals with diminished cognitive and social skills. A cross-disciplinary examination of research in economics, developmental psychology, and neurobiology reveals a striking convergence on a set of common principles that account for the potent effects of early environment on the capacity for human skill development. Central to these principles are the findings that early experiences have a uniquely powerful influence on the development of cognitive and social skills and on brain architecture and neurochemistry, that both skill development and brain maturation are hierarchical processes in which higher level*

functions depend on, and build on, lower level functions, and that the capacity for change in the foundations of human skill development and neural circuitry is highest earlier in life and decreases over time. (p. 10155) [133]

These findings lead to the conclusion that the most efficient strategy for strengthening the future workforce, both economically and neurobiologically, and improving the quality of life for workers is to invest in the environments of disadvantaged children during the early childhood years [133].

Trauma Touches Everyone

The likelihood is exceedingly high that anyone reading this book has not only experienced adversity in childhood but will endure a traumatic event at some time in his or her life [134–136]. Epidemiological studies define a traumatic event conservatively as *"an extreme traumatic stressor involving direct personal experience of an event that involves actual or threatened death or serious injury, or other threat to one's physical integrity; or witnessing an event that involves death, injury, or a threat to the physical integrity of another person; or learning about unexpected or violent death, serious harm, or threat of death or injury experienced by a family member or other close associate"* (pp. 218–219) [17].

But an arguably more useful definition is one that sees trauma as occurring when external and internal resources are inadequate to cope with an external threat [13]. People's internal resources include their bodies, minds, and spirits. Their external resources include everyone else. This kind of a definition helps to determine why some people respond to an event in very different ways than other people. However, it is clear from many studies that interpersonal violence is more likely to have long-term consequences than natural disasters or accidents. People who have had adequate childhood development, current social support, a normally reactive central nervous system, and are without any other psychological disorders are likely to recover relatively well from a single incident, adult-onset traumatic event, particularly in the absence of interpersonal violence. But someone whose exposure begins early in life, occurs repeatedly over an extended period of time, is highly invasive, is associated with a great deal of stigma, and is interpersonal is far more likely to experience long-term consequences of a traumatic event. It is this latter complexity that differentiates posttraumatic stress disorder as it is usually described from more complex problems that are the typical presentation of many of the clients who seek services in the human service delivery systems [137].

Currently, efforts are underway to expand our understanding of the complexity associated with exposure to repetitive and overwhelming stress that usually begins in childhood by using different terms such as "complex posttraumatic stress disorder (PTSD)" or "developmental trauma disorder" [137–139]. These terms embrace a wide variety of interactive problems that include the following: alterations in the ability to manage emotions; alterations of identity and sense of self; alterations in ongoing consciousness and memory; alterations in relations with the perpetrator; alterations in relations with others; alterations in physical and medical status; and alterations in systems of meaning.

The bottom line is that there is no clear dividing line between "us" and "them"—between the people who need our help and the people that offer that help. Frequently, the helpers are themselves "wounded warriors" of a different sort. In the next section we will look at the aspects of workplace stress that add—often unnecessarily—to the physical, emotional, and moral burdens of caregiving.

Workplace Stress: Definitions, Scope, and Costs

The National Institute for Occupational Safety and Health (NIOSH) defines job stress as the *"harmful physical and emotional responses that occur when the requirements of the job do not match the capabilities, resources, or needs of the worker"* (p. 6) [140]. Workplace stress is created by uncertainty along with a lack of control over important factors at work [141]. The job demands for human service workers are significant, particularly when there is a mismatch between the work that is often difficult and uncertain, and the individual's resources. Exposure to childhood adversity and to other traumatic experience complicates and compounds normal workplace stress and workplace stress itself can become toxic.

The ways in which individuals respond to workplace stress is multidetermined by sources specific to the individual, the job, and the organization [85]. There are many indicators of individual stress, including an increase in unexplained absences or sick leave, poor performance, poor time-keeping, increased consumption of alcohol, tobacco, or caffeine, frequent headaches or backaches, withdrawal from social contact, poor judgment/indecisiveness, technical errors, constant tiredness or low energy, and unusual displays of emotion [142].

A large body of research has accumulated about the impact of stress on the individual. In general, it has been found that too much stress is bad for our psychological well-being [143], hurts our bodies [144] and our mental health [145], decreases job commitment [146], increases a sense of threat and anxiety at work [147], lowers nonwork satisfaction [148], and reduces job involvement [149]. Workplace stress contributes to a three-fold risk for heart and cardiovascular problems while stressed employees are two to three times more likely to suffer from anxiety, back pain, substance abuse, injuries, infections, cancers, and obesity [150]. A recent study found that 54% of workers leave work feeling fatigued and at least 10% percent of workers are too tired to even enjoy their leisure time. The result is that one out of five workers is at risk for stress-related health problems—and all of this research was performed before the economic downturn of 2008.

Let's look more closely at the issue of substance abuse. Alcoholism alone causes 500 million lost workdays annually. Absenteeism among alcoholics or problem drinkers is 4 to 8 times greater than for nonalcoholics and up to 16 times greater among all employees with alcohol and other drug-related problems. Family members of alcoholics and substance abusers use 10 times as much sick leave and have higher than average health care claims than family members of nonalcoholic and other substance-using families [150].

According to the NIOSH, job stress has become a common and costly problem in the American workplace, leaving few workers untouched while 40% of workers report that their jobs are very or extremely stressful. In fact, one-fourth of employees view their jobs as the number-one stressor in their lives; three-fourths of employees believe the worker has more on-the-job stress than a generation ago. Problems at work are more strongly associated with health complaints than are any other life stressor, more so than even financial problems or family problems [140].

As for the cost of workplace stress, one authority has estimated that 60%–90% of medical problems are associated with stress and one large insurance company estimates that 45% of corporate after-tax profits are spent on health benefits [151]. But that only reflects a portion of the actual cost. A true analysis must include absenteeism, job turnover, replacement cost for employees who leave the job, accidents, workplace injuries (and in the worst cases, death), the long-term health and social consequences of tobacco, alcohol, and drugs, as well as the costs of quality control, administration, and customer service problems related to stress. The American Institute of Stress claims that chronic stress actually adds over $300 billion each year to cover associated health care costs and absentee rates. That represents a cost of over $600 to every "stressed" worker—an investment of dollars that gives no return on investment. Meanwhile, the cost for health insurance of a single employee doubled over the last few years and is still rising [150].

"Normal" Sources of Workplace Stress

We have labeled this discussion of workplace stress as "normal" because these sources of problems are so widespread as to be virtually universal, at least in the human services. These chronic sources of stress then provide the context within which the dramatic and traumatic experiences of workplace violence and traumatic bereavement in the workplace (which we will focus on in Chapter 5) create situations of chronic crisis.

Stress becomes toxic when it is unrelenting, has multiple origins, is unavoidable, and occurs in the context of relative powerlessness. According to experts, the top 10 workplace stressors include "the treadmill syndrome" where employees have too much or too little to do; random interruptions, such as telephone calls, walk-in visits, demands from supervisors; pervasive uncertainty as a result of organizational problems, unsatisfactorily explained and unannounced change; funding changes; mistrust, unfairness, and vicious office politics; unclear policies and no sense of direction in the organization; career and job ambiguity resulting in feelings of helplessness and lack of control; no feedback, good or bad; no appreciation; and lack of communication up and down the chain of command, leading to decreased performance and increased stress.

The greatest perceived stressor for people is a lack of control over their participation or the outcome of their work [151]. It is important to note that these sources of stress appear to have very little to do with the work itself. Instead, the main sources of stress on workers are the ways in which organizations operate and the nature of the relationships that people experience within the work setting.

Downsizing and Turnover

Research on downsizing has shown an array of negative results and minimal positive results for organizations, confirming a decline in job satisfaction and organizational commitment among those who survive the layoff. Nine studies published since 1994 reported actual turnover data for rather diverse segments of the behavioral health workforce in the United States. The findings ranged from a low turnover rate of 13.2% to a high of 72.6% in a single year. Addiction treatment programs have turnover rates, according to one study, of 50% in frontline staff and directors [61].

Children's programs face similar dilemmas with potentially more dire results. Studies indicate turnover rates that hover near 50% [152]. *"In its simplest terms that means that children who have faced rejection and abandonment by so many adults in their lives are waking up in the morning to a new worker caring for them over and over again,"* said Jim Purcell, executive director of the Council of Family and Child Caring Agencies [153]. The GAO did a survey and report of child welfare agencies and found that turnover rates are about 30%–40% nationally and that the average tenure for child welfare workers is less than 2 years. The dominant reasons include low salaries, combined with a high risk of violence, staff shortages, high caseloads, administrative burdens, inadequate supervision, and inadequate training [154].

These high turnover rates are also an important barrier to any kind of organizational change. No sooner are workers trained in a new methodology or an evidence-based practice than they move on to a new job and it is necessary to start all over with someone new [155]. Not only does this have hugely negative consequences for the organization, but since one of the main etiological forces behind childhood problems is disrupted attachment, high turnover rates negatively impact children's treatment as well.

We have learned through decades of solid research that relationships and attachment are the crux of change and at the heart of the repair work that needs to happen for children and adults whose lives have been disrupted. This cycling of both clients and staff in and out of treatment settings is an excellent way of guaranteeing that change will not occur. It sets up a child—or a troubled adult—for repeated failure and reenactment of previous disrupted attachments and defeats the very purpose of intervention.

As Brian describes:

Many years ago in our residential program we began to struggle with turnover. We lost a couple of workers unexpectedly. Under the stress of open positions we made several quick, but flawed, hiring decisions. The workers we hired were ineffective and inexperienced, which further stressed the system. Workers who had been in place and were rock solid suddenly felt overtaxed, began looking for alternatives, and often left abruptly. Suddenly two vacancies became four and then six. Every new worker seemed to become the senior worker on the shift within 3–6 months, if he or she lasted that long. More experienced staff and managers became inordinately stressed. During that year our turnover, normally hovering around 10%–20%, ballooned to almost 50%. The cascade of events caused by the initial loss threw us off for over a year. We were able to eventually pull out of this, but it was a very difficult phase.

Severe funding cutbacks in the social services have resulted in cutbacks in most social service providers and therefore the loss of jobs and key personnel. In the case of frontline workers, this often means the loss of someone upon whom you have depended for a sense of safety, not just for collegial relationships. In dealing with volatile, sometimes dangerous clients in situations that are highly emotionally charged, social support is likely to be the only attenuating factor that helps staff members manage difficult situations in a constructive way. As Brian reports:

One real problem with human service organizations is that funders and donors do not support overhead. Somehow overhead is seen as taking dollars away from clients. But to be successful, organizations need strong infrastructure for finance, human resources, data compliance, and information technology. These overhead costs are seen as wasteful by funders but are key components to developing a strong organization. More and more mandates around reporting and compliance require increases in overhead costs, but the mentality about overhead has not changed much. The lack of support for overhead ensures nonprofits will always be limping along, never really able to invest in the kind of innovation and expansion of services that our clients actually need. This is one place where we could use more and better business practices. A factory that makes widgets cannot produce—and cannot compete in the marketplace—without adequate infrastructure support and neither can we.

In any organization, usually because of a lack of transparency, staff members are unlikely to know the entire story when one person or a group of people are laid off. They do not see the financial statements and have no idea whether the organization is in real trouble. They worry about their own position and livelihood. Some staff may increase their productivity to make themselves more indispensable, but many become gripped by fear and worry and may instead become less productive.

When team members are laid off or leave because of adverse working conditions, this vital network of social support is eroded and the team members left behind may experience an acute sense of loss. The impact of these losses on teamwork, communication, and emotional management is frequently devastating to the total environment. Despite the fact that there are far fewer people necessary to do the work, no individual will be held any less responsible or legally liable should someone fall through the cracks and suffer harm as a result. The media attacks will still come; the lawyers will still seek damages. The impact on every remaining member of the social service sector who must pick up the slack and therefore ration services, which often means rationing attention that very distraught children or adults desperately need, will also be extremely stressful [156].

When there are high turnover rates it is difficult for staff to form and maintain the relationships necessary to really work effectively together. We need to be able to rely on our coworkers if a team is to be effective, and constant disruptions as a result of turnover make a difficult job even more difficult. Tight bonds develop between coworkers in social service organizations, mirroring the bonds between people who have served together in the military or in law enforcement, related to the shared exposure to danger and stress. Sometimes it may reflect a similar kind of "trauma bonding" because of how difficult, demanding, and frequently frightening it is to provide care for psychologically damaged and sometimes violent children and adults. It is not uncommon to go to a party at someone's home and see only coworkers there—none of their friends from college or childhood, just coworkers—and what they are talking about is work. With little time left for debriefing in the workplace, workplace issues erode into and may even come to dominate personal time.

Workload and Job Complexity

Another major contributor to stress-related problems is workload: both too heavy and too light a workload can be stressful. However, in the case of the social service system, conditions leading to too light a workload are presently difficult to imagine. On the contrary, research has demonstrated that a lack of adequate staffing is the main stressor reported by staff. Qualified nurses reported significantly higher workload stress than less professionally developed staff in acute care settings, resulting in high levels of burnout and emotional exhaustion [157]. A recent review of research on workload issues by the National Association of Social Workers shows that increased caseloads negatively impacts case outcomes and is a major cause for a high rate of turnover which is financially expensive in many social service areas [158].

And it is not just the workload itself. The fact that the situation can change almost instantly from one that is relaxed and comfortable to one that is filled with threat and even danger is also a major stressor. Life is not predictable when you are working with troubled children or adults who are responding to external events but also to their own internal stimuli. For instance, a childcare worker is quietly watching a movie with the kids in a cottage, where everyone seems relaxed and calm, and then suddenly a fight breaks out. As chairs are being thrown around, the formerly calm worker is thrown into his own fight–flight reaction, but he has to get the situation under control to prevent any damage to the kids, property, and himself. Remember that sometimes these "kids" are 250 pounds and 6'2". Most parents can relate to the emotional climate in the home when two kids are squabbling, but then extend that to the impact of having 20 or 30 kids in a small space, many of whom are likely to have difficulty controlling their impulses and are easily frustrated. That's part of what we mean by workload.

It's not just working with kids that creates these demands. Here is an example from one of our colleagues, Dr. Lyndra Bills, from the first day of her first job, just out of her psychiatric residency training.

My first day on the unit will always stand out vividly in my memory. I was freshly out of my residency and eager to start my new job. …But the first few moments of that first day prepared me to reevaluate my decision. As I opened the door, I looked down a long, dimly lit, drab hallway. The sound of women's screams filled the air and as I stared, halted in my progress for a moment, a chair flew across the hallway and crashed to the floor, and then a large woman, presumably a patient, came up behind a staff member and began to pound the nurse on the head. Several other staff members rushed up, grabbed the patient's arms, and began to talk to her. Only later did I learn that this was routine behavior for that patient. During the brief period of calm that ensued, I discovered that there were four rooms with staff posted on chairs outside because those four patients required one-to-one supervision for 24 hours a day and one room with two staff posted outside because their patient required two-to-one supervision for 24 hours per day. Even with this close contact, however, the staff would rarely talk to the patients to whom they were assigned, but every 15 minutes they would carefully note the status of the patient on the clipboard that accompanied them throughout their long and tedious shifts. When they were not assigned to this kind of supervisory duty, the staff members would gratefully retreat behind a raised plexiglass wall at the nursing station which separated the staff from the patients. The nurses were clear that the job they had been instructed to do was to observe, record, and report. Talking to the patients, engaging in a therapeutic dialogue, was considered beyond their abilities. The nursing staff did not necessarily always follow this dictate, but it was clear that if they wished to do so, such a policy would be backed up by the normative expectations of the institution (p. 350) [159].

Job complexity is another established source of stress. It is difficult to conceive of a subject more complex than trying to help someone recover from the long-term effects of multiple traumatic and abusive experiences in a limited period of time with radically reduced resources. Yet that is what virtually every human service worker is trying to do. This is the notion that lies at the heart of the movement to make services "trauma-informed." This demand is particularly challenging for staff in children's programs and child welfare agencies, since the child is still developing and the outcome of intervention may—or may not—alter a child's destiny. Child welfare workers must deal with the demands for permanent placement of the children in their care, even though finding adequate placement for these children can present overwhelming challenges. Here Brian describes some of the difficulties with job complexity:

Job complexity in many of our positions is stunning. Some years back I remember being quite confused by JCAHO [The Joint Commission on the Accreditation of Heathcare Organizations] focus on competency-based job descriptions. The intent of the standard appeared to be that organizations should ensure that employees had the knowledge, skills and competencies to safely perform their jobs. The standard suggested that for every position there should be a list of necessary competencies, methods for how to assess that the members of the workforce possesses those competencies and processes to insure that staff who pull up short are brought up to speed. While this is a useful concept in principle we found the practice to be quite something else. Expecting staff to make the right choice when confronted with a very difficult child often requires that they do things that are counter-intuitive, even when under a great deal of stress and strain. That is a very tall order. There are other sources of constant stress and strain with line staff that become very complicated in organizations like ours. Childcare staff are generally among the lowest paid staff in the organization and as a result frequently work an excessive amount of overtime to make ends meet. This group of staff are also overwhelmingly black and Latino; they tend to be young and supporting young families. They work long hours and at times their work entails providing one-to-one staffing with some of our most challenging, threatening and troubled children. These assignments would try the patience of our most rested and patient workers, but it is not uncommon that staff members accept these difficult assignments after having just worked a full shift. They will, at times accept overtime assignments day after day and week after week, sometimes working 100–120 hours in a pay period. The worse the staff shortages and the more rapid the staff turnover, the more likely it is that an organization will have to use overtime staff to provide enough staff coverage.

Role Definitions

Role overload is determined by how many different roles a person has to fulfill; it is stressful because it creates uncertainty, ambiguity, and conflict about an individual's ability to perform. This becomes particularly important when people's lives and safety are at stake [85]. In mental health settings, it is at the level of the frontline staff that problems with role overload, role ambiguity and conflict, and the burden of role responsibility are most likely to surface. Direct care staff in residential settings are assigned to clients for 8–10 hour shifts at a time, constantly accompanying the clients to a much greater extent than any other professionals in the setting. In childcare settings, each childcare worker—whose training is likely to have been minimal—must serve as parent-surrogate, educator, therapist, disciplinarian, caretaker, nurturer, and security guard, often within the space of a single shift. This level of extreme role ambiguity can be a constant source of stress. Additionally, given the low pay scale, as Brian described earlier, many frontline workers must work more than one job or volunteer constantly for overtime in order to make ends meet at home, while shift work is well established as a significant workplace stressor [85]. Brian details the role complexity of his workers:

Our line staff have to play many different roles, even in the span of one 8–10 hour shift. They must be able to manage basic routines and activities of daily living with the children. They must be able to assess risk for suicidality and various sorts of perpetrator behavior, including sexually inappropriate behavior, fire setting, and homicidality. They must know how to use behavioral support techniques. They must understand the basics of group work. They must understand trauma and have a strong understanding of each child's history and how that history impacts the child's current behavior. They must understand a variety of Microsoft Office applications. They need to know lock-up procedures, food handling procedures, and sanitation requirements. They need to know whom to call for what. They need to understand the basics of pharmacology, pediatrics, first aid, parenting skills, activity planning, fashion, music, and art. They need to be ready for anything and everything, and they need to do it with a smile on their face and a song in their heart, for 8 to 10 hours at a clip with some of the most challenging children in the county. And they are supposed to do this with (for some) a bachelor's degree or at least the start of it or (for others) with little more than a high school education.

Child welfare workers, as another example, are often beset by conflict in what is expected of them. Are they to help families? Investigate abuse?

Police families? When a child known to a public agency dies, society, the child's family, the press, and the agency often hold the caseworker responsible for the tragic death. When interviewed for a study on burnout in child welfare workers, child protection workers blame themselves for situations for which they could in no way be responsible. *"What did I do wrong?" asked one worker. "I am programmed to think there is a deficit in me"* [160]. As astute observers of child welfare practice have noted: *"The decisions caseworkers make every day would challenge King Solomon, yet most of them lack Solomon's wisdom, few enjoy his credibility with the public, and none command his resources.... Child care workers are expected to somehow straddle the two core values of U.S. society—the protection of children and respect for the privacy of the family. CPS is accused of both 'unwarranted interference in private life' and 'irresponsible inaction' when children are truly threatened"* (pp. 4–5) [161].

There may be a poor fit between the personality of the individual and the role requirements of the workplace, but when jobs are scarce people may find themselves taking jobs in social service settings without being fit for the role, without a prior understanding of the responsibilities that are going to be expected of them, and without clear notions of the roles they will be expected to fill. In areas where there is fierce competition for qualified workers but limited resources to compete, or in rural areas where there are simply not many available employees, organizations may hold on to employees who are minimally capable of responding to the complex roles demanded of them.

In response to all of the external stressors we are describing, the internal response of the system is usually to oversimplify or "dumb down" the demands made on staff. As a result, over time the role of the mental health technician, childcare worker, or child protection worker may become more clearly defined, but the role definition becomes too simple to reflect the needs of these very troubled children and adults. In this way, programs that may have formerly engaged in more complex team treatment and supervision may deteriorate into a system that has frontline workers doing little except enforcing rules and meting out punishments. This practice then inadvertently sifts out anyone capable of the more complex role demands that should be fulfilled in order to help clients recover. It is not unusual to encounter an inpatient or residential mental health or other social service program where the direct care staff lack any training in mental health assessment, evaluation, or treatment. They may not ever participate in any team discussion or get a chance to discuss what they are seeing and experiencing with anyone who has extensive expertise—which is the way frontline staff used to learn how to understand complex problems. Because of this deterioration in training, supervision, and expectations, it is a common practice to withhold vital clinical information from direct care staff on the spurious grounds of "confidentiality." This absence of information or case formulation leaves them without any way to even begin to understand the complex behavior of the children, much less respond to it with consistently therapeutic approaches.

What this really means is that clinical information is withheld because managers are afraid that frontline staff will use the information irresponsibly simply because they have not had the training to know how to understand that information or they lack a theoretical construct that allows them to make sense of it. Without this, the fear is that the staff member will use the information in some way to hurt the child and therefore further jeopardize the child's ability to trust adults. The lack of strong middle managers in many human service organizations makes it very difficult to keep frontline staff aligned with the overall mission. At the same time, imagine you are a childcare worker in this situation, having total responsibility for the safety and well-being of a child about whom you know virtually nothing. *That* is stressful. Brian recalls an event he experienced while at a conference:

> *One time I was doing a training on situational leadership, and I told the group that you want to make sure that staff who have low motivation and low skills are either not getting hired or are being counseled out of your organization. One of the participants, who was a manager at a residential program, raised his hand and said, "What if those are the only staff you have?" I really didn't know how to answer that one, but it was quite a sad commentary on the state of the industry.*

In outpatient settings, support staff have often been cut in response to funding cuts. As a result, highly trained clinicians do the clinical work and documentation but also may have to do time-consuming administrative tasks that they despise and for which they are not particularly well suited. Whatever time is spent doing paperwork and other administrative tasks is time taken from supplying direct client care. As Brian recalls,

> *This was a major problem at the outpatient mental health program when we merged with it, and it had to do with role definitions. After the merger when I started seeing how the organization worked, I saw that the pressure on clinicians was incredible. Clinicians did the clinical work and documentation but also did their own authorizations, arranged client transportation, did their own scheduling, negotiated sliding scale fees, and on and on. This was a double-edged sword: The clinicians had an enormous amount of power and an enormous amount of autonomy. They set fees, waived fees, continued to see people who could not pay, decided when they would take another case, when they would discharge a case. At the same time, they were hopelessly overworked, doing tasks that clinicians really should not be doing and are not particularly suited for.*

Relationships, Diversity, and Health Disparities

Relationships at work, such as those with supervisors, colleagues, and subordinates, are key ingredients to either attenuate stress or increase work stress. Negative interpersonal relationships and a lack of social support from others in the workplace have been established as significant stressors [85]. Organizational-level stressors can produce changes in the bureaucratic structure that then negatively affect individuals, such as when supervisors are stressed and take it out on workers, when colleagues leave, when there is inadequate time to resolve interpersonal conflicts, or when subordinates blame supervisors for problems attributable to larger forces. All of these can contribute to an atmosphere that is not only stressful because of the failure of interpersonal relationships but also because those relationships are the only source of buffering against the other difficulties inherent in mental health and social service delivery.

Interpersonal conflict is a serious source of job stress and has been demonstrated to interfere with job performance. Conflict can arise between a manager and a staff member when the manager communicates what the staff member perceives as mutually incompatible expectations such as "you must always treat the patients with kindness and respect" and "it is your responsibility to guarantee safety and order." It may be possible to both promote safety and respect, but to do so may require a degree of skill that a worker lacks. There may be conflicts between one's own expectations and the values of the organization: "These children are sick and you need to understand their behavior" and "These kids are just bad—they need more discipline." Mental health settings are fundamentally rife with conflicts for several reasons: because that is the nature of the work—the clients end up in treatment because of intrapsychic and interpersonal conflicts they have not been able to resolve within the scope of their own resources—and because there is a lack of agreement at a theoretical level about what good treatment actually is. Managing conflict while creating and sustaining a healthy relational network is a critical component to helping people recover, but this relational network is extremely vulnerable to the impact of workplace stress.

The quality and nature of relationships and interpersonal conflict in mental health and social service settings is further complicated by issues of race, ethnicity, gender, age, and sexual orientation. It is clear from many national reports, including The President's New Freedom Commission on Mental Health [162], the Surgeon General's report on culture, race, and ethnicity [84], and the Institute of Medicine's *Unequal Treatment: Confronting Racial and Ethnic Disparities in Health Care* [163] that there are serious disparities in the quality of health care received by African Americans, Asian Americans, Native Hawaiians and other Pacific Islanders, Latinos, Hispanics, and First Nations Native Americans. These disparities get played out in social service settings that are almost solely dependent on mutual communication skills to provide effective service. When there are no native speakers, when there is a lack of understanding of the multiple ways in which background and culture interact with problem presentation, then misdiagnosis, inappropriate treatment, and premature treatment termination are all more likely to occur.

There is a notable lack of racial and cultural diversity among the mental health disciplines. The vast majority of professionals are non-Hispanic whites, often exceeding 90% of discipline composition. Studies indicate that from 70% to 90% of substance use disorder treatment personnel are primarily older, female, and Caucasian, while their clients are predominantly young, male, and represent ethnic minorities [61]. The racial split can be easily perceived in many treatment settings in various parts of the country. In many programs the direct care staff members are largely drawn from minority populations, while the clinical, education, and management staff are Caucasian. In other cases, particularly where a facility is located in a rural area, the entire staff may be Caucasian, while the clients are sent from urban areas and are mostly from racial minorities. However, despite these obvious disparities, race and ethnicity are rarely a central focus of conversation and in fact, such conversations are likely to be actively avoided by everyone, as if the mere presence of a diverse workforce nullifies past or present issues related to discrimination, racism, and structural violence [164].

Homophobia and social stereotypes about gay, lesbian, and transgendered people continue to be a source of stress for LGBT employees and are rarely directly addressed in the workplace. Long-standing discriminatory practices and sentiments may be supported in some programs by religious and personal beliefs that are not overtly disclosed, or if disclosed, not addressed in the social services' version of a "don't ask, don't tell" policy. All may be fine until a gay staff member mentions his or her sexual orientation to the clients. This is when other staff members and managers often react negatively, as though it is acceptable to be gay only if it is kept as a secret among staff. With notable exceptions, programs are not directly addressing the needs of LGBT children, adolescents, or adults [165].

Inadequate Training and Career Development

As the New Freedom Commission on Mental Health pointed out in their final 2003 report, training in the mental health sector—and by extension other components of the social service network, including addictions treatment—is inadequate [166]. The problems are legion: delays in translating science into services; educational systems emphasizing the teaching of specific practices and focusing on teaching "content" as opposed to teaching and instilling in students a *"process of continuous, lifelong, real-world learning; training in behavioral health (and other social services) occurring in disciplinary or sector silos; little cross-disciplinary training or emphasis on competency development exists"* [61].

This is so extreme that one authority has noted that *"frontline human service workers in child welfare, childcare, education, or juvenile justice are often not recognized as part of the mental health workforce"* (p. 168) [167]. This is an astonishing reality since children in these populations that do not need these services, especially in child welfare and juvenile justice, are the exception, not the rule. People routinely seem to believe that children who go into the custody of a child welfare agency because they have been abused or neglected and are therefore removed from their parents also get treatment. This is not the case. Unless they pose enough problems for whatever system that has to deal with them, they probably will not get any treatment. Our system remains under the illusion that simply taking children away from "bad" parents will automatically heal their wounds—a profoundly wrong-headed assumption.

The Annapolis Coalition, a group convened by the Substance Abuse and Mental Health Services Administration (SAMSHA) to examine and report on the serious workforce issues that surround the delivery of mental health services, noted multiple paradoxes that exist at the training and education level for practitioners. They have pointed out that graduate students and residents are trained for a health services world that no longer exists. For the most part, continuing education programs are utilizing teaching strategies that are ineffective. The people who spend the most time caring for people—adults and children—receive the least training and the people receiving the services, including involved families, receive little education [168–169].

The career paths of many mental health professions have radically changed. Reflecting the general trend of shrinking inpatient hospital utilization, the numbers of social workers in hospitals fell from 19.2% to 11.3%. This decline in social work employment in hospitals represents a long-term decline since 1989, when 20.8% of social workers were in hospitals [170]. The numbers, however, do not accurately reflect what has been lost. In health, mental health, and social service systems, social workers traditionally have played a linking role with other service providers, serving in many settings as the official or unofficial communication channels, the "glue" in the systems. The result of the decline in social work roles has been not just a decline in direct service, but the increased fragmentation of an already fragmented service delivery system [171].

Over the past two decades, the rate of growth in the number of clinically trained psychiatrists has decreased and in fact the number of psychiatric residents has remained relatively constant since 1990. There has, however, been significant growth in the number of international medical graduates entering psychiatric residencies [170]. Again, the numbers do not tell the human story. Psychiatrists, previously trained in a wide variety of modalities, and frequently experienced in running a multidisciplinary team, no longer have the time—and in many cases, the training—to provide leadership within inpatient or outpatient settings. Existing language barriers result in a deepening emphasis on intervention strategies that do not depend on complex communication strategies. Psychiatric shortages in many areas of the country create situations where patients cannot be properly medicated and where there is a decreasing systemic knowledge base about the complex interactions between mind, body, and social adjustment.

Students are seldom educated about the complex and competing demands that shape physical or behavioral health care and the intriguing challenges and dilemmas that face all human service delivery sectors [172]. Among all disciplines that provide mental health care to children, there is a striking trend toward the use of professionals who lack specialty training in child mental health. The bulk of psychotherapy—such as it is—as well as behavioral therapy is provided by mental health workers, many of whom lack child-specific training. Most prescriptions for psychotropic medication for children are written by pediatricians and family physicians, not psychiatrists. Child psychiatrists are in exceedingly short supply. The federal Bureau of Health Professions projects that just to maintain the current utilization rates of psychiatric care, and considering that currently most children who need care do not get it, by 2020 the nation will need 12,624 child and adolescent psychiatrists but is expected to only have 8,312 [173]. As a result, many adult and child psychiatrists, regardless of their inclinations or training, are compelled to do nothing except check medications, see a number of patients in every hour. This significantly diminishes the possibility that utilization of medications will be integrated within an overall complex treatment process. This may be good for the pharmaceutical industry, but is not a good outcome for children, adults, families, or communities.

Then there is the pressing issue of training for direct care workers in adult and children's human services. Direct care staff do not have advanced professional degrees; they may have a bachelor's degree, they may have attended some college or taken courses, but likewise, they may have no formal education except for a high school diploma. They may be referred to by a number of different titles: paraprofessionals, psychiatric technicians, aides, mental health workers, child care workers. Direct care personnel without advanced professional degrees comprise nearly 40% of care staff in mental health organizations, and more than 60% of client care staff in state and county psychiatric hospitals [174].

The orientation and training programs for these providers are often minimal and frequently limited to the topics that regulatory and accrediting bodies insist they have so that there is little time to give them the vital training and supervision they need to actually engage in therapeutic work with very disturbed adults and children [172]. And then there is the extremely disturbing issue of turnover that we mentioned earlier, particularly turnover of frontline staff, so that no sooner are people trained then they are leaving and going to another job.

The slow translation of science into practice is particularly striking in areas of evidence-based practice, an understanding of the widespread exposure to adversity in childhood and what it means for evaluation and treatment; attachment-based research; addictions; and recovery. A large body of knowledge about the impact of traumatic experience and disrupted attachment on a wide variety of psychological, physical, and social problems has been researched and is by now well established, yet there is still relatively little application of this science to standard practice.

What is also strikingly absent from many entrenched social services is good management training. Good people are put into positions of management because they were good at what they were trained to do in their most recent position—usually some form of social work or medical/nursing specialty—not because they necessarily had *any* management skills. There appears to be an unexplored underlying assumption that if you are working in any form of social services you are then, by necessity, "good with people" and that alone qualifies you to be a manager. Unfortunately, that turns out to be a dangerous and foolhardy assumption. Good management requires skills that not every human service worker has acquired and does not necessarily have anything to do with professional degree. But once given the authority and the responsibility, it can be very difficult to admit that you simply do not know how to properly wield that authority. For many people, moving into management positions isn't really a choice—it is the only way to get ahead and make a decent salary. Most frontline positions are capped at a low wage. For instance, your talent may lie in providing direct care for very troubled children or adults, but if you stay doing what you are best at doing—and what is desperately needed—you are unable to support your own family. Human service delivery represents a near-perfect example of the famous "Peter principle," which asserts that *"in a hierarchy every employee tends to rise to his level of incompetence"* (p. 25) [175].

Career development issues also play a substantial role in determining the way an individual manages other kinds of stressors in the environment. Job insecurity, perceived underpromotion, overpromotion, and a general sense of lack of achievement are all established sources of workplace stress [85]. Studies have shown that managed care practices are having a significant impact on mental health practitioners' incomes, their level of fulfillment in their jobs, the nature of the practice in which they engage, and their morale [51; 55; 176–178]. And as the Annapolis report points out, *"we do not plan systematically to recruit or retain staff, once hired, there is little supervision or mentoring that is provided, career ladders and leadership development are haphazard and service systems thwart rather than support the competent performance of individuals"* [168]. It is important to recognize that none of these activities—recruitment, training, supervision, mentoring—are billable activities. In a closed system, if you spend time on these activities, time is taken away from activities that bring in money.

As a result, with less and less capital in the system, these are the activities that are the first to go.

Regulation, Paperwork, and Corporate Compliance

The Annapolis Coalition also noted that people working in behavior health *"routinely struggle with the ambiguity of the rules, regulations, standards, and procedures that govern service delivery, and which sometimes conflict with one another. These rules may not be grounded in an evidence base. They often limit professional judgment, and can constrain efforts to tailor interventions to individual need. Productivity is reduced because of administrative burdens, most notably those involving extensive and often repetitive documentation"* (p. 9) [61]. Increases in paperwork were among the five most significant toxic changes noted by social work practitioners across all behavioral health settings [179]. Brian knows firsthand about the difficulties inherent in keeping up with compliance standards:

> *As the Chief Operating Officer I am particularly tuned in to compliance issues. The insistence on corporate compliance has become an increasingly important consideration in recent years. Just like our administrative approach to systemic problems within our programs is often a punitive and coercive pseudosolution, regulatory bodies often approach systems that seem out of control by focusing on punishment that rarely seems to really solve the problems. Organizations are expected to comply with literally thousands of pages of rules and regulations that change almost daily. Failure to comply can result in enormous fines that can cripple an organization. The process is so complicated that even the most well-intended organization cannot possibly avoid all the potential risks and pitfalls. Worse yet, recently compliance regulations have encouraged staff in organizations to turn in their organization for compliance problems by offering a cut of the money taken back from the organization and the fines levied. These practices serve to increase the stress levels in the organization and promote secrecy, but they do little to improve service delivery.*

Professional Values, Ethical Conflicts, and Burnout

Many studies have examined the consequences of a lack of congruence between the personal characteristics of employees and the attributes of the organization at which they are employed [180]. This assumption has been supported by research demonstrating that a conflict between the characteristics of the employees and their organizations is related to job dissatisfaction, low organizational commitment, substandard job performance, job stress, and turnover [181–182]. Empirical investigations have explored conflicts between employees and their organizations on a variety of characteristics, including conflicts in values, attitudes, needs, and goals [183].

One way of understanding person–organization fit is to look at the congruence between organizational values and personal beliefs and preferences [184]. A mismatch in values occurs when the organization makes choices that are inconsistent with the employee's core values. The greater the mismatch between a person's values and the organization's, the more burnout the person will experience, the more time the person will spend on activities not related to work, and the more likely that the person will leave as a result of job dissatisfaction [185–187]. But in a tough employment environment and when turnover is high, managers become focused on just filling the job slots rather than assessing the job–person fit, often with detrimental outcomes for everyone. Research has shown that employees who are pressured to engage in what they consider to be unethical work activity are less likely to be committed to the organization and are more likely to leave [188].

Ethical conflicts are one of the most underestimated, but chronically unrelenting sources of stress in today's human service delivery environment. As examples, relationships with managed care companies can present professionals with significant ethical dilemmas over the issue of patient confidentiality. As examples, this can occur when the managed care company demands access to client records, including detailed information about intimate aspects of the client's history, presenting problem, course of treatment, and documented outcomes as a condition of authorizing services [189]. Managed care policies may impinge on the practitioner's capacity to act on clinical knowledge appropriately because of multiple barriers to practice that are established in service of cost-cutting methods [48]. Entry into the system can only be achieved by applying a diagnostic label that is likely to become a part of the client's permanent record and therefore accessible to anyone who has access to the records from that point forward [48]. At least one study has demonstrated that intervention methods in a managed care environment are dictated not necessarily by what the practitioner believes the client needs but by limitations on the number of visits that are covered. Managed care requirements become a significant mediating factor in treatment planning and although clinicians feel strongly that the choices they must make are "unethical," they make them nonetheless. As the authors of the study note, *"widely accepted ethical principles may be rationalized in practice in regard to either what is in the best interest of the client, or perhaps, on the basis of the inherent 'unfairness' of the managed care system"* (p. 209) [166].

In this way, there is nothing new about health care rationing, which has been in place for years, decided by who will fund what when and under what circumstances. But the decisions about who gets health and mental health care, how much they get, who they get it from, and what they get are determined by people with various levels of professional training and experience—sometimes very little at all—based on financial incentives to minimize costs. As one social worker has written:

> In the meantime, my next client arrives, one of 14 for the day, for his 30 min-
> utes of positive reframing. I work with my client to help him change cognitions
> that evoke psychic discomfort, yet I seem unable to do much about my own.
> Hopelessness dominates after I realize my indoctrination into a culture of com-
> pliance with the dictates of managed care. I have become an assembly line
> worker who quickly ushers clients in and out of therapy to clear operational
> costs. Ironically, in this way mental health workers have become enforcers of
> the managed care system rather than advocates for systemic change. We
> have successfully used our expertise to normalize the injustice of managed care
> and operationalize program dictates despite seeing the inhumanity of it all.
> (p. 364) [190]

In order to help their clients or prevent harm from being done, practitioners will sometimes purposely misdiagnose clients or distort their activities and reports in such a way that the written information is relatively useless going forward. For instance, since decisions about hospital course may be made by reviewers who have little experience and are motivated to save money for the company, if a hospital employee reports that a previously suicidal patient is no longer suicidal, these will be grounds for immediate termination of benefits if the patient is not discharged. On the other hand, rarely is a patient truly sui-cidal one day and nonsuicidal the next in any absolute or clinically viable sense, and yet charts will reflect this unlikely phenomenon simply because it is may be the only way to keep someone who is still quite dangerously fragile, but not openly expressing suicidal ideation, in a hospital setting. It is also an expedient way to discharge a client who is in some way being bothersome to the staff— "Your insurance company says you have to leave."

Such a Catch-22 situation puts the clinician in profound professional and personal ethical conflict. Is it more wrong to lie on the record and to the reviewer or risk being compelled to discharge a patient who is still not truly safe? Is it more wrong to put the financial stability of the hospital at risk or the financial stability of the patient if one tells the truth and the patient's benefits are termi-nated? As discussed by two social work academics, "When a clinician must lie or omit crucial information in order to ensure that appropriate services are pro-vided, the secondary conflict is clearly one of a legal-ethical nature. The profes-sional in such a situation must violate the principle of integrity in order to provide what is clinically necessary for the client" (p. 47) [48].

Inpatient providers may be faced with repetitive and frustrating dilemmas because they have so little control over decisions impacting their work. For inpatient services, Dr. Glen Gabbard points out that a big roadblock has been the existence of a *"largely mythical treatment model designed for a mythical psychiatric patient"* (p. 27), for whom rapid pharmacological stabilization is followed by discharge with no regard for the actual complexities of a person's problems, the psychodynamics of noncompliance, and the nature of decompensation episodes [191]. People simply do not get better, become less depressed, suicidal, or homicidal on a managed care deadline.

One investigator has expressed her concerns about the far-reaching implications this could have on clinicians as they adapt to the demands of managed care. She suggests that *"the meaning of managed care for this group of clinicians lies in the prospect of being gradually, unknowingly, and unwillingly reprofessionalized from critics into proponents simply by virtue of continuing to practice in a managed care context, and in losing a moral vision of good mental health treatment in the process"* [192].

During the same period in which managed care has come to dominate mental health treatment, many psychiatrists have moved away from doing little except medication management. Older psychiatrists, trained in a very different way of doing things, may be acutely and depressingly aware of the ethical dilemmas they are situated within. Younger psychiatrists, trained in no other methodology, may consider their professional conduct entirely acceptable and are sometimes trained to believe that managing medications is the primary and sometimes sole responsibility of a psychiatrist. As a result, integrated forms of treatment are, in many cases, a thing of the past. If all a psychiatrist knows to do is how to administer drugs, then every person he or she sees is likely to be diagnosed with a problem that is said to respond to medications in a self-reinforcing loop. If the only reimbursable form of treatment is a brief medication check by a psychiatrist, then every person that the psychiatrist sees will assuredly have some problem for which he or she is given a medication, while the psychiatrist may be sincerely trying to do the best thing possible for the patient.

Complicating all this is the fact that, as we noted in Chapter 1, in the entire human service delivery field there has been relatively little emphasis on results. Professionals providing care have opinions, which may or may not be sound positions, about what "works" and what doesn't. There are plenty of people in human services who know what they are doing, are competent, and successfully help their clients—at least by the current variable criteria of what "success" means in every component of the system. There are other people who are poorly trained, poorly supervised, and basically incompetent but who are scared to admit it or just do not care as long as they keep getting paid. Without a system that competes internally and externally based on results—and results consistent with the mission of the organization, not just money—it is impossible to raise the standards of care. Managed care is not responsible for all of these problems that long predate changes in the health and social services funding streams. Managed care simply has applied unsustainable pressure to an already vulnerable and broken system.

The literature clearly demonstrates that the combination of uncertainty and the likelihood of change, both favorable and unfavorable change, produces stress and, ultimately, affects perceptions and judgments, interpersonal relationships, and the dynamics of the work itself [193]. In the mental health field for the last two decades, change has been steady and certain only in its tendency to be unfavorable to the practice of the health, mental health, and social service professions and therefore to the clients they serve. Brian notes that:

It always has to be balanced and it always has to be acknowledged that ethical standards come with a price—a price we all have to be willing to pay in an organization. If I decide I am not going to get an authorization before I render a session, then I have to be willing to shoulder some of the consequences. It is easy to have high ethical standards when someone else pays for them. We end up fighting with each other for the scraps that are falling off the plate of managed care companies. I am a clinician looking at a kid in crisis, but I have not gotten an authorization, or I have already seen the kid today, or this week. Perhaps I could get an authorization, but that might take 30 to 60 minutes waiting on the phone with some anonymous reviewer who does not know me or the kid, and I have other clients I need to see as well. So I say, "Ms. Johnson, just bring your boy in." I see the boy and now someone in billing might be stuck sorting out what to do with this claim. The people in billing then are frustrated and take it out on the clinician who may appear irresponsible but, in fact, is just trying to do the right thing for the client. The clinician and the billing staff end up in a steel-cage-death-match over this $70 claim. The managed care company and its draconian processes, designed not to manage care but to refuse it, gets off the hook and we duke it out amongst ourselves. The system, designed to limit care, is successful at doing that, but is also doing a hell of a job making us want to kill each other. It's just another secondary result of a really broken system.

Disruption in the Organizational Operating System

As we mentioned in the Introduction, we see the organizational culture as being the "operating system" for organizations; therefore, disruptions in the culture cause problems at every level interactively. Organizational culture is an astonishingly powerful force that affects all of us who function within organizational settings, all of the time. But it is also the most overlooked force because it works indirectly and frequently at the level of nonverbal communication. Organizational culture can be defined as a *"pattern of shared basic assumptions that a group has learned as it solved its problems...and that has worked well enough to be considered valid and taught to new members"* (p. 29) [194] or "how we do things around here." Organizational culture matters because it determines so many underlying assumptions about our strategies, goals, and direction.

Organizational culture arises out of the history, memory, experiences, and formal structures and personnel of the organization and helps to determine the health and well-being of the individual worker. As organizational research has demonstrated, uncertainty is a main contributor to the perception of stress, and there is nothing so uncertain in corporate life as organizational change. As one author from the world of business has noted:

> the combination of economic scarcity, the recession of the late 1980s and early 1990s, the widening gap between demand and resources in public services such as health and education, and the rampant influence of technological change has produced a deeply uncertain organizational world which affects not just organizations in their entirety but groups and individuals at all levels of the organizational matrix. (p. 253) [195]

When there are organizational problems that create toxic organizational cultures, everyone suffers: the employees, the administrators, and the clients [196]. Because the delivery of human services is so utterly dependent on empathic human relationships, human communication, and human cognitive and emotional responses, a negative organizational climate may have an even more profound impact than it does on other employment sectors. This is true regardless of whether we look at the nonprofit, governmental, or for-profit service delivery sector; or at the acute care psychiatric, residential, child protection, shelter, health, juvenile justice, domestic violence, outpatient, or other social service setting. It is true for services directed at children, adults, or families. Negative workplace cultures create negativity in employees and this inevitably affects the care that people receive [197–200].

As an example, in a study of child protection workers and their exposure to vicarious trauma, researchers found that all of the participants in the study cited the agency and office working conditions as significant stressors [160]. Given the enormous organizational complexity that we have been describing thus far, it is easy to see how an organization and the people who are trying to direct its course, can become confused and lose their way. It is easy to see how an organization could lose sight of its original mission in dealing with every new crisis and economic downturn. In a larger, more complex organization it becomes quite challenging to share new information and ensure it is built into your information sharing systems so that all new staff members receive what they need. Failing to build a robust orientation process means important information will eventually seep out of the organization.

Lack of Mission Clarity

What have been termed "mission-driven organizations" focus on the customer, and the mission depends on the exact product or services that the organization intends to provide to its customer [201]. This raises two obvious questions: What is the mission of each human service, and who exactly is the customer?

The mission of health care, of course, is to save lives, but without a focus on prevention we seem to always be closing the barn door after the horse has already left. Only recently have consumers become directly involved in trying to influence the mission of the mental health system, raising voices that insist on inclusion in decision making, empowerment, and nonviolent, trauma-informed care. But for several hundred years, a fundamental mission of the mental health system and all social services that attend to the poor—sometimes freely admitted and sometimes glossed over—has been to exclude the poor and the mentally ill from social view. The actual goals of treatment have not been tied to successful outcomes and even "success" has yet to be clearly defined. And, of course, prevention depends on preventing the social causes of most mental illness: exposure to childhood adversity, discrimination, lack of support for families, and exposure to violence.

Similarly, the substance abuse field initially had sobriety as its criterion for success. But as it has become clear that so many people entering rehabilitation settings have "co-occurring" disorders, their mission has had to expand to include greater complexity. The mission for child protective services remains clouded in confusion. Is the mission to protect children or to reunite families, and what happens to the mission when these two goals are contradictory? The mission for domestic violence advocacy was originally social and political in its aims but has become more confused in recent years as the women and children who enter shelters often have co-occurring substance abuse as well as mental health problems and because the issues that pertain to structural violence remain largely unaddressed by the society as a whole.

And who is the customer? In many cases, the customer of health and mental health services used to be the consumer. That is no longer the case. The consumers of services rarely get anything to say about service delivery options once they have signed up for a coverage plan. There are grievance procedures, of course, but in reality, the consumer no longer has much power in the situation. To survive, hospitals and care providers must please the insurance companies or close.

Lack of Innovation and Stagnation

Although an extensive research base has been documenting the enormous implications of previous exposure to trauma, violence, and abuse to the physical, emotional, and social health of the nation for several decades, only now is the issue of trauma beginning to be addressed by both the private and public health systems. This is largely due to the insistence of the consumer recovery movement and some very diligent and persistent mental health providers and administrators [202–204]. Most mental health programs and substance abuse programs are only minimally addressing the issue of trauma, and public systems are only now receiving pressure to become trauma informed. Although, there are other reasons for resistance to incorporating the issue of trauma, particularly because it is so fundamentally disturbing to the underlying mental models upon which mental health practice is based, the most obvious cause for this resistance is the lack of innovation and creativity that is typical of both stressed individuals and stressed systems.

The human service delivery system as a whole and each individual element of that system have had all they could manage to simply contend with the enormity of the changes they have undergone. The capacity to innovate, experiment, evaluate innovations, and tolerate the uncertainty of trying new things is extremely difficult under the conditions we describe in this book. Worse yet, innovation that was burgeoning in the private psychiatric system in the 1990s was almost completely eliminated by the managed care environment. Dozens of programs specializing in the treatment of psychological trauma were created in the early 1990s and almost all were closed by the beginning of the new century—not because of a lack of clients seeking services but because the loss of beds and the tightening of budgets meant that beds could be filled with far less expense by eliminating all specialty care [62]. More recently, many isolated examples exist of exemplary programs but as a recent Bazelon Center report illustrates, these are rarely brought to scale and made available to significant numbers of people in need. These successful programs, often funded with demonstration dollars for limited periods, are overshadowed by the disintegration of the system as a whole [100]. Is there any other sector of the economy that can function with little to no research and development funding?

Conclusion

In this chapter we have described the incidence and universality of exposure to overwhelming, repetitive, and toxic stress in the workplace. Community violence in our urban areas is epidemic. Gun ownership has skyrocketed. Domestic violence has not waned. Child abuse is a national shame as is the rate of incarceration, as we imprison more of our own citizens than any other country on earth. We think that understanding what happens when people are exposed to adversity and overwhelming experiences is as critical to a new understanding of and response to violence as being able to recognize microbes was 200 years ago. In Chapter 3 we will look more closely at what exposure to unrelenting stress does to the bodies, minds, and actions of individuals and groups, and then in Chapter 4 we will describe the parallel processes that occur in organizations and systems as they become increasingly organized around responding to the stress, often at the expense of aiding in the recovery of their clients.

Chapter 3

When Terror Becomes a Way of Life

SUMMARY: *If we are to solve the multiple crises facing human service delivery systems—and humanity for that matter—we need a different way of understanding human nature and human dysfunction, but one that incorporates 150 years of accumulated scientific knowledge and clinical wisdom. To understand what we are going to "diagnose" and "prescribe" for our troubled social service and mental health organizations, you will need to have a working knowledge about the psychobiology of trauma and adversity, what it does to individuals, particularly when trauma is repetitive, occurs in early development, and is a result of interpersonal violence. Computers are modeled on the brain and every computer runs on an "operating system," and all the software applications must be compatible with that operating system. We believe that attachment is the human operating system, the master program that allows other human functions to work. Trauma disrupts attachment and, like a computer virus, wreaks havoc in unpredictable ways, with the total life experience of the person involved. The younger the person is, the more powerful the disruption to this human operating system. In this chapter we describe and summarize some of those impacts on individuals and groups. Only when we understand the nature of psychobiological adaptation are we able to truly embark on creating trauma-informed cultures because doing so requires what is often radical change in thinking, behavior, and attitudes. These changes are beginning to describe what it really means to have a "trauma-informed culture."*

Attachment: The Human Operating System

The social nature of our brains is hardwired; it is online at the time of birth. Newborns begin imitating facial gestures when they are only 41 minutes old, so early imitation is not about learning; it is innate. Autobiographical memory—the memory that we use all the time once we enter childhood, when we know where we are, who we are with, what we are doing and thinking—does not function when we are born. A vital structure in the brain, the hippocampus, must mature before we can integrate all these different pieces of memory, which begin as separate elements, into a whole. Because emotions are so vital to our ability to respond to danger, emotional memory is with us at birth, controlled largely by another structure called the amygdala. Even before we have names for things, we are associating important experiences with significant emotions aroused by those experiences [205]. Every negative and positive experience with our primary attachment figures is creating an emotional worldview that colors how we see the world, what our expectations are of other people, whether the world is a good place or a bad place, long before we have words to explain any of this. These early experiences can likewise color the experiences and interpretations of the adults we ultimately become and can have significant impact on our home lives and our work lives.

Some researchers believe that it is this ability to imitate that is the moving force differentiating humans from all other species, and this is the basis for why we call attachment the human operating system or what the "grandfather" of attachment studies, Dr. John Bowlby called the "internal working model" [206–207]. Since World War II, attachment scientists have laid the scientific groundwork for understanding how we become human in the intricate dance that goes on in infancy and early childhood between children and caregivers, setting the patterns we are likely to follow for the rest of our lives. Bowlby and many other attachment researchers have said that the internal working model forms the basis of each person's personality the *"rough-and-ready blueprints for what should be expected and what is likely to occur in different kinds of inter-actions with attachment figures"* (p. 7) [208]. These early attachment experiences then determine how one views the lovability and worthiness of the self, what it means to be cared for and care about others, what to pay attention to and what to forget, how to manage emotions and how to behave, what to expect from other people [209–211].

Thanks to the work of John Bowlby, Mary Ainsworth, Mary Main, and many others, we now have a framework for understanding how the sense of individual self emerges out of the transactions between the individual and others, how the self and social development are inextricably bound together [211–215]. Human social life originates with the evolution of parental care and the mother–infant bond. The behavior between mother and infant, and later between father and infant, establishes the foundation for adult bonding, friendliness, and love—all of which are at the heart of social organization [216].

Mirror Neurons: Wired at Birth for Social Relationship

The brain areas for the brain system that we use to begin imitation of others at birth is called the mirror neuron system and were first localized in primates. The discovery of this mirroring system was made accidentally by laboratory researchers studying monkey behavior. As Daniel Goleman tells the story, the monkeys were hooked up to machines that were reading their brain waves.

When a research assistant came back from lunch eating an ice cream cone, the monkey saw the cone and a part of his brain lit up in response to watching the lab assistant eating the ice cream (p. 41) [217]. In further investigation, this part of the brain became known as the mirror neuron system. And so great discoveries are made!

In the last 10 years functional magnetic resonance imaging (fMRI) has been available to study the human brain, and the result of that advance in technology is a revolutionary advance in understanding the social brain. Researchers around the world are currently developing maps for how the human brain responds to other people in a wide variety of ways. Because of fMRI research it is possible to see the brain in action, to look at not just the structure of the brain, but the brain in action. And it's not just in monkeys that we can see the mirror neuron system. According to neuroscientists like Dr. Marco Iacoboni, the part of the human brain that also lights up while watching someone eating an ice cream cone is called the mirror neuron system. Like our monkey friends, mirror neurons in our brains are activated when we watch other people in action. If we see someone grasp an object, the motor area of our brain that would perform the same action, is also activated, even if we don't move. We are all probably a bit aware of this when we watch a sports event or some very demanding physical activity that someone else is performing. You may find your own muscles activated when the batter swings or the pitcher throws, particularly if you have ever played baseball. As Dr. Iacoboni explains it,

> The initial automatic mirroring of the facial expressions of babies triggers a whole cascade of other automatic simulative brain responses that reenact interactions between mother and baby in real life. This constant automatic stimulation and reenactment has the purpose of making us ready when action is needed. This is probably especially true in the domain of empathy, where one of the defining elements is the ability to respond compassionately to another person's distress. In the case of maternal empathy, this ability surely reaches its highest possible expression. (pp. 128–129) [218]

But human beings have mirror neurons all over our brains because we don't just mirror motor actions. We mirror emotional expression, tone of voice, gestures, mental images when we talk to someone, and facial expressions, and in doing so we come to know what someone else's intentions are and what another person is feeling. As Dr. Iacoboni writes, "When we see someone else suffering or in pain, mirror neurons help us to read her or his facial expression and actually make us feel the suffering of the pain of the other person. These moments are the foundation of empathy and possibly of morality, a morality that is deeply rooted in our biology" (p. 5) [218].

Another component of the social brain, the spindle neurons, also called Von Economo neurons, are situated directly behind our eyes and connect to our emotional centers. These cells, so vital to social development, grow connections after birth and allow us to keep track of our interpersonal interactions and guide snap decisions. There are indications that these neurons are impacted by abuse and neglect. Currently, another area of research is investigating whether the mirror neuron system and the Von Economo neuronal system may be involved in the autistic spectrum disorders in which children have serious problems with their ability to engage with other people.

From an evolutionary perspective, human infant safety is dependent on the protection of the mother and then of the entire social group. This behavior originates in the infant–mother bond, and the need to seek closeness with each other is innate. As children, our only safety is to be found in the protection of others. Tactile communication is extremely important among primates and humans and has a calming, positive effect. Researchers looking at the origins of language have suggested that language between humans developed as a way of maintaining a similar form of "grooming" behavior with larger groups of people [216].

The National Scientific Council on the Developing Child is a multidisciplinary collaboration of leading scientists in early childhood and early brain development whose mission is to bring sound and accurate science to bear on public decision making affecting the lives of young children. In one of their review publications on children and relationships they have said:

> *The initial emotional duet created by mother and baby—with their complementary interweaving of smiles, gestures, and animated vocalizations in social play—builds and strengthens brain architecture and creates a relationship in which the baby's experiences are affirmed and new abilities are nurtured. Children who have healthy relationships with their mothers are more likely to develop insights into other people's feelings, needs, and thoughts, which form a foundation for cooperative interactions with others and an emerging conscience. Sensitive and responsive parent–child relationships also are associated with stronger cognitive skills in young children and enhanced social competence and work skills later in school, which illustrates the connection between social/ emotional development and intellectual growth. The broader quality of the home environment (including toys, activities, and interactions within the family setting) also is strongly related to early cognitive and language development, performance on IQ testing, and later achievement in school. (p. 2) [219]*

The need to attach to others, to seek protection from other people when we are frightened, and to be powerfully influenced by other people's emotions are innate to the human species and accompany us throughout our lives from cradle to grave. This need to attach is as important to our work lives as it is to our family lives, and it is particularly relevant in the human service professions because of the repetitive exposure to fear that our clients endure and because so many of our clients have had experiences of disrupted attachment.

Attachment in Adults

Adult attachment has been defined as *"the stable tendency of an individual to make substantial efforts to seek and maintain proximity to and contact with one or a few specific individuals who provide the subjective potential for physical and/or psychological safety and security"* (p. 8) [220]. The bonds of adult attachments appear to have their roots in childhood attachment bonds. This does not mean an absolute one-to-one correlation. It simply means that early attachment experiences set the tone for future attachments. They are likely to determine the kinds of partners with whom new attachments are formed most easily and the developmental course of new attachments [221].

Thus, over the long haul, attachment styles appear to organize emotional and behavioral responses [211–213; 222–223]. Bowlby's theory was that they do this through the creation of an *internal working model* that guides us to re-create the original attachments throughout a lifetime, a sort of cookie-cutter pattern into which we jam anything that doesn't quite fit the mold. Then, in the form of a self-fulfilling prophecy, the more we make new relationships replicate the old, the more we become convinced that our relational models and assumptions are correct. The result: If we are lucky, we have loving parents, we establish secure relationships with them throughout childhood and adolescence, and when we have children we become loving parents who establish secure relationships with our own children. But what if luck is against us? What if we experience a traumatic loss or traumatic betrayal of parental care? Then we are likely to have difficulty in meeting our children's basic needs for love, security, and affirmation unless something or somebody changes the patterns of relationship that we have already established. That's where other people come in; that's the place for therapeutic change.

Social Support

What role do other people play throughout our lives, for better or for worse? Let's take a look at what we know about the elusive quality called "social support." The whole idea of social support dates back to at least the nineteenth century when, in 1897, the sociologist Emil Durkheim wrote one of the first books to show a marked increase in concern for the physical and mental health of modern society. Considered the founder of scientific sociology, Durkheim tried to understand the unconscious sources of social existence as Freud was trying to understand the unconscious sources of personal existence. For Durkheim, society is the source of morality, personality, and life itself at the human level. Durkheim saw modern societies as being sick, and a sign of the sickness was not only the rising suicide rate but also the appearance of a growing cynicism and despair [224]. In his classic study on suicide he discussed the way suicidal behavior evolves out of diminished social connections to family, friends, and community. According to Durkheim, when an individual does not feel that he is a part of a group, when he recognizes no higher purpose or meaning, and has few social supports, suicidal behavior becomes more likely [225]. His conclusion was that the social conditions that underlie the rising suicide rate and other forms of social pathology *"result not from a regular evolution but from a morbid disturbance which, while able to uproot the institutions of the past, has put nothing in their place"* (p. xxix) [226].

Social support theory provides a direct line of connection between childhood attachment, adult attachment, and social connectedness. Caplan described support systems as an enduring pattern of social ties that play a major role in maintaining the psychological and physical integrity of the individual [227]. This sense of being cared about is possible because of the human capacity for attachment, emotional resonance, and empathy.

Attachment to the Group

Throughout the last two centuries, historians, sociologists, philosophers, and psychologists have wrestled with the question of how the individual relates to the group. George Mead, another social philosopher of the late nineteenth century, saw human group life as an essential condition for the emergence of consciousness. He described the dialectical relationship between the individual and society, pointing out that the development of individuality and the development of social institutions are both part of human evolutionary experience and that individuals change and are changed by social institutions [228]. By the end of the nineteenth century, while Freud and his followers were developing a complex theory of individual development and pathology, other thinkers were focusing on the massive social disruptions of the Industrial Revolution. In doing so, they were compelled to look at the connection between individual maladjustment and social forces.

Just prior to World War I, sociologist Charles Cooley declared in 1909 that human nature cannot exist separately in an individual but is, in fact, a "group-nature," a "social mind," and that wherever there is an individual aspect of human function there must also be a social fact [229]. In 1920, McDougall asserted that *"We can only understand the life of individuals and the life of societies, if we consider them always in relation to one another. . . each man is an individual only in an incomplete sense"* (p. 6) [230]. John Dewey, one of America's most influential philosophers, saw the individual as so embedded in the social milieu that mind is capable of operating only by the continual stimulus of the social group and that the origins of the self lie within the social context [231].

Similarly, the famous philosopher Alfred North Whitehead noted that philosophy has been haunted by a misconception throughout the centuries, the notion of independent existence: *"There is no such mode of existence. Every entity is only to be understood in terms of the way it is interwoven with the rest of the universe"* (p. 3) [232]. William Alanson White, an influential early-twentieth-century psychiatrist observed, *"Society, while it is composed of individuals, reflects its degree of development in each individual psyche, so that man and society occupy relations of mutual interdependence, each profoundly affecting the other"* (p. v) [233].

Another psychiatrist, little remembered today, was named Trigant Burrow. He helped found the American Psychoanalytic Association in 1911 and became its president in 1926. His work has been largely ignored mainly because he took a radical turn away from individual psychoanalysis and toward a study of the group that was unfashionable at the time. In his papers and books from 1914 on, he developed the idea that the neurotic elements that Freud had identified in individual patients were embodied in the entire society. He gathered around him a group of colleagues, family members, and patients, and they formed the nucleus of a group of investigators that remained together in an experimental community for more than 30 years. In this group setting, called the Lifwynn Foundation as of 1927, they spent their time observing interrelational processes through their own interactions, using themselves as the laboratory agents.

Burrow regarded conflict, alienation, crime, and war as major public health problems that could be solved through science [234]. *"Man is not an individual,"* he said. *"His mentation is not individualistic. He is part of a societal continuum that is the outgrowth of a primary or racial continuum"* (p. 349) [235]. Later he presciently warned, *"My researches clearly indicate to me ... that with the enhancement of individualism the balance in favor of group survival has been placed in serious jeopardy. Today the very existence of the species is threatened because the antagonisms characterizing man have been largely divorced from his biological needs and actualities"* (p. 55) [236].

In 1936, Lawrence K. Frank, considered to be the originator of the child development movement in the United States, wrote: *"Today we have so many deviations and maladjustments that the term 'normal' has lost almost all significance. Indeed, we see efforts being made to erect many of the previously considered abnormalities into cultural patterns for general social adoption. . . . The disintegration of our traditional cultures, with the decay of those ideas, conceptions, and beliefs upon which our social individual lives were organized, brings us face to face with the problem of treating society, since individual therapy or punishment no longer has any value beyond mere alleviation of our symptoms"* (p. 335) [237].

Researchers today emphasize the collapse of the "relational milieu" that characterizes modern society. As Dr. Bruce Perry has pointed out, until quite recently, humans had spent at least 150,000 years living in multigenerational, multifamily groups where the ration of mature individuals to young children was roughly 4:1, meaning four adult caregivers for every child. It is this rich group environment that our brains need to develop properly and is precisely what our children today, for the most part, are not receiving [238].

Group Cohesiveness

In studies of reasonably healthy people, each of us seems to see ourselves in three dimensions: our personal or intimate self, our social or relational self, and our collective self—a broader social identity that is linked to larger social groups [239]. Cohesiveness is a scientific term meaning the strength of the relationships linking group members to one another and to the group itself. Research has shown that cohesiveness at the level of the group reflects the "we-feeling" that joins people together to form a single unit. Highly cohesive groups are known to have more enjoyment and satisfaction, more frequent communication, more participation, and less absence. People in cohesive groups experience heightened self-esteem and lowered anxiety, apparently because the group provides a source of security and attachment similar to the original childhood parental attachments [240].

Trauma Disrupts Attachment

To understand the profound impact of trauma and adversity, we need to understand the way in which trauma disturbs the human operating system by disrupting attachment relationships. As we mentioned in the Introduction, a computer virus is a small piece of software that piggybacks on real programs. Each time the program runs, the virus has a chance to spread and to wreak havoc on the entire computer. It is contagious, virulent, hard to diagnose, unpredictable, may shut the whole system down or have peculiar and individual effects, is difficult to treat, may masquerade as other things, and like so much violence, it is self-replicating, with no other purpose than to create more violence. Trauma and adversity create toxic stress; when this begins in childhood, in particular, it does to the human operating system what a computer virus does to the computer operating system. It wreaks havoc unpredictably, contagiously, and virulently with the attachment system and spreads through intergenerational contagion. Trauma disrupts attachment.

Because children are dependent on their caretakers for safety and the fulfillment of their basic needs, any traumatic situation has the potential to disrupt the child's primary attachments and sense of basic trust. This disruption is particularly profound when the source of the trauma *is* the primary caretaker. Mary Ainsworth and her colleagues have taken advantage of normal stranger anxiety to discover the different ways in which children attach to their caregivers [214]. The typical patterns of normal attachment are well organized and consistent over time with that particular caregiver, although a very different pattern of relationship may develop with a different caretaker. Longitudinal research has begun to show that these patterns of attachment are predictive of a child's behavior in school, at home, and in social situations to at least the tenth year.

Considerable evidence suggests that an individual's relationship history is an important variable determining parental behavior [21]. A child's attachment style is also consistent with future parenting characteristics and parental attachment style [220]. In other words, we tend to raise our children similarly to the way we were raised. This does not mean that maltreated children inevitably maltreat their children in the same way, but the risk of doing so is disturbingly increased. Even without actual maltreatment, what can be repeated, down through the generations, are attachment styles that become organizing themes of relationships.

The attachment style of the greatest concern related to a past history of trauma has been called the disorganized/disoriented attachment [18]. This style is characterized by a lack of coherent strategy of relating to the caregiver. The behavior of these children is inconsistent and contradictory without the usual sequencing of behavior and with the addition of quite unusual behaviors such as freezing and hand flapping. These children appear to be caught in a dilemma; their attachment figure is also the source of fear. They respond to this conflict with mental, emotional, and behavioral disorganization and confusion. This style of attachment has been found to be highly correlated with parents who have unresolved traumatic loss in their own backgrounds. The parent's state of continuing fear and the behavioral components of this fearful state frighten the child [18].

The Young Brain Organizes Around Trauma

Children's brains are still forming. We can now see neural cells from the brains of young animals as they actually reach out and make the cellular connections that are the basis of new learning. But, the release of powerful neurohormones like norepinephrine, serotonin, cortisol and beta-endorphin, particularly during critical and sensitive moments in development, is thought to have such a profound impact on the developing brain that the brain may organize itself around the traumatic event. Sustained or frequent activation of the hormonal systems that respond to stress can have serious developmental consequences, some of which may last well past the time of stress exposure. For example, when children experience toxic stress, their cortisol levels remain elevated for prolonged periods of time. Both animal and human studies show that long-term elevations in cortisol levels can alter the function of a number of neural systems and even change the architecture of regions in the brain that are essential for learning and memory (p. 3) [241].

We are only beginning to understand how the effects of chronic stress set the stage for long-term physical as well as emotional and social problems [123; 242]. Epigenetic research is demonstrating that environmental factors, including exposure to toxic stress, may influence gene expression and thereby extend the effects of stress through the generations. *"Animal studies have shown that the quality of the mother–infant relationship can influence gene expression in areas of the brain that regulate social and emotional function and can even lead to changes in brain structure. The nature of the relationship also can have long-term influences (into adulthood) on how the body copes with stress, both physically and emotionally"* (p. 3) [219].

Attachment Trauma and Betrayal Trauma

Clinically, the people who have the most problems are those who have experienced traumatic attachments. Attachment trauma is defined as *"a fear-provoking threat to the self that is accompanied by a perceived threat to the availability of the attachment figure"* (p. 389) [243]. Attachment trauma occurs whenever there are disruptions in which an attachment figure is perceived as unavailable as the result of a substantial unplanned separation, which may happen when a parent is mentally ill, physically ill, a substance abuser, or imprisoned.

When the attachment figure is the source of the trauma, *betrayal trauma theory* asserts that children are more likely to dissociate important memories of the abuse because of the great conflict between the need for closeness, safety, and trust and the awareness that the people they are attached to are not safe [244]. Attachment trauma is more likely to occur in situations of child physical or sexual abuse, emotional or physical neglect, domestic violence, and abandonment. Attachment injuries can occur when an individual feels abandoned by an attachment figure at a time of crisis, as when a car accident injuring mother and child creates a prolonged separation, and attachment trauma occurs when a child loses an attachment figure through death.

Disrupted Group Attachment Threatens Survival

Research on attachment and disrupted attachment connects our understanding of the individual with that of the group. In our evolutionary history, being separated from our group would have meant a death sentence. Other important work has related the effects of social support and stress on physical health. Certainly, as a result of the research that is being done in the field of posttraumatic stress we are beginning to understand how social support, to the extent that it helps people deal more effectively with stress, can lower the amount of hyperarousal, thereby changing the internal biochemistry of the stressed person and, in so doing, positively affect the immune system [245]. In study after study, social isolation increases the risk of developing coronary disease and other life-threatening illnesses, and among people who already have coronary disease, people who are socially isolated have a two- to five-fold higher death rates than those observed in nonisolated patients [246]. This is particularly problematic in our current cultural context because of the measurable trends showing a decline in social connection in America. As Dr. Bruce Perry points out, in 1850, the average household size in the West was six people while today it is three or fewer. A full quarter of Americans live completely alone [238].

Throughout our lives, this connection between attachment, stress, social support, and trauma will influence how well we cope with stressors at home, at work, and in our community. Support provided by key people and groups in a person's life are seen as playing a significant role in cushioning or "buffering" the individual against both the physical and psychological consequences of stress [247–248]. At the same time, many forms of stress also cause major disruptions in social ties, which then exacerbate the stress, creating a vicious downward spiral and put people at risk for the development of longer terms problems [249–250].

Deindividualization and Ostracism as Disrupted Attachment

So deep is this neurorelational wiring that ostracism, social exclusion, and rejection from the social group triggers physical pain. Neuroimaging studies have localized where we actually register rejection as physical pain in our brain [251–252]. Since social disconnection undermines our ability to think clearly and to regulate our physiology and maintain emotional equilibrium, ostracism is dangerous to our well-being physically, emotionally, socially, and spiritually [252].

Separation from one's group comes at too high a risk to tolerate easily. But perhaps as a result, circumstances can occur when a person attaches so pathologically to a group that the person submerges his or her own individual feelings, thoughts, and values. This is known as *deindividuation* [253]. First described as a psychological state in which inner restraints are lost and individuals are not seen or paid attention to as individuals, anonymity is particularly known to promote this pathological state. Studies have shown that individuals who believed their identity was anonymous are more likely to act aggressively and punitively toward others if that is in line with the group expectations. It is not a coincidence that in so many cultures across time and geography warriors have masked their identities before going into battle, thus hiding their individual identities, combining with a group identity, and permitting more violence [254].

Disrupted Attachment, Stress, and Trauma

The key to understanding the remainder of our theoretical premises is recognizing the connections we make between attachment as the basic survival mechanism for human beings *and* human groups. Therefore, anything that disrupts attachment between and among people "from cradle to grave," as Sir John Bowlby put it, threatens our survival. Traumatic experience disrupts attachment and, in doing so, disrupts relationships with individuals and with groups. To understand the nature of this disruption and lay the groundwork for how this can manifest in whole organizations, we need to understand the human stress response acutely. Then we can see what happens when people are exposed to chronic and toxic levels of stress and the ways in which groups are similarly affected.

The Human Stress Response: What Does Everyone Need to Know?

Like other animals, humans have formed a highly effective protective system that evolved in our original evolutionary environment when human beings lived in small groups of family members and were threatened by hungry predators. This defensive action system is a total body mobilization, driven by the powerful neurochemicals that flood our brain and body. To survive, we must pay attention to any information from the environment that might help us, so many of our senses become more acute—eyes dilate, hearing improves, smells sharpen. Whenever threatened, our attention becomes riveted on the potential threat, and we become hypervigilant to what is going on in our surroundings. Peripheral details are screened out as our brain filters in only the most relevant information about the threat. This state is called "hyperarousal" [255]. Below the level of our conscious awareness, we choose appropriate survival-based action: fight, flight, freeze, appease. If we survive the threat, recuperation follows, which is characterized by rest and isolation, wound care, and gradual return to daily activities [16].

Emotions can be seen as sensitive mental radar alerting us about the significance of things that happen to us externally or within our bodies [256]. This has important survival value because without emotion we would be unable to pick out important information from the myriad forms of experience and objects that surround us. Emotions automatically activate tendencies to act in preset ways that are evolutionarily designed to help us cope with environmental challenges. Fear and anger are the dominant emotions when we are under threat. Fear prepares us to flee the situation and mobilizes our protective defenses. Anger prepares us to fight an enemy. There are only four emotionally based strategies that animals have available to deal with danger: withdrawal (flight), immobility (freeze), defensive aggression (fight), or submission (appeasement) [257]. Emotions, not rational thought, help us determine which strategy is most likely to keep us alive.

But feeling too much emotion can be fatal—our emotions are hardwired through our autonomic nervous system to such an extent that it is possible for us to die of fright. When we are in acute danger, if we were to focus on our mortality we could easily become nonfunctional. Fear of dying would prevent us from saving ourselves. A certain amount of denial and avoidance of reality is healthy, particularly in the face of imminent death. Under such conditions, our central nervous system is buffered by an automatic "failsafe" mechanism called "dissociation" which is defined as the loss of integrated function of memory, sensation, perception, emotions, and identity. In a dissociated state the person may grow calm, with a lowered heart rate and an apparent invulnerability to fear, panic, or pain. Acute dissociation, commonly called "shock," helps to temporarily reduce the overwhelming nature of the stress response and allows us to stay to function in an emergency situation rather than experience over-whelming emotions [14; 258–259]. Additionally, since extremely heightened physiological states can be associated with sudden death, acute dissociation can be life saving [260–261]. Because they are helpless and because they dissociate more readily than adults, children who are exposed to traumatic events are particularly prone to dissociation [15]. In a very basic way dissociation allows us to lie to ourselves, to buffer our central nervous system by parceling out just how much reality we can deal with in manageable pieces. Too much reality is sometimes simply too much to bear [262].

Our capacity to think clearly changes radically when we are under stress. When we perceive that we are in danger, we are physiologically geared to take action, not to ponder and deliberate. In many situations of acute danger, it is better that we respond immediately without taking the time for complicated mental processing so that we respond almost reflexively to save our lives or to protect others. Our ability to recall data from memory, to analyze and reason, and to make decisions all may be seriously impaired under conditions of fight-flight because whatever is threatening demands our full attention. This can appear as cognitive tunnel vision, as our perceptions become narrowed and focused and we lose the background context of the situation. In this cognitive mode we are responding only to short-term goals. Problems that lie further down the road may not be anticipated, even though we would be able to anticipate future consequences if we were not stressed. In this state, we look for simple solutions and these solutions will be largely determined by emotion, not reason. There is a narrowing of the perceptual field so that it becomes more difficult to engage in complex thinking, to see interconnectedness or interrela-tionships between bodies of information, to develop themes and integrate information. Learning new information becomes difficult when we are very stressed. Under stress we plan less and revert to automatic reactions and rules.

"Under stress, people tend to do what they know best rather than what would be best" (p. 109) [263].

Decision-making abilities change as a consequence of these stress-related changes in mental processing. Under these conditions, our decisions tend to be based on impulse and on whatever will immediately lower tension and fear. As a consequence these decisions are likely to be inflexible, oversimplified, directed towards action, and often are very poorly constructed [264]. We stop being able to think creatively and become more dogmatic, focusing on solutions to problems that have worked in the past rather than trying something new. There is often an increase in cautiousness, perseveration, and stereotyped thinking, and an unwillingness to question the existing status quo [265].

Our method for remembering things, processing new memories, and accessing old memories is radically changed when under acute stress. Although our cognitive function may be oriented entirely toward the present emergency, our associational brain guarantees that we can make hundreds, even thousands of associations to any event, and the more dangerous the event, the more likely that we will make a multitude of interconnected associations. A growing body of evidence indicates that there are actually two different memory systems in the brain—one for verbal learning and remembering that is based on words, and another that is nonverbal.

The memory we consider our "normal" memory is a system based largely on language. Under normal conditions, the two kinds of memory function in an integrated way. Our verbal and nonverbal memories are thus usually intertwined and complexly interrelated. However, the human verbally based memory system is particularly vulnerable to high levels of stress. Like our animal ancestors who lacked verbal communication, we become less attentive to words and far more focused on threat-related signals in the environment—all of the nonverbal content of communication. As fear rises, we may lose language functions altogether, possibly mediated by the effect of rising levels of cortisol on the language centers of the brain [259; 266–268].

Without words, the mind shifts to a mode of cognition characterized by visual, auditory, olfactory, and kinesthetic images, physical sensations, and strong emotions. This system of processing information is adequate under conditions of danger because it is a more rapid method for assimilating information. By quickly providing data about the circumstances surrounding the danger and making rapid comparisons to previous experience, people may have a vastly increased possibility of survival in the face of threat. Later, traumatic memories may be triggered by any reminder of the previous threat experience [269].

Communication with others of our kind is likely to immediately increase under threat as we try to convey messages about the immediate danger. We are a social species and part of the stress response is to call out to others as a warning and to solicit help [20]. The alarm call is evident in all primate species and the crying of a child can be so persistent and arousing (as anyone knows who has been on a small airplane with a crying infant) because the crying is itself an alarm response alerting parents that a helpless child is in danger. Communication richness and complexity, however, are reduced under these conditions. Rumors fly and information is spontaneously and rapidly conveyed verbally and nonverbally under conditions of threat. We perceive someone else's threat responses without even knowing it—body posture, erect hair follicles, the smell of fear. During times of immediate danger, we are likely to put aside conflicts with each other in favor of individual and group survival. The feeling of well-being with the group we are affiliated with is enhanced while danger is located in an external source.

This state of extreme "hyperarousal" serves a protective function during an emergency, preparing us to respond rapidly to any perceived threat, preferentially steering us toward action and away from the time-consuming effort of thought and language. Taking action appears to be the only solution to this extraordinary experience of tension. As a result, we respond today with a response that compels us to act on our impulses to aggressively defend ourselves or to run away, even when the threat may be one to our self-esteem, not to our physical well-being.

Animals and children that are defenseless against a predator may automatically adopt a different strategy in the face of threat—the freeze component of the stress response, like a deer in the headlights of your car on a country road. Only when the immediate danger has passed are they then able to release the tension by running away, as the deer does if you have managed not to hit it. If an adult, particularly an adult male, freezes in the face of threat, the consequences for later self-appraisal can be very negative. Appeasement is an innate strategy that many young animals employ to deal with fear aroused by a larger and more dominant and dangerous animal of their own kind in all hierarchical species.

Recently another strategy has been recognized in primates and humans, particularly among females that holds out significant hope for the survival of the human species. "Tend and befriend" is described as an inclination to address the threatening other with an offer of something they might want and therefore changes the emotional dynamic away from immediate danger, while allowing the threatening other to remain in control of the situation [270]. Research suggests that, by virtue of differential parental investment, female stress responses have selectively evolved to maximize the survival of self and offspring. As a result, females are more likely to respond to stress by nurturing offspring, exhibiting behaviors that protect them from harm and reducing neuroendocrine responses that may compromise the health of their offspring (the tending pattern), and by affiliating with social groups to reduce risk (the befriending pattern). Researchers of social animals and humans hypothesize that females create, maintain, and utilize social groups, especially relations with other females, to manage stressful conditions and that these attachment processes chemically counteract the negative impact of the stress hormones [270].

As a result of the automatic emotional and arousal systems that we have described, we either survive the experience and gradually calm down, or not. Animals in the wild, who may be routinely threatened by predators, do not appear to develop posttraumatic stress, presumably because the brain systems that prepare them for action are effective in that they do take action and they survive to meet another day. The situation is quite different, however, for animals and for us, when the threat is repeated and when no survival action is possible.

When Terror Becomes a Way of Life

The problem we currently face as an entire species is that, for the most part, we no longer occupy the same evolutionary niche as we once did as small groups of vulnerable primates. In fact, the exposure to a wide variety of stressors that are not actually life-threatening but are characteristic of modern life leaves us vulnerable to the repetitive and unnecessary triggering of this physiological stress response. The pace of life and the pace of change have increased exponentially over the last few centuries, leaving many of us psychologically "breathless."

Individualism, the Common Good, and Modern Day Stress

In the last few decades, massive social movements have produced radical shifts in family structure, a problem since the family for most of human evolutionary history has been our main source of support. These changes have occurred against a philosophical background of what can be thought of as extreme individualism, defined as a *"political doctrine which declares that the aim of a political order should ultimately be to satisfy individual needs, wants, and goals, rather than the common good, the general will, or the public interest"*. When applied to the social sciences individualism asserts that *"scientific explanations must be grounded in the actions of, or facts about, individuals: that is, the actions of social collectivities must be ultimately decomposable into acts, intended or otherwise, of individuals"* (pp. 376–377) [271]. Individualism is a fundamental characteristic of capitalist American society, and as interpreted today, actively discourages collective bonding for the common good. Meanwhile, financial restructuring of the entire global economy is presently causing enormous and unrelenting stress on most of the population. The accumulation of wealth has become so unbalanced that according to some sources, 1% of the U.S. population now own 90% of the wealth and undoubtedly, social divisions are widening [272–273]. Levels of interpersonal and intrafamilial violence in the most stressed families and communities have become precariously high, endangering our shared social stability, welfare, wealth, and system of government. Since we evolved to depend so much on social support under stress, the widespread loss of social support does terrible damage to our bodies, our minds, and our relationships with each other, while our primitive fear responses leave us extremely vulnerable to political and economic manipulation.

Our bodies cannot keep up with the changes that our social environments demand. Stress-related physical problems are widespread and include cardiovascular problems and a wide range of other physical problems, sleep disorders, emotional difficulties, and behavioral problems. Physiologically we are still in the Stone Age, while socially we live in the Information Age. It is absolutely necessary to our continued survival that we learn how to more effectively manage our primitive, fear-based threat responses at home and at work. We believe we take the first step in that management when we understand what actually happens to us, both individually and in groups, under conditions of chronic stress so that perhaps we can come to depend on each other for better self-control.

Loss of Basic Safety and Chronic Hyperarousal

As we have discussed, we are all capable of responding to a threat to survival with the fight-flight-freeze-appease response. Some of us respond with fight, others with flight, or with freeze, and some with appeasement and a heightened inclination to care for others. But whatever the response, minor frustrations should not trigger an alarm response. What we know now, from decades of research on people suffering from various manifestations of posttraumatic stress, is that if we are exposed to danger repeatedly, our nervous systems become unusually sensitive so that even minor threats can trigger a sequence of physical, emotional, and cognitive emergency responses—a state termed *chronic hyperarousal* [274].

Each episode of danger connects to every other episode of danger in our minds, so that the more danger we are exposed to, the more sensitive we become to any kind of threat—even minor threat [275]. With each experience of fight-flight-freeze, our mind forms a network of connections that is triggered with every new threatening experience. As a result of this change in the central nervous system, people who have become chronically hyperaroused may feel safe in only very constricted situations or they may no longer ever feel safe at all.

We know from neuroimaging studies of the brains of people suffering from chronic hyperarousal that reminders of a traumatic event activate regions of the brain that result in intense and distressing emotions. At the same time, traumatic reminders inhibit the parts of the brain that allow us to translate experience into language. But it is language that allows us to communicate with ourselves and others [276]. When hyperarousal stops being a state and turns into a trait, human beings lose their capacity to accurately assess and predict danger, leading to avoidance and re-enactment—repetition of the same dysfunctional behavioral pattern—instead of adaptation and survival [13]. Prolonged hyperarousal can have disastrous physical effects as biological systems become progressively exhausted.

Loss of Emotional Management

This experience of repetitive, overwhelming terror destabilizes the internal system that regulates emotional arousal. Usually, people respond to a stimulus based on the level of threat that the stimulus represents. People who have been traumatized frequently lose this capacity to modulate arousal and manage emotions. This can look like too much emotion, the expression of inappropriate emotion, or too little of an emotional response, and this loss of control can negatively impact on a number of important functions. Emotional management is critical to learning and the capacity to exercise reasoned judgment. Emotional numbing alternating with periods of high arousal is characteristic of posttraumatic stress disorder (PTSD) and is often mistaken for depression.

The failure to develop healthy ways of managing emotional arousal interferes with the development of healthy relationships. Mature emotional management endows us with the abilities to interpret the meanings that emotions convey regarding relationships, to understand complex feelings, and to recognize likely transitions among emotions. We learn how to express how we feel to others and can find words for emotions within ourselves. The gradual acquisition of this emotional intelligence allows us to monitor emotions in relation to ourselves and affect the emotions of others. As we mature we gradually learn how to manage emotion by moderating negative emotions and enhancing pleasant ones without repressing or exaggerating the information they convey.

Children who are exposed to repeated episodes of overwhelming arousal do not have the kind of safety and protection that they need for normal brain development; therefore, they may never develop normal modulation of arousal and this severely compromises their capacity to self-regulate. As a result, they may be chronically irritable, angry, unable to manage aggression, impulsive, anxious or depressed. Compromised emotional management interferes with learning and the development of mature thought processes, reasoning, and judgment [277].

Under any circumstances, people will seek out some way to manage distress and to a large extent that will depend on what resources are available. If trustworthy others are able to help, then a sense of belonging, a need to be part of a group, and trust in the self-soothing of others may be the result. If instead, people are not available or if available, not trustworthy, then it is more likely that the chronically hyperaroused, distressed individual will turn to drugs, alcohol, smoking, sex, criminal activity, or risk-taking behavior—any activity that relieves the unrelenting, emotionally driven, repetitive distress.

Difficulties With Learning, Memory, and Decision Making

Dissociation at the time of a traumatic event appears to be a significant risk factor for the development of PTSD. After a one-time, consensually validated traumatic experience such as an earthquake, people are likely to be compassionate toward someone in "shock." This state of speechless terror is a result of a change in the brain's capacity to process information in a normal way under the influence of extreme stress. But under normal circumstances, over the next few hours, days, or weeks the environment will provide many opportunities and cues providing the affected person with opportunities to gradually get back in touch with what has really happened and begin to order, organize, and integrate the sensory experiences with the overwhelming emotions associated with the event.

Dissociation, a coping skill that can be life saving at moments of peak fear, appears to interfere with this organizing and integrating capacity. When this happens, our minds will not let us rest. The cognitive imperative refers to the *"drive in man, other mammals, and birds to order their world by differentiation of adaptively significant sensory elements and events, and to the unification of these elements into a systemic, cognitive whole"* (p. 10) [278]. We are subject to this cognitive imperative, but we have a special dilemma that does not appear to plague our mammalian or avian cousins: There is a great deal about reality that we simply cannot bear. How does one place into a meaningful and ordered scheme the idea of one's own death? *"The human brain evolved in such a way that it became capable of arriving at greater order than it perceives"* [279]. Under conditions of extreme stress, our minds cannot grasp the magnitude of what has happened or is repeatedly happening to us. At the same time, the arousal of our normal responses to danger continues to arouse bad feelings and this draws our attention to the contradictory information until the mind has managed to put the confusing information into a more comfortable mental "box." Conditions of high stress may impair the capacity to order reality normally due to the profound effects of stress hormones on the verbal capacities of the brain [262; 280].

Formerly well-adjusted adults usually fare better than children who have been traumatized. They at least have some memory of events, some idea of what normal is or was. The situation is quite different for children. The ease with which children automatically dissociate makes it likely that they will dissociate under conditions of stress as an automatic defense to protect themselves from becoming emotionally overwhelmed [281]. Given the powerlessness and defenselessness of children, dissociation is often the only thing they can do to protect themselves.

When the trauma does not stop, or when it is too severe for anyone to deal with, or when it is a secret trauma that no one else is allowed to know about, the gap between everyday reality and traumatic reality can continue to increase. The child cannot deal with the traumatic experience because it continues to pose some kind of life threat and the culture cannot or will not help the child come to terms with the experience. This may leave the child unable to establish a coherent and consistent sense of identity because the traumatized self is directly in conflict with the normal self. The child may then be unable to establish a comprehensive and flexible meaning system or philosophy of life because he or she harbors too many internal contradictions. Under these circumstances dissociation becomes a way of life, and the disintegration of the person's life is likely to continue.

The end result of chronic dissociation in childhood may be a serious inability to understand or contend with consensual reality even as an adult. Most childhood abuse is hidden and denied. On the surface, some nonviolent forms of sexual abuse may not even appear to be traumatic. It is not necessarily the pain or terror that is the most traumatic aspect of a childhood experience but the betrayal that is so damaging [282]. Children are helplessly dependent on their caregivers. In order to survive, they must trust those on whom they depend. When those caregivers turn out to be untrustworthy, children must deny this reality. Often this betrayal is denied or minimized by the perpetrator as well as by other family members and other members of the child's community. This means that the experience of individual reality becomes increasingly divergent from cultural reality. The individual symptoms are related to the child's or adult's attempt to individually make sense of a distorted reality [262]. The child, in such a situation, must make a choice. Deny your own individual reality and fit into the culture, or defy the cultural beliefs and end up alone and eccentric or even "crazy." It is an impossible choice.

Children who are traumatized do not have well-developed coping skills, a developed sense of self, or a developed sense of self in relation to others. Their ability to make sense out of their world is still immature. As a consequence, all of the responses to trauma are amplified because they interfere with the processes of normal development. Many children lack a concept of what is normal or healthy because traumatic experience has become their normative childhood experience. Raised in abusive, violent, and/or neglectful homes, they have never learned how to think in a careful, quiet, and deliberate way. They have not learned how to have mutual, compassionate, and satisfying relationships that help them differentiate between right and wrong. They have not learned how to listen carefully to the messages of their body and their senses. Their sense of self has been determined by the experiences they have had with caretaking adults, and the trauma they have experienced has taught then that they are bad, worthless, ineffective, a nuisance, or worse.

Dissociation of emotions often takes the form of emotional numbing. In his book about the impact of trauma on the lives of young African American boys, Dr. John Rich, a public health physician, describes the impact of unrecognized dissociation of emotions that is a frequent accompaniment of the violence these young men are exposed to. He quotes James, a boy whose best friend and cousin was murdered in a drive-by shooting: *"It's like they just took some emotions that I used to have. That nervous feeling, that scared feeling? It's gone,"* James said clearly. *"I think I lost emotions over this whole thing. I lost emotions. I think my heart got a little stone in it now"* [283]. James, and so many like him, is more likely to put himself in harm's way because the dissociative response that is so life saving in the short term does not just automatically resolve. Instead, the person may remain numb to emotions that are vital to us if we are to avoid danger and if we are to enjoy life and create sustaining relationships.

When feelings are not well managed, thinking—and therefore learning—can be impaired. Recent scientific advances have shown how the interrelated development of emotion and cognition relies on the emergence, maturation, and interconnection of complex neural circuits in multiple areas of the brain, including the prefrontal cortex, limbic cortex, basal forebrain, amygdala, hypothalamus, and brainstem. The circuits that are involved in the regulation of emotion are highly interactive with those that are associated with executive functions (such as planning, judgment, and decision making). Neuropsychological and neuroimaging research has shown that traumatized people have difficulty with focusing their concentration and this plays a role in their learning difficulties [276].

During the preschool years these circuits are critical to the development of good problem-solving skills. In terms of basic brain functioning, emotions support executive functions when they are well regulated but interfere with attention and decision making when they are poorly controlled. Children who are chronically hyperaroused have significant difficulties in learning any information that is not tied to immediate survival, so they tend to do poorly in school. The emotional health of young children—or the absence of it—is closely tied to the social and emotional characteristics of the environments in which they live, which include not only their parents but also the broader context of their schools, families, and communities.

Our very complex brains and powerful memories distinguish us as the most intelligent of all animals, and yet it is this very intelligence that leaves us vulnerable to the effects of trauma Exposure to trauma can alter people's memory, producing extremes of remembering too much—intrusive flashbacks, posttraumatic nightmares, and behavioral reenactments—and recalling too little—amnesia. Unlike other memories, traumatic memories appear to become etched in the mind, unaltered by the passage of time or by subsequent experience [284].

But without verbal content, traumatic memories fail to be integrated into the narrative stream of consciousness but instead remain as unintegrated fragments of experience that can then intrude into consciousness when triggered by reminders of a previous event.

A flashback is a sudden intrusion of a fragment of past experience into present consciousness. A flashback may take the form of a visual image, a smell, a taste, or some other physical sensation, including severe pain, and is usually accompanied by powerful and noxious emotions. Even thinking of flashbacks as memories is inaccurate and misleading. When someone experiences a flashback, he or she does not remember the experience, but relives it. Time is not as linear as we perceive it to be and without verbal integration of an experience to form a completed narrative, the experience is trapped in the ever-present moment of "now," not a memory but a haunting reenactment. Often the flashback is "forgotten" as quickly as it happens because it has not really been "re-membered"—put altogether into a completed narrative form—because the two memory systems of implicit or nonverbal memory and explicit or narrative memory have become disconnected from each other. Every time a flashback occurs, the complex sequence of psychobiological events that characterize the "fight-flight-freeze" response is triggered, resulting in a terror reaction to the memories themselves. The result is a vicious cycle of flashback-hyperarousal-dissociation that further compromises function. As the survivor tries to cope with this radical departure from normal experience, he or she is more likely to do anything to interrupt the vicious cycle—substance use and abuse, a preoccupation with violence and risk taking, even self-mutilation—all of which can temporarily produce an interruption. But each in its own way compounds the individual's growing problems [266; 285].

Miscommunication, Conflict, and Alexithymia

Communication between people is frequently challenging—just recall the children's game "Whisper Down the Lane"—and how readily verbal communication can go awry. After all, communication between people is conveyed through at least three channels simultaneously: nonverbal information, emotional information, and verbal content [8]. The more stressed a child has been, the less likely the child is to have developed the skills required for good communication, or had the social context within which good communication skills could be practiced. When you are chronically hyperaroused and unable to effectively manage emotions, then vital aspects of interpersonal communication are radically skewed and you are likely to be grossly misinterpreted. The difficulties in communication will make it unlikely that chronically hyper-aroused people will develop good conflict management skills; in fact, they may precipitate themselves into many conflicts because they misinterpret other people's messages and are misinterpreted by others.

Our dependence on language means that wordless experiences cannot be sufficiently integrated into consciousness and a coherent sense of identity, nor will those experiences rest quietly. When exposure to toxic stress occurs in childhood, children's identity may not solidify around a solid core [281; 286]. Instead it remains fragmented, and the fragments are separated from and inaccessible to each other. Critical brain functions do not become properly integrated and organized [287]. The most extreme cases are now called "disso- ciative identity disorder." Each separated fragment is constituted by an array of associated memories, feelings, and behaviors that remain chaotic, disordered, and emotionally charged. Experiences of speechless terror thus may lead to amnesia for the traumatic event—the memory is there, but there are no words attached to it, so it can be neither talked about nor thought about, though it may be expressed through behavior and physical symptoms [266; 285].

In this way the survivor becomes haunted by an unnarrated past. *"The trauma of language creates a parceled body, a sense that the body is in pieces. Language divides the subject from the organism, it breaks into our bodies and writes on our flesh"* (p. 263) [288]. Since the sense of self refers to a verbally based identity, experiences that have not been encoded in words are not recog- nized as a part of the "self." People for whom this has been the case may not have developed words to identify emotions and are therefore unable to think about their own emotional experience—a state termed *alexithymia*, first used in reference to survivors of the Holocaust but later described in virtually all trauma survivor groups [289].

Lacking an ability to talk to themselves—an internal dialogue that is going on for most of us all the time—the trauma survivor finds it exceedingly diffi- cult to control impulses and to extend their imagination out into the timeline of the future so that they can anticipate the future consequences of their actions. Children, and the adults they become, who experience compromised emotional management are likely to experience high levels of anxiety when alone and/or in interpersonal interactions. Without an ability to manage overwhelming feelings, they will understandably therefore do anything they can to establish some level of self-soothing and self-control. Under such circumstances, people frequently turn to problematic behaviors, all of which help them to calm down, at least temporarily, largely because of the internal chemical effects of the sub- stance or behavior [290]. Human caring, including human touch, could serve as a self-soothing device, but for trauma survivors, trusting human beings enough to tolerate healthy human touch may be too difficult.

Impaired communication skills that accompany the inability to manage the emotional aspects of communication are one mechanism of intergenerational transmission of traumatic effects since under healthy conditions these skills build up over time in the interaction between parent and child. A parent who has compromised emotional management skills will be unable to provide the important emotional learning experiences that their children require. Instead, the children will adapt to the parental style of communicating about emotions and then when they become parents themselves, they are likely to pass on these same styles—for better or worse—to their children.

Authoritarianism and the Danger to Democracy

Interpersonal trauma is usually associated with the abusive use of power. Not surprisingly, people who have been exposed to violence and/or abuse have difficulty contending with how to use their own power and what that power means in the context of their own social and political lives. Power is relational and therefore how we exercise power as adults depends a great deal on how the powerful people in our lives used their power with—or against—us when we were children. There is reason to believe that people who are exposed to chronic stress, abuse, and victimization, particularly beginning in childhood, may be more likely to adopt authoritarian characteristics [291]. People who score high on authoritarianism have been found to be more susceptible to perceive the world as a threatening and dangerous place and people tend to become more authoritarian when they are exposed to threat. Research on terror management theory strongly suggests that death anxiety, which is frequently aroused by traumatic experiences, moves people to become both more conservative and more intolerant of differences [292]. There is even some indication that taking authoritarian positions may help alleviate mental distress and provide a buffer against negative emotions, making it more likely that chronically frightened people may turn to authoritarian modes of interacting with others [293].

Authoritarianism and democracy are usually viewed as polar opposites for good reason. In his books on combat trauma, psychiatrist Jonathan Shay discusses the connection between trauma and democracy: "*Unhealed combat trauma—and I suspect unhealed severe trauma from any source—destroys the unnoticed substructure of democracy, the cognitive and social capacities that enable a group of people to freely construct a cohesive narrative of their own future*" (p. 181). He goes on to warn that "*unhealed combat trauma diminishes democratic participation and can become a threat to democratic political institutions. Severe psychological injury originates in violation of trust and destroys the capacity for trust. When mistrust spreads widely and deeply democratic civic discourse becomes impossible*" (p. 195) [294].

The effects of trauma and adversity, particularly when it originates in childhood, can be seen as the opposite of what is required for democratic participation. Democracy requires the ability to manage emotions, even in the face of conflict, and to exercise good impulse control. It requires process and patience; using words as a substitute for action; trusting others enough to share in decision making; a willingness to listen, demonstrate fair play, exercise influence wisely and flexibly; and the willingness to compromise and negotiate. All of these are advanced social skills which may be severely impaired by exposure to chronic stress [295].

Learned Helplessness

It is well established that human beings deplore being helpless. Placed into situations of helplessness, we will do anything to escape and restore a sense of mastery. But helplessness is a hallmark characteristic of a traumatic experience. Helplessness in the face of danger threatens survival and our carefully established sense of invulnerability and safety. Worse yet, repetitive exposure to helplessness is so toxic to emotional and physiological stability that in service of continued survival, survivors are compelled to adapt to the helplessness itself, a phenomenon that has been termed *learned helplessness* [296]. Like animals in a cage, with enough exposure to helplessness people will adapt to adversity and cease struggling to escape from the situation, thus conserving vital resources and buffering the vulnerable central nervous system against the negative impact of constant overstimulation. Then later, rather than change situations that could be altered for the better, they will change their definitions of "normal" to fit the situation to which they have become adapted. For them, even when change is possible, the formerly adaptive response of simply buckling down and coping can create a serious obstacle to positive change, empowerment, and mastery. This then may contribute to the dynamic of revictimization which is so much a part of exposure to sustained and unavoidable adversity [297].

As a result of this adjustment, people who have had repeated experiences of helplessness are likely to exhibit a number of apparently contradictory behaviors. On the one hand they may demonstrate "control issues" by trying to control other people, themselves, their own feelings—anything that makes them feel less helpless. The threat of or use of violence is a way to control other people that is frequently effective. At the same time, they are likely to be willing to turn over control to substances or behaviors that are destructive or to people who cannot be trusted. They may have difficulties discriminating between abusive and healthy authority and may be willing to give up control to abusive authorities or abuse their own authority, a problem well documented in the historical appraisal of notorious persecutory figures like Adolf Hitler and Saddam Hussein [298].

Punishment, Revenge, and Injustice

In the course of normal development, children learn how to modulate and manage the desire to "get even" for hurts to their bodies, their sense of identity, and their cherished beliefs. Psychobiologic inhibitory responses to anger develop in the context of an empathic relationship with caretakers. In interaction with family members and peers, children learn the rules of fair play, the role of apology, and how to cooperate with others [299].

Some people who have suffered developmental insults in their early years may not only have reasons for feelings of vengeance toward others but may also be biologically predisposed to react violently when provoked as a result of chronic hyperarousal. The brain is a delicate organ, and any damage to the brain can also damage the development of normal inhibitory pathways created over time in the context of healthy caretaker relationships. If children's attachment relationships are disrupted, as is the case with exposure to trauma, abuse, and neglect, they may fail to develop normal biological and psychological mechanisms that inhibit retaliatory behavior. If they come from violent and abusive homes, children learn that violence is a viable and effective means of solving problems. Because abusive adults were often exposed to abuse and/or neglect as children, an important way of viewing the intergenerational cycle of abuse is through the lens of displaced revenge. In part due to their own level of hyperarousal, parents who have been abused are likely to be more easily provoked and feel very threatened by what may be a child's normal rejection of authority, and if they have not worked this out for themselves, may end up repeating the same vicious cycle that was inflicted upon them.

In clinical populations and in literature we can see many examples of the deep connection between shame, grief, and the desire for vengeance. People prone to experience overwhelming shame in response to disrespect are most likely to become angry, violent, and retaliatory when shamed and may direct their anger at the person who has hurt them, at innocent others, or at themselves [300]. Under the guise of a quest for justice, an ongoing desire for revenge may also serve as a defense against completing the tasks of mourning and thus impede therapeutic progress and improvement in life adjustment [301].

In practice, most victimized, chronically hyperaroused people probably present with combinations of beliefs and behaviors about justice, injustice, punishment, and revenge. Failures in healthy development may lead to failure in the ability to successfully evolve a personal system of justice that is fair, meaningful, and satisfying [302]. Developmental arrests in the process of developing healthy notions of reciprocal behavior can lead to psychopathological behavior and relationships [303].

Criminals are often unconsciously trying to exact revenge for past injuries and injustices that have not been rectified. Bullying in a child or an adult is abusive behavior that the bully experiences as justified and right. As a result, the victim becomes the perpetrator in a cycle of revenge that has no prescribed limits. The original perpetrator rarely perceives that what he or she did to the victim was as bad as the victim experienced it to be. So when the victim responds, the perpetrator experiences the response as an escalation of aggression, creating another cycle of revenge. When the original perpetrator is not the target of the revenge, the satisfaction that vengeance can give is a sense of dominance over the original perpetrator through the mechanism of displacement, while an innocent person becomes the victim, thus arousing the cycle of vengeance in yet another. Since the desire for vengeance is tied to unresolved loss, acts of revenge tend to escalate violence rather than healing the individual or social condition.

According to large surveys, most parents in America hit their children, doing to their children what would be criminal were it between two adults. The universality of this behavior has made it difficult for pediatricians to take a firm and unequivocal stand on corporal punishment because punishing children, and punishing them physically, is an accepted social norm [304]. The risk to the child's health and well-being and the general welfare, however, is significant [305]. Corporal punishment, the deliberate infliction of pain as retaliation for perceived wrongdoing, puts children at risk for engaging in many forms of displaced retaliatory behaviors. Research has shown that children who are physically punished are more aggressive as adults, are more likely to be depressed, to abuse substances, and stand a higher likelihood of engaging in criminal acts. And it's not just physical punishment that matters. Studies have shown that "power-assertive punishment," meaning hitting, scolding, threatening, and privilege removal were found to be long-acting risk factors for child psychopathology [304; 306].

Studies of delinquent and prison populations demonstrate the high correlation between criminal behavior and a previous history of childhood abusive behavior [300]. It is possible that many of the symptoms manifested in various mental disorders and the behaviors that we associate with violent criminal activity originate in a frustrated sense of righteous indignation and the search for justice and culminate in acts of vengeance against self and others. Dr. James Gilligan, former director of the Center for the Study of Violence at Harvard Medical School and former medical director of the Bridgewater State Hospital for the criminally insane, has written movingly about the connection between violence, vengeance, and justice. He has pointed out that the motives and goals that underlie violent crime are the same as those that motivate the pursuit of justice: seeking justice by retaliating against those whom the criminal perceives have punished him unjustly. The criminal is trying to exact revenge for past injuries and injustices through violent means. As Dr. Gilligan writes,

The first lesson that tragedy teaches . . . is that all violence is an attempt to achieve justice, or what the violent person perceives as justice, for himself or for whomever it is on whose behalf he is being violent . . . Thus, the attempt to achieve and maintain justice, or to undo or prevent injustice, is the one and only universal cause of violence (pp. 11–12) [300].

Addiction to Trauma, Trauma-Bonding, and Traumatic Reenactment

The endorphins are substances that are chemically related to morphine and heroin and are part of our natural attachment system, producing powerfully soothing and comforting feelings. When we feel safe and socially supported, endorphins are elevated. But because they are powerful analgesics, circulating levels of endorphins are increased as a part of the stress response so that in case of injury we can continue to self-protect and not experience what otherwise could be paralyzing pain. At least in part as a result of this, exposure to chronic severe stress may be so disruptive of the attachment system that stress—instead of social support—becomes associated with anxiety relief and soothing emotions, an outcome known as *addiction to trauma*.

Under these conditions each subsequent experience of trauma may further damage the attachment system, creating an increased likelihood that people will turn to self-destructive behavior, addictive substances, violence, and thrill seeking as a way of regulating their internal environments when their own chemical responses are insufficient [274; 297; 307]. Even more ominous for repeatedly traumatized people is their pronounced tendency to use highly abnormal and dangerous relationships as their normative idea of what relationships are supposed to be [139].

Trauma bonding describes a relationship based on terror and the twisting of normal attachment behavior into something perverse and cruel [281]. Relationships to authority also become damaged. Human beings first learn about power relationships in the context of the family. If we experience fair, kind, and consistent authority figures, then we will internalize that relationship to authority both in the way we exert control over our own impulses and in the way we deal with other people. If we have been exposed to harsh, punitive, abusive, inconsistent authority, then the style of authority that we adopt is likely to be similarly abusive. Once we have become bonded around issues of trauma and abuse, these are the relationship patterns that we tend to reenact.

Traumatic reenactment is the term we use to describe the lingering behavioral enactment and automatic repetition of the past. The very nature of traumatic information processing determines the reenactment behavior. The traumatized person is cut off from language, deprived of the power of words, trapped in speechless terror. Trauma demands repetition—what Pierre Janet, Sigmund Freud, and so many others observed when they noticed the compulsion to repeat in trauma survivors. As Freud wrote, *"He reproduces it not as a memory but as an action; he repeats it without, of course, knowing that he is repeating ... he cannot escape from this compulsion to repeat; and in the end we understand that this is his way of remembering"* (p. 271) [308].

But why is this the case? Why does trauma demand repetition? Probably because of the inherent conflict between what the brain does to manage overwhelming stress at the time of an overwhelming event and the later effects of this loss of integration. The mind has shattered into fragments and yet the cognitive imperative asserts itself, demanding that all aspects of reality and experience are integrated into a meaningful whole. Imagine then, how damaging traumatic experiences are when they occur in childhood, when the brain itself is not yet sufficiently organized to manage such internal conflict.

Robert Lifton, a psychiatrist who has made an intensive study of various traumatized and traumatizing populations, has talked about the *failed enactment* that occurs at the time of a traumatic event [309]. This failed enactment is associated with profound feelings of helplessness, which is a fundamental characteristic of any traumatic experience. He has found that at the time of the trauma, there is some beginning, abortive image toward acting in a way more positive than can actually happen at the time. This schema for enactment is never completed and was in most instances impossible to achieve in the first place. Nonetheless, the person feels guilty about not having completed the successful act, even though it was impossible in reality. Lifton and others believe it is this failed enactment that probably helps to propel the reenactment behavior, as the person unconsciously attempts repetitively to do the situation differently, unwittingly becoming traumatized over and over again.

Reenactment behavior, therefore, seems to also be biologically based, part of the innate and programmed behavioral repertoire of the traumatized person. We can look at the trauma victim as someone who is signaling through behavior what he or she cannot verbally discuss with his or her social group. From this point of view, then, traumatic reenactment demands repetition because the cognitive imperative demands that the individual order his or her memories, emotions, feelings, and perceptions, but the person cannot do that without the safety and narrative engagement of the social group. The child who experiences trauma may just be learning to talk, to use language appropriately, to make sense out of his or her experience, and to organize information and all of these functions may be radically compromised when traumatic experience causes further disorganization in a developing brain.

The role of the social environment is to engage enough with the story to understand the script but then to change the automatic roles that are being cued for by the client so that the story changes instead of being repeated. Unfortunately, as audience, we have largely lost the capacity for nonverbal interpretation, and we have ceased to take the time to examine and understand repetitive patterns of behavior. As a result, these symptomatic "cries for help" fall on deaf ears. Instead, the society and its representatives judge, condemn, exclude, and alienate the person who is behaving in an asocial, self-destructive, or antisocial way without hearing the meaning in the message. Trapped in a room with no exit signs, the person hunkers down and adapts to ever-worsening conditions, unaware that there are many opportunities for change and terrified that taking any risk to get out of this dilemma could lead to something even worse.

Traumatic reenactment can be seen in the shifting roles that clients and staff assume on the "rescuer-victim-persecutor" triangle originally known as the "Karpman drama triangle." First described in the 1960s by transactional analysis therapist Stephen Karpman [310], it started as a bunch of doodles that Karpman was drawing while he tried to figure out basketball and football fakes [311]. But it turned out to be a powerful tool in understanding some of the more perplexing of human behavior. Karpman described three dramatic roles that people act out in daily life that are common, unsatisfactory, repetitive, and largely unconscious. When playing the "persecutor" role, we are operating from a position of some kind of power, and we tend to bully, find fault, accuse others, lead by threats, and are often blaming and shaming. When in the "rescuer" role, we are working hard to "help" someone else but are often feeling martyred, guilty, angry under the surface, and may be considered meddlers by others. In the "victim" role, we become helpless, incompetent, oppressed, and hopeless. Here is a case example of behavioral reenactment, taken from an Andrus story that helps to explain traumatic reenactment and the reenactment triangle:

> A little girl was admitted because she had impulse control problems and she could not be managed in public school or in foster care. She was placed in foster care after it was discovered that she was being sexually abused by a family member. She came to the attention of the Andrus administrators because she was being restrained every night around bedtime. When an administrator met with the staff to discern the pattern of what was happening, it turned out that every night, before bed, she would start moving furniture in her room. The staff would try to get her to stop doing this since she was angling the furniture in a way that posed a fire hazard. She would refuse to stop, however, and the situation between the child and the staff member would escalate until she ended up down on the floor, being held down by a staff member who was usually a male. She was totally unaware of the repetitive pattern, but in conference the staff were able to realize that she was—with their help—repeating her traumatic scenario every evening. Her uncle had held her down and raped her at night when she was isolated in her bedroom. The staff realized that in moving her furniture she was trying in her own way to barricade her room so no one could get to her, but at some point in the sequence, probably when she was prevented from self-protecting, she entered an altered, dissociative state. In that state, she perceived the staff member as her uncle and although she tried to fight him off each time, ultimately her small size meant she was overwhelmed. Every night she went from "persecuting" the staff to being "victimized," while the staff member who was her "rescuer" ended up himself being "victimized" (with punches, kicks, and scratches) and then in restraining her immediately became her "persecutor."

When we are trapped in any one of these roles, the roles can shift quickly and dramatically, and being trapped in one inevitably means being trapped in all three. Rotating around the reenactment triangle means that problems will not be solved but will instead be endlessly repeated, and everyone involved will feel more or less "jerked around." When a client is reenacting a violent experience, then playing any of these roles can lead to disaster.

Grief, Reenactment, and Decline

Living beings are meant to be in constant flux, changing and adapting all the time. Reenactment behavior flies in the face of this adaptive ability, endlessly repeating a relational style that brings only more disappointment, despair, and trauma. In this way, reenactment behavior can be seen as a sign of unresolved grief. The person continually reenacts what he or she has not been able to resolve. Under normal circumstances, the human ability to form healthy attachments to other people allows us to successfully transit through the process of grieving after a loss. But people who have disrupted attachment experiences and experiences with traumatic bereavement have difficulties with grieving. To grieve a loss, we need to be able to manage overwhelming feelings. People who have compounded losses have often become emotionally numb. New losses tend to open up old wounds that never heal. Arrested grief is extremely problematic because it is impossible to form healthy new attachments without first finishing with old attachments. In this way, unresolved loss becomes another dynamic that keeps an individual stuck in time, unable to move ahead, and unable to go back. Compounded and unresolved grief is frequently in the background of lives based on traumatic reenactment [312].

As this process of prolonged hyperarousal, helplessness, emotional numbing, disrupted attachment, and reenactment unfolds, people's sense of who they are, how they fit into the world, how they relate to other people, and what the point of it all is can become significantly limited in scope. As this occurs, they are likely to become increasingly despairing. The attempt to avoid any reminders of the previous events, along with the intrusive symptoms, like flashbacks and nightmares, comprise two of the interacting and escalating aspects of posttraumatic stress syndrome, set in the context of a more generalized physiological hyperarousal. As these alternating symptoms come to dominate traumatized people's lives, they may feel more and more alienated from everything that gives their lives meaning: favorite activities, other people, a sense of direction and purpose, a sense of spirituality, a sense of community. It is not surprising, then, that slow self-destruction and decline through addictions, or fast self-destruction through suicide, may be the final outcome of these syndromes. For other people, rage at others comes to dominate the picture and these are the ones who end up becoming significant threats to other people as well as themselves.

Children who are repetitively traumatized have not yet had an opportunity to develop adequate, mature coping skills, and the results may negatively impact their developing sense of self, self-esteem, and self in relation to others. Their schemas for meaning, hope, faith, and purpose are not yet fully formed. They are in the process of developing a sense of right and wrong, of mercy balanced against justice. All of their cognitive processes, most importantly, their ability to make decisions, their problem-solving capacities, and learning skills are still being acquired. As a consequence, the responses to trauma are amplified because they interfere with the processes of normal development. Living in a system of contradictory and hypocritical values can impair a child's development of conscience, of faith in the possibility of justice, and of a belief in the pursuit of truth.

We are meaning-making animals. We must be able to make sense out of the things that happen to us, and this often includes creating order out of chaos and structuring our reality. Traumatic experience robs people of a sense of meaning and purpose. It shatters basic assumptions about the nature of life and reality [313]. Close contact with traumatic death or threats to our own mortality cannot be accepted but can only be transcended, and trauma dramatically interferes with our capacity to grow, to change, and to move on. Shared cultural beliefs largely determine the way human beings cope with the terror of inevitable death, and traumatic experiences disrupt the individual's sense of individual and cultural identity [292; 314]. Losing the capacity for psychic movement, they may deteriorate into a repetitive cycle of reenactment, stagnation, and despair.

The end result of this complex sequence of posttraumatic events can be repetition, stagnation, rigidity, and a fear of change all in the context of a deteriorating life. As emotional, physical, and social symptoms of distress pile upon each other, victims may try desperately to extricate themselves by using the same protective devices that they used to cope with threat in the first place: dissociation, avoidance, aggression, destructive attachments, damaging behaviors, and addictive substances. The response to threat has become so ingrained and automatic that victims experience control as beyond them and as their lives deteriorate, their responses become increasingly stereotyped and rigid.

The Germ Theory of Trauma and Public Health

> *We would all like to believe that the world is fundamentally a logical, well-managed place. Since the evidence against this is overwhelming it is inevitable that we seek a defense against finding it so frighteningly unsafe.* (p. 129) [315]
>
> Oberholzer and Roberts, *The Troublesome Individual and the Troubled Institution*

Whole fields of current endeavor are devoted to the study of the myriad ways toxic stress, trauma, and disrupted attachment disrupt the minds, bodies, and spirits of individual victims of overwhelming, prolonged, repetitive stress. These last few pages have just been a simple introduction to the concepts at the heart of chronic stress, adversity, and trauma. But before moving on to the group impact of these same experiences, let's speculate about why the study of these subjects is so important.

Louis Pasteur, a nineteenth-century French scientist, is a seminal figure in the history of public health because he is considered one of the fathers of microbiology and our understanding that microbes (aka germs) are the source of infection (i.e., the germ theory). Before Pasteur's discovery that it was microbes that were causing infections, the general beliefs were that the sources of disease were to be found within the diseased person as a manifestation of inner corruption, the result of punitive wrath of God, or demonic possession. These beliefs had been firmly entrenched for centuries and therefore were given up only with great resistance, including resistance from the medical community of his day. The greatest significance of Pasteur's observations was that he was able to establish a cause-and-effect relationship between pathogens and disease. Once a causal connection could be established, efforts could be undertaken to combat the causal agent and to increase the resistance of the host to disease. The germ theory showed that the infectious agent came from outside the person and if the person was vulnerable an infection would ensue [316–317]. As the science of microbiology grew, it became apparent that some bacterial agents were so virulent that they could overwhelm the defenses of virtually everyone and that some social conditions like poor nutrition and improper sanitation were known to increase the likelihood of infection universally. The public health profession grew upon the premise that infectious agents killed and maimed both the innocent and the guilty and could only be kept at bay by the enforcement of public policy that applied to all. Protecting the health of the nation's most valuable resource—human labor—was considered a social, moral, and economic responsibility.

We believe that our growing understanding about the impact of adversity, toxic stress, disrupted attachment, and trauma is the psychological version of the germ theory. It is the scientific discoveries that relate to the effects of these that give "legs" to the biopsychosocial model of illness. We now have an understanding of the connection between pathogenic forces in the external world and the internal pathology of the person. We know a great deal about how the body, mind, and soul of the victim interact with the body, mind, and soul of the perpetrator. Trauma theory proposes that the origin of a significant proportion of physical, psychological, social, and moral disorder lies in the direct and indirect exposure to external traumatogenic agents. Psychological trauma can cause chronic, infectious, multigenerational, and often lethal disease. Although some traumatic events are highly likely to create posttraumatic effects in anyone, the more usual interaction is between the strength and persistence of the stressor and the vulnerability of the stressed. Certain environments are clearly more likely to provide a fertile breeding ground for traumatogenic events than others.

Just as bacteria and viruses are the usual infectious agents, the perpetrators of violence are the carriers of the trauma infection: the more destructive the perpetrators, the lower the chances of survival for their victims; the more intense the level of contact with violence, the greater the likelihood that victims will suffer from the long-term consequences of the infectious nature of violence; the poorer the health of the victim—physical, psychological, social, and moral—the greater the likelihood of exposure. The infection even takes on a pseudo-genetic form of transmission, as the effects and patterns of violence are passed from parents through children via the attachment relationship, both through what is done that is negative and what is not done that is positive. And the latest research indicates that there may in fact be a genetic transmission of the effects of violence through alteration in epigenetic factors that then get passed on via the genome down through the generations [318].

Over 15 years ago, after recognizing the enormity of the connection between human dysfunction and past exposure to adversity and trauma, Sandy wrote:

> The human balance of power with our "violence microbes" has been lost. It is as if the infectious agent carrying violence has mutated and the infection has become so virulent that it no longer serves any master except the Grim Reaper. The causes for this increased virulence are complex—increasing world population, diminishing resources, loss of frontiers, urbanization, increased destructive power of weapons, globalization, increasingly complex civilizations—some of the same circumstances that lead to the increase in other forms of disease as well. Whatever the cause, at present we do not appear able to contain the infection, as we even do such violence to the environment that we may be past the point of saving ourselves and the planet. People are coming down with the disease faster than we can treat them, and for many the damage is so profound that our best efforts to save them are stymied. Our entire society has been infected by an AIDS-like virus that has destroyed our capacity to resist violence. In fact, we long for it, seek it, profit from it, enjoy it, get sexually aroused by it, and deliberately expose our children to it. The social forces that previously held violence to sustainable limits have been shattered in this century. Our capacity for violence has outstripped our ability to limit it. The infection is out of control and we now have an epidemic. It is not enough to look for increasingly potent antibiotics—we cannot afford to imprison or kill the large percentage of the population that it would be necessary to isolate from others if we were to focus on perpetrator behavior alone. While we try to contain the most virulent strains and take steps to decrease the virulence of the rest, we must provide the conditions that improve our ability to resist the infection of violence. This is a public health emergency (p. 263) [316].

Unfortunately, although fifteen years has passed, relatively little has been done to address this particularly problematic public health problem. That is because to change our attitude and behavior toward violence virtually every-thing about our culture must change. And change is fundamentally frightening to us.

Time-Binding Animals

Much of human existence derives from the protective mechanisms of our minds and bodies that help us adapt to a dangerous world. But even as we have grown far away from our primeval roots, we have not yet truly committed ourselves to creating a safe world, where everyone can live in peace. It seems that fear and the defenses against fear continue to dominate our existence. Where does this fear originate? It appears to be a result of the enormous com-plexity of the human mind. Humans can be considered to be "time-binding" animals [292]. Unlike the other animals around us, we do not just live in the present. We are able to reflect on the past and to anticipate the future. This is a greatest strength/greatest weakness issue because our early experience in infancy with total helplessness is something we struggle with throughout our lives. And being able to anticipate the future, we *know* we are helpless and ulti-mately that we will die as will everyone else we care about. This existential awareness fuels the terror that lies at the heart of every one of us [319]. As social psychologist Ernest Becker pointed out long ago, "*The thing that makes man the most devastating animal that ever stuck his neck up into the sky is that he wants a stature and a destiny that is impossible for an animal; he wants an earth that is not an earth but a heaven, and the price for this kind of fantastic ambition is to make the earth an even more eager graveyard than it naturally is*" (p. 96) [320].

Existential Terror and Terror Management Theory

Strongly influenced by Ernest Becker's work, terror management theory is the study of how humans cope not with the imminent threat of extermination but with the awareness that such threats are ubiquitous and will eventually succeed. It concerns the impact that the awareness of the inevitability of death has on how we live our lives. A vital role of culture and the institutions that support the culture is to protect us from this awareness, to assist us in constructing beliefs about the nature of reality that mitigate the horror and dread of what inevitably will confront us. All cultural worldviews serve an important anxiety-reducing function by providing shared meaning and purpose and a way of achieving symbolic or literal immortality. "*Psychologically, then, the function of culture is not to illuminate the truth but rather to obscure the horrifying possibility that death entails the permanent annihilation of the self*," wrote Becker (p. 22) [292]. This helps us to understand why any disturbance in the culture, including the organizational culture, arouses anxiety that is not necessarily commensurate with the change that is being required.

Cultural reality—organizationally and socially—is a fragile construction that can be easily disturbed. We are repeatedly being confronted by the reality of our own mortality, which is called "mortality salience" in the research literature. Modern communication with twenty-four-hour-a-day news, instant communication around the world, and a deluge of information everywhere bombards us with reminders that terrible things happen to people who are more or less like us. And cultural ideas and values are constantly being disturbed by the seemingly incompatible ideas and values arising from people representing different cultures, particularly in the melting pot that is the United States. As a result, the anxiety buffer that culture represents can be easily threatened by the diversity of ideas, opinions, worldviews, and lifestyles represented in a multicultural society.

Terror management theory hypothesizes that human awareness of the inevitability and possible finality of death creates the potential for existential terror, which is controlled largely in two ways: (a) faith in an internalized cultural worldview, and (b) self-esteem, which is attained by living up to the standards of value prescribed by one's worldview. Research has in fact demonstrated that when the fear of death, or mortality salience, is triggered, even outside of conscious awareness, people tend to become more fearful, less tolerant, more prejudiced, more socially conservative, more supportive of leaders who support their worldview, more fundamentalist, and more punitive toward those who are disrupting or who threatened to disrupt their worldview [292]. To date, over 300 experiments, conducted in 15 different countries, have provided support for terror management theory hypotheses [321].

Social Problems are Preventable

This helps to explain why changes in organizational culture can be so disorienting and so strongly resisted by staff members, even when the changes appear to be in their interest. If we control this fundamental existential terror largely through faith in our cultural worldview and our own self-esteem, then whenever either or both is threatened, these terrors are unleashed. Incorporating knowledge about the traumatic experiences that underlie most of child and adult psychopathology is terribly threatening to the existing worldview and the mental models upon which human service delivery is built. People in all branches of the human service delivery system deal day in and day out with the army of people who have been the victims of *largely preventable* social ills. Psychologically injured children and adults fill our homeless and domestic violence shelters, acute care psychiatric units, psychiatric hospitals, residential programs, group homes, foster care agencies, juvenile justice facilities, jails, and prisons.

The closer we are to loss, trauma, and the specter of death, the greater the mortality salience and therefore the more powerful a role these automatic and unconscious defenses will play in any environment. In treatment environments where the causes of the clients problems lie in the tragic nature of human existence, the greater the likelihood that even those who are supposed to be helping them will instead consciously or unconsciously blame the victims to distance themselves from this awesome reality. But understanding the complex problems that develop as a result of exposure to trauma, childhood adversity, and disrupted attachment helps us to make sense out of many of the dynamics we see in individual clients and families. As we will see, it can also help us understand what goes on in organizations.

Many of us come into human service work with our own stories of trauma and adversity and we bring these to the workplace. When things happen in the workplace it is easy to slip into the victim role, to feel powerless, hopeless, and helpless. The growing understanding about the neurobiology of stress and traumatic stress has fundamentally changed everything about the way we think about the work we do. We now understand that our primary role is to change the trajectory for the clients we serve. Many of the children and adults we work with have suffered terrible injuries and events. Those who have not been abused or neglected have lived in a world that has been quite unkind. All of them have learned that the world is not a very safe place; they have often felt misunderstood and mistreated. We know now that these experiences have been etched on their brains when they were very young, and we know that traditional treatment approaches, at least those based on control and coercion, serve only to dig these channels deeper and reinforce established dysfunctional patterns.

Who Deserves Empathy?

For thousands of years, human beings have based decisions on who gets help and who gets punished or neglected on group and cultural determinations about who is deserving of empathic regard and who is not. In part, these decisions have been and still are made based on age, gender, race, religion, class, and a wide range of social and philosophical determinants. Individuals, subgroups, and cultures vary greatly as to how they define who is worthy and deserving. Those determinations are likely to be applied everywhere—in parenting practices, schools, workplaces, and even health care, mental health care, and social services. Western culture has historically placed a significant emphasis on free will, the extent to which people are able to exercise control over their choices in the world, in deciding who is deserving of empathy and who is not. But even within philosophical schools of thought there are wide variations in just how "determined" every person's life is by forces outside of rational thought and control. As a result, when society makes a decision that the action of an individual was freely chosen with a negative result as defined by that society, then that person is thought to be responsible for doing wrong and is therefore deserving of punishment, not compassion.

Progress in achieving human rights can be seen as a widening of who deserves compassion, not punishment. A widening circle of empathic inclusion can be viewed as the greatest achievement of humanity thus far. All human societies have evolved from family and then tribal groups who feared and often killed outsiders. Not too long ago, if you lived in the United States and you were a person of color, or a woman, or suffered from any number of disabilities, you could be deprived of rights based solely on that component of your identity. We still have a long way to go to include children and the mentally ill as deserving of fully human rights, although progress has certainly been made in the last half century. And in our present cultural milieu, people who break the law—regardless of whether they commit violent or nonviolent acts—are definitely not seen as deserving of anything but punishment. These decisions about who deserves our concern and who deserves are wrathful vengeance are at the heart of all violence, all warfare, all killing. If we are to survive as a species, we will have to unite to save the planet. That means we will have to radically extend the circle of empathic regard to be virtually all inclusive, and we need to do so quickly. We are in a race with doom and doom may be currently winning.

Science: Enemy or Ally?

In the last three decades, our knowledge about stress, traumatic stress, development, resilience, psychosomatic influences, and the brain–body interface have all grown at an astonishing pace. Technological advances allow us now to see the brain and the body in action, changing with different provocative influences, altering in real time. Advances in understanding neurotransmission and neurohormonal influences have helped us to recognize how automatic neurobiological response are activated far below the level of a person's conscious awareness. Intensive studies of infants, children, and adolescents have revealed facets of human development not previously recognized, while the ability to see the brain in action has led us to recognize the wide variety of circumstances that influence actual brain development—everything from genes to television. Thousands of research studies looking at the effects on various survivor groups of exposure to adversity, toxic stress, and trauma have given us an inside look at how the brain and the body respond to different events in a wide variety of ways. Scientists around the world are linking together nature and nurture so that we know both are interactively vital in understanding the nature of human nature.

As we stand now, science can be an enemy in the race against catastrophe or our best ally. Scientific progress has brought us the Industrial Revolutions and therefore pollution and climate crisis. But science has also brought us improved health and longer lives. The psychobiology of trauma and our expanding knowledge about development and disrupted attachment are teaching us that many of our feelings, thoughts, choices, and actions are determined or at least powerfully influenced by forces we are unaware of and that our voluntary control is more illusion than reality. But at the same time, it is at the junction between knowledge and ignorance that free will has a starring role. The central question of the next few decades is this: Can we choose to get out of our own evolutionary shadows and decide to launch ourselves onto a different trajectory?

So we believe it is critically important that everyone—child and adult, manager and frontline worker, business person or social service professional, policy maker and legislator—in every domain of human endeavor should gain a working knowledge about how stress, toxic stress, and traumatic stress affect human thought, feelings, and behavior. Likewise everyone needs to know how important attachment, empathy, and loving regard are for healing, recovery and most importantly, the survival of the human species.

Social historian Jeremy Rifkin has claimed that *"empathy is the very means by which we create social life and advance civilization"* (p. 11) [322]. Trauma theory combined with attachment theory provides us with a fundamental shift in addressing individual and group dilemmas retaining several centuries of biological, psychological, social, and spiritual knowledge gained, but providing an integrative framework and a scientific grounding for that knowledge. By better defining what goes wrong, we are in a much better position to decide both how to help and what results we should see if our help is effective. Perhaps most importantly, our understanding of the relationship between stress, chronic stress, traumatic stress, and disrupted attachment offers the possibility of expanding our capacity to empathize with a wide variety of people who have sustained psychological and social injuries.

Conclusion

Thanks to scientific advances of the last few decades, we now know a great deal about the impact of trauma and adversity on individuals. The conclusion we can draw is that violence is not unlike a contagious virus that is permeating our culture at a disturbingly rapid rate. Now we need a new framework—a trauma-informed framework—for understanding what happens to groups and entire organizations that are trying to contain the distress, frustration, and often overwhelming suffering of the clients and the staff. This framework also needs to help us understand what happens when an entire organization is itself traumatized. In Chapter 4 we will pursue what it means to become a trauma-informed system through understanding the impact of trauma and chronic adversity on groups and organizations. We will also focus on the largely unconscious processes that occur in large groups that we call "parallel processes" from which sometimes emerge "trauma-organized systems."

Chapter 4

Parallel Processes and Trauma-Organized Systems

SUMMARY: *Organizations are living complex systems and as such are vulnerable to the impact of trauma and chronic stress. In this chapter we will explore how groups respond to stress and suggest that as a result of acute and chronic organizational stress, destructive processes occur within and between organizations that mirror or "parallel" the processes for which our clients seek help that we covered in the last chapter. The result for them is "sanctuary trauma" and "sanctuary harm," while the result for providers of service is a collective kind of trauma as the organizations within which we work cease fulfilling a fundamental social role, that of containing anxiety in the face of death, suffering, defeat, and uncertainty. In such cases, social defense mechanisms come to dominate whatever therapeutic activity is supposed to be occurring in the social service environment. However, these parallel processes can be named and understood within the context of our present knowledge of individual and group psychology.*

Organizations as Complex, Adaptive, Emergent Systems

There is a different way of looking at and operating organizations—a different mental model than the one we have become accustomed to. The newer model is that of organizations as alive, possessing the basic requirements of living systems and therefore are capable of adapting to changing conditions [6; 323]. In the business world, unlike the social service sector, this new mental model has been itself in part due to the enormous pressures of globalization. Some strong proponents of this emergent point of view have claimed that *"the 20th century gave birth to a new species—the global corporation... a life form that can grow, evolve, and learn"* (p. 6) [324]. In this new paradigm, individual consciousness becomes even more—not less—important, so that *"the key challenge is to apply inner knowledge, intuition, compassion and spirit to prosper in a period of constant and discontinuous change"* (p. 6) [325].

The Concept of Groupmind

A key question underlying our belief in organizations as living systems is, Can a group take on an identity that is some way distinct from the individuals that comprise it? Can a group develop a "groupmind"? Is there something else, something more than the simple sum of individuals, that is real and not just a metaphor used whenever a journalist refers to the "soul" or the "heart" or the "character" of the nation?

Groupmind is the word that has been used to describe the concept of a supraindividual nature and independence of the collective mind of a social group. The concept goes back at least to the German philosopher Hegel, who felt that individual minds are active participants of a larger social mind, concepts that later influenced Marx and Engels (and these latter two influences may help explain why this concept has evoked such controversy over the years) [230; 326]. It was Durkheim who first used the term "groupmind" to refer to collective consciousness. He suggested that large groups of people sometimes acted with a single mind and that rather than being merely collections of individuals they were linked by some unifying force that went beyond any single individual, a force so strong that the will of the individual could be completely dominated by the will of the group [240]. William McDougall, a psychologist at Harvard and one of the first social psychologists, was convinced that a society is more than the mere sum of the mental lives of its units, "*a complete knowledge of the units, if and in so far as they could be known as isolated units, would not enable us to deduce the nature of the life of the whole*" (p. 7) [230].

General Systems Theory

General systems theory is an important scientific and philosophical conceptual framework that emerged in the twentieth century out of quantum physics and cybernetics but profoundly influenced the ecological movement and psychiatry as well [7]. The main premise is that every individual component of any system influences and is influenced by every other component. General systems theory provides a theoretical underpinning for some of the observations that were central to the lessons that psychiatrists took from their involvement in World War II. Psychiatry came to recognize that individuals could be understood and helped only in the context of understanding their family system, their cultural framework for constructing reality, and the larger systems within which they lived and worked—school, workplace, friendship patterns—as well as the network of connections that comprised each individual's personal and cultural history [327].

Living systems are not nearly as predictable as machines, and they require living processes in order to function properly. The system you work in is, probably at most, about a hundred years old and in all likelihood much younger than that, may be located in different physical locations, and is interactively impacted if not guided by thousands of brains. Systems are, on the one hand, indispensable in a complex society. On the other hand, systems—all systems that have not been shaped by Nature but by humans—are notoriously difficult to manage, move, start, stop, or change. John Gall, author and retired pediatrician, expressed it best in his work on "Systemantics":

> *Systems are seductive. They promise to do a hard job faster, better, and more easily than you could do it by yourself. But if you set up a system, you are likely to find your time and effort now being consumed in the care and feeding of the system itself. New problems are created by its very presence. Once set up, it won't go away, it grows and encroaches. It begins to do strange and wonderful things. Breaks down in ways you never thought possible. It kicks back, gets in the way, and opposes its own proper function. Your own perspective becomes distorted by being in the system. You become anxious and push on it to make it work. Eventually you come to believe that the misbegotten product it so grudgingly delivers is what you really wanted all the time. At that point encroachment has become complete... you have become absorbed ... you are now a systems person!* (pp. 127–128) [328]

Unlike a machine, like your car or your vacuum cleaner, your body and every organization that delivers human services are living systems—they are open, complex, and adaptive. Living systems are *open systems* because they accept input from their environment, they use this input to create output, and they then act on the environment. Living systems are adaptive because they can *learn* and based on that learning, they can adapt to changes in their environment in order to survive. As a living system, the human service system and every component of that system has an identity, a memory, and has created its own processes that resist changes imposed from above but will evolve and change naturally if the circumstances are conducive to change.

The mental health system is complex because it is comprised of other complex adaptive systems: the staff, administrators, and boards, the clients, and their families. It is rooted within health, public health, and social service systems of a county and state, and all are set within a country, a country that is embedded within a global civilization. And all these components are complexly interactive with each other. The past history of any service program, like the histories of the individual clients and staff, and the systems they are embedded within, continue to determine present behavior and in every moment, present behavior is playing a role in determining the future. All of these components—individual, group, organization, local government, national government, global influences, past, present, and future—all are interacting with and impacting on each other in complicated ways, all of the time. That's what makes things so *complex*. It is this complexity that arouses anxiety because there is no sure way of being certain that what you do will change anything. The anxiety associated with uncertainty then compels the usual oversimplification that occurs whenever an individual or a group of individuals encounters the apparently overwhelming complexity of changing systems.

Living systems are not entirely controllable by top-down regulation. Like the human body, a living system functions through constant feedback loops, flows of information back and forth. In the body, there certainly are hierarchies, but these hierarchies are "democratic hierarchies"; power distribution is circular [329]. Regulation comes through feedback mechanisms and changes constantly over time, adjusting and readjusting to internal circumstances that have been altered and reacting and adjusting to external changes in the environment. Information from below in the hierarchy has as much influence as control mechanisms higher in the hierarchy. If you find this difficult to believe, just try focusing your own sophisticated intellectual attention on something else when even your little toe is throbbing with pain.

A living system evolves, regenerates, and self-organizes to adapt to changing circumstances. Complex adaptive systems change constantly, but the change is self-organized change, a process by which a structure and pattern emerge without that change being directed from outside [330]. Living systems learn and use that new information to alter present and future behavior. A living system is constantly balancing and rebalancing to maintain homeostasis. And in a living system there is no such thing as an absolute state of "health"—health is a relative term. You cannot feed a living system and then leave it alone; it must be fed and maintained all the time. Unpredictable things happen in complex adaptive systems—things that could not be predicted ahead of time because of the phenomenon known as *emergence*.

Living Systems Are Characterized by Emergence

The simplest way of understanding emergence is that it occurs whenever the whole is greater than, or smarter than, the sum of the parts. It is about understanding how collective properties arise from the properties of parts and the relationship between them [331]. As neuroscientist John Holland described it, *"we are everywhere confronted with emergence in complex adaptive systems—ant colonies, networks of neurons, the immune system, the Internet, and the global economy, to name a few—where the behavior of the whole is much more complex than the behavior of the part"* (p. 2) [332]. The idea of *emergence* is behind the concept of collective intelligence, a vibrant area of exploration; the Internet, cell phones, social networking, and all communication technologies are wiring together people from around the globe in unexpected and unpredictable ways; and a long list of hard-core scientists have been demonstrating the relational and molecular substrate for social interactions that takes us out of the realm of speculation or science fiction and plunges us right into brain science [333].

Emergence helps to explain how collective phenomenon can arise and be different than the components that comprise it, which, by the way, is what true teamwork is all about. Just as neurons interconnect in networks that create structured thoughts beyond the ken of any individual neuron and what emerges is consciousness, so people spontaneously organize themselves into groups to create emergent organizations that no individual may intend, comprehend, or even perceive [334].

Not Sick or Bad, But Injured

A corollary of thinking about the organization as a living body not entirely unlike our own leads also to using the same parallels to think about the impact of adversity and trauma on the human organization, parallel thinking that can be served by our deepening understanding about the ways in which adversity impacts the human body, mind, and soul. We look at human service organizations at the present time as badly *injured.*

An injury model of understanding human systems—systems as small as one individual or very extended and comprising thousands of people—leads to very different kinds of thinking and behavior than a sickness model and reflects another significant change in mental models. Right now, there are basically three explanations for problematic human behavior: people are thought to be "sick," and if so they are usually sent to the mental health system; they are "bad," and they are relegated to the justice system; or they are both, and no one wants to deal with them, so they shuttle back and forth between the two systems. It has been difficult for individual clinicians and the system as a whole to have any kind of an integrated point of view about people who have significant problems—that people in the mental health system can do very bad things *and* that people in the criminal justice system can have significant mental health problems.

The attitude toward troubled organizations swings between these two poles as well. People within the organization often view their system as "sick," frequently irredeemably so, and people outside of the organization view it as "bad," frequently irredeemably so. This is part of what makes the whole study of the complex biopsychosocial impact of adversity and trauma so very important—that it is all about *injury,* and that you can injure a human being, and human organizations, in an almost infinite variety of ways and it can look like everything from physical illness to moral corruption.

An injury model connects the injured person to his or her environment; injuries always occur within an interpersonal and social context. Injury implies recovery and rehabilitation, even with a possible long-lasting handicap. Injury requires the active participation of the injured party; injured parties must do what they can to help themselves heal and not do anything that will make their injuries worse. They are personally and socially accountable for the healing of their injuries, although the social context within which the injuries occurs may make it impossible to fairly locate "blame." In an injury model we should pay a great deal of attention to injury prevention and universal precautions that prevent injury. Injury can be physical, psychological, social, and moral, and all these forms of injury are recognized as being interactive and complex. Injuries can result from too much of something or too little, as in neglect, deprivation, and developmental insult. An injury model implies a process of recovery and rehabilitation that is mutual and may require a long-term commitment to that recovery. And such a commitment requires an actively collaborative relationship between the helper(s) and the injured party (ies). It leads interactive exploration away from that sickness/badness dichotomy expressed as "What's *wrong* with you?" to a very different question of "What *happened* to you?" [2]. Such a change in focus provides a framework for addressing problems that everyone can relate to; we have all suffered physical, emotional, social, and moral injuries. A thorough notion of injury brings those who have been dehumanized back within the scope of human concerns and empathic regard. Such a change in basic stance simultaneously increases compassion and increases expectations for everyone.

Living Systems With Visible and Invisible Groups

In looking at organizations as living systems and not as machines, we are required to understand that human beings and human organizations of all sizes have a dual existence at all times—conscious and unconscious realities— and that quite frequently they are in conflict with each other. This is a situation that gives rise to great complexity. Every individual member of the organization is motivated by conscious and unconscious forces. Individual consciousness is a relatively recent evolutionary development. Conscious awareness is layered atop eons of unconscious individual and group processing. Consciousness can be thought of as the beam of light in an otherwise dark room. The dark room is all that we are unaware of at any moment in time. Freud called this the "unconscious mind," the storehouse of instinctual desires, needs, memories, and psychic actions that direct the thoughts and feelings of the individual from this darkened realm. Advances in neuroscience have shown that very clearly, there are thousands, even millions of unconscious processes operating all the time and that though we can become conscious of some of them, our consciousness or awareness occurs after the unconscious processes occur.

Group theorists have long recognized that when people come together and form a group, there are also conscious and unconscious components to group life. We are born into groups, also known as families, and we are involved with many groups throughout our lives. The roles we assume in groups are often unconsciously driven by previous experiences that have been with us since childhood, and then we relate to colleagues in an organization based on those early experiences. Like a family, every group and every organization has its own values, beliefs, norms, and behaviors that are affirmed and transmitted to every new member.

In every organization, there are many visible subgroups and invisible subgroups that we, as individuals, move in and out of routinely, while the organization as a whole also develops a conscious and an unconscious identity [10; 335–337]. Just as it is possible to understand the multiple levels of an individual human being, it is also possible to work within the complexity of human systems. But problems arise when we fail to grapple with this complexity. Past and present leaders have significant influence over these conscious and unconscious forces within an organization. But because living systems are complexly interactive, leaders are also constrained by these same forces [337]. Mythology often develops around the central moments of an organization's history and those myths may help to determine how new members, most importantly new leaders, become socialized to the organizational culture. If we are to explore the notion of parallel processes, it is important that we first look at some basic concepts about the evolutionary mechanisms that groups of people evolved to cope with danger and stress.

Group Stress Responses

Group Emergency Responses to Threat

In our evolutionary past, the development of extended social networks increased the likelihood that vulnerable offspring would be protected and in combination with our expanding intelligence, made hunting and food gathering far more successful. Human beings could accomplish much more in groups than any one individual could on his or her own. Part of the evolved response to stress that built on our capacity for attachment was a strong inclination to gather together in groups whenever threatened [240]. This inclination to "tend and befriend," which we mentioned in Chapter 3, has been described as another important component of the stress response that may be more dominant in females than in males because of the evolutionary necessity of childcare responsibility falling largely to women [270].

Under severe stress, emotional arousal becomes so intense that if emotional responses are not buffered by others through social contact and physical touch, our central nervous system is left exposed to unrelenting overstimulation. The result can be long-lasting harm to our bodies as well as our psyches. Our capacity to manage overwhelming emotional states is shaped by our experience with early childhood attachments and is maintained throughout life via our attachment relationships. The human species survived largely because we form astonishingly powerful social attachments not only to our caregivers for a limited period of time, as do all mammals, but also to groups of people through bonds that last throughout our lives and sometimes beyond.

Under threat, human beings will more closely bond together with their identified group, close ranks, and prepare for defense of the group. Human groups under stress tend to become less democratic and more hierarchical and authoritarian, a group structure that lends itself to rapid response. But this rapidity of response sacrifices the more complex group processing of information that is typical of democratic interactions. A leader rapidly emerges within such a group, another complex process that is an interaction between the individual characteristics of the leader, the needs of the group, and the contextual demands of the moment. Under such conditions, the vast majority of human beings become more suggestible to the influence of a persuasive, strong, assertive, and apparently confident leader who promises the best defense of the group, thereby containing the overwhelming anxiety of every member of the group [338]. A leader who is attempting to be thoughtful and cautious may instead be considered equivocating or weak when he or she fails to adequately channel the group's anxiety by taking action. Likewise, a leader who drives the group toward action, regardless of how ill considered may be lauded as strong, noble, and courageous.

Decisions are made quickly and the process of decision making is characterized by extremist thinking, a deterioration of complex processes into oversimplified, dichotomous choices. Decisions are often made autonomously by the leader with relatively little input, and the input that he or she receives is likely to be significantly colored by the pressure everyone feels to conform to standards of group cohesion and unanimity. As stress increases, the leader is compelled to take action to reduce the threat, while the followers simultaneously become more obedient to the leader in order to insure coordinated group effort.

The development of human moral reasoning and our desire for justice can be recognized in early evolutionary development as well. Social relationships are built on the logic of reciprocity, or "tit for tat," probably the basis of all cooperative relationships [339]. Out of betrayed reciprocal relationships comes the natural desire for retaliation or revenge [301]. Our need to achieve satisfaction for injury and eventually our uniquely human system of laws designed in part to contain and channel vengeance emerges out of this innate desire for revenge [340]. Under stress, cohesion among the group increases as does a need to protect what the group perceives as its territory. The desire for retaliation for real or imagined violations is increased. Internal conflict and dissent from the will of the group is actively suppressed, while projection of hostility onto an external enemy and dehumanization of that enemy is encouraged. These powerful influences combine to produce a cohesive and organized group that is prepared to fight and kill whomever is designated as the group enemy [341–342].

Under these influences, longstanding interpersonal conflicts within the group seem to evaporate and everyone pulls together toward the common goal of group survival, producing an exhilarating and even intoxicating state of unity, oneness, and a willingness to sacrifice one's own well-being for the sake of the group. This is a survival strategy ensuring that in a state of crisis decisions can be made quickly and efficiently, thus better ensuring survival of the group, even while individuals may be sacrificed.

When Threat Becomes a Way of Life: Parallel Processes Emerge

Group responses to stress are measures that may be extremely effective during an acute state of crisis. However, chronic and recurring threats to the group can lead to states as dangerous for a family, an organization, or a nation as chronic hyperarousal is to the health and well-being of the individual. When a group atmosphere becomes one of constant crisis, with little opportunity for recuperation before another crisis manifests, the toxic nature of this atmosphere tends to produce an increased level of tension, irritability, short tempers, increased needs for command and control, and abusive, controlling behavior.

The urgency to act in order to relieve this tension compromises decision making because group members are unable to weigh and balance multiple options, arrive at compromises, and consider long-term consequences of their actions under stress. Decision making in such groups tends to deteriorate over time with increased numbers of poor and impulsive decisions, compromised problem-solving mechanisms, and overly rigid, extremist and dichotomous thinking and behavior. Interpersonal conflicts that were suppressed during the initial crisis return, often with a vengeance, but conflict resolution mechanisms, if ever in place, deteriorate further under the influence of chronic stress [264].

Unable to engage in complex decision making, group problem solving is compromised making it more likely that the group will turn to, or continue to support, leaders who appear strong and decisive, and who urge repetitive but immediate action that temporarily relieves tension and may even bring a sense of exhilaration. Leaders may become increasingly autocratic, bullying, deceitful, and dogmatic, trying to appear calm and assured in front of their followers while narrowing their circle of input to a very small group of trusted associates. As the leader becomes increasingly threatened, sensing the insecurity of his decisions and his position, these small groups of associates feel increasingly pressured to conform to whatever the leader wants and are more likely to engage in groupthink [343]. In this process, judgment and diversity of opinion are sacrificed in service of group cohesion and as this occurs, the quality of decision making becomes compromised, progressively and geometrically compounding existing problems.

Escalating control measures are used to repress any dissent that is felt to be dangerous to the unity of what has become focused group purpose.

This encourages a narrowing of input from the world outside the group. Research has demonstrated that when threatened by death, people will more strongly support their existing cultural belief systems and actively punish those who question those belief systems [292]. Any subgroups that attempt to protest against unfolding events are likely to be harshly punished. As a result, all forms of dissent are silenced.

If group cohesion begins to wane, leaders may experience the relaxing of control measures as a threat to group purpose and safety. They may therefore attempt to mobilize increasing projection onto the designated external enemy who serves a useful purpose in activating increased group cohesion while more strenuously suppressing dissent internally. This cycle may lead to a state of chronic repetitive conflict externally and escalating repressive measures internally.

This entire process tends to increase, not decrease, the sense of fear and insecurity on the part of everyone within the group. As leaders focus exclusively on physical security, the group may be willing to sacrifice other forms of safety and well-being in order to achieve an elusive sense of physical security that remains threatened. In doing so, the group may endorse rapid changes that result in the creation of new rules without considering the unintended consequences that may include the widespread loss of rights, liberty, and freedom. In order to restore the illusion of safety that can then only be secured through an endless escalation of hostility, aggression and defense, projection onto an enemy, suppression of internal conflict, and demands for greater group loyalty all intensify. Group norms shift radically but insidiously, the changes cloaked within a fog of what appears to be rational decision making.

As time goes on and the recurrent stress continues, the group will adapt to adversity by accepting changed group norms. Although this adjustment to changed group norms feels normal, actual behavior becomes increasingly aberrant and ineffective. When someone mentions the fact of the changed norms, about the differences between the way things are now and the way they used to be (when the group was more functional), the speaker is likely to be silenced or ignored. As a result there is an escalating level of acceptance of increasingly aberrant behavior.

Like individuals, groups can forget their past and the more traumatic and conflicted the past the more likely it is that groups will push memories out of conscious awareness. Critical events and group failure change us and change our groups, but without memory we lose the context. As in families, so too in organizations and in whole societies, past traumas are frequently known and not known—historically recognized but never really talked about, mourned, or resolved [344–346]. This is particularly true when the past traumas are also associated with guilt. Studies have shown that institutions do have memory and that once interaction patterns have been disrupted these patterns can be transmitted through a group so that one "generation" unconsciously passes on to the next norms that alter the system and every member of the system. But without a conscious memory of events also being passed on, group members in the present cannot make adequate judgments about whether the strategy, policy, or norm is still appropriate and useful in the present [347]. This process can present an extraordinary resistance to healthy group adaptation to changing conditions.

Groups that have experienced repeated stress and traumatic loss can also experience disrupted attachment. In such a system there will be a devaluation of the importance of relationships. People are treated as widgets, replaceable parts that have no significant individual identity or value. There is a lack of concern for the well-being of others as the group norm, perhaps under the guise of "don't take it personally—it's just business." In groups with disrupted attachment schemata, there is a high frequency of acceptance or even active encouragement of addictive behavior, including substance abuse. There is also an unwillingness and inability to work through loss so that people leaving the group are dealt with summarily and never mentioned again. The result is that the group becomes more stagnant and disconnected from a meaningful environment, group loyalty plummets, and productivity declines.

A group that cannot change, like an individual, will develop patterns of reenactment, repeating the past strategies over and over without recognizing that these strategies are no longer effective. With every repetition there is instead further deterioration in functioning. Healthier and potentially healing individuals may enter the group but are rapidly extruded as they fail to adjust to the reenactment role that is being demanded of them. Less autonomous individuals may also enter the group and are drawn into the reenactment pattern. In this way, one autocratic and abusive leader leaves, only to be succeeded by another.

When guilt is involved, it is common to find projection and displacement of unpleasant realities onto an external enemy. The continued use of projection over time causes increased internal group splitting and a loss of social integration. Absent a language that engages feeling and the multiple narratives of history, a group cannot heal from past traumatic events and is therefore compelled in overt or symbolized ways to repeat those events.

Similar to a chronically stressed individual, as group stress persists, a pattern of group failure begins to emerge. Unable to deal with the increasing complexities of an ever-changing world because of the rigidity and stagnation of problem solving and decision making, the group looks, feels, and acts angry, depressed, and anxious but is helpless to effect any change. There is an increasing rate of illness, addiction, and antisocial acts among the individuals within the group. Burnout, personality distortions, and acting-out behavior all increase. Conflicts arise repeatedly and are not resolved or even addressed.

As this deterioration continues, group members feel increasingly demoralized and hopeless, concerned that the group mission and value system have been betrayed in countless ways.

Alienation begins to characterize the social milieu and evidence for it can be seen in increased internal splitting and dissension, rampant hypocrisy, a loss of mutual respect and tolerance, apathy, cynicism, hopelessness, helplessness, loss of social cohesiveness and purpose, loss of a sense of shared social responsibility for the more unfortunate members of any population, and the loss of a shared moral compass. Alienation is the end result of an unwillingness or inability to work through the fragmentation, dissociation, and disrupted attachment attendant upon repetitive traumatic experience. Increasing feelings of alienation are symptoms of severe degradation and stagnation and signal that the time for systemic change is at hand if the organism is to survive. System-wide corruption, systematic deceit, empathic failures, increasingly punitive laws, hypermoralism, hypocrisy, and a preoccupation and glorification of violence are all symptomatic of impending group bankruptcy or system failure [348–351].

Sanctuary Trauma

We first started calling our inpatient psychiatric program "The Sanctuary" around 1986 after reading a description of something termed "sanctuary trauma." First described by Dr. Steven Silver in one of the first papers about the inpatient treatment of Vietnam War veterans, he defined "sanctuary trauma" as that which *"occurs when an individual who suffered a severe stressor next encounters what was expected to be a supportive and protective environment"* (p. 215) and discovers only more trauma [352]. The concept of the Sanctuary spring-boarded from this idea when we recognized that many patients who had come into psychiatric facilities expecting help, understanding, and comfort had found instead rigid rules, humiliating procedures, conflicting and often disempowering methods, and inconsistent, confusing, and judgmental explanatory systems. This led to a rethinking of the basic assumptions upon which we base treatment and a formulation of our treatment approach as "The Sanctuary Model" requiring radical changes in our mental models for understanding our work and the world around us [1].

Sanctuary Harm and Collective Trauma

The concept of "sanctuary harm" has been applied to events in psychiatric settings that do not meet the formal criteria for trauma but that involve insensitive, inappropriate, neglectful, or abusive actions by staff or associated authority figures and invoke in consumers a response of fear, helplessness, distress, humiliation, or loss of trust in staff [353–354]. In Chapter 2, we provided evidence that the incidence of sanctuary trauma is considerable. It is interesting to wonder how many people come into health, mental health, and social service environments expecting emotionally intelligent, caring environments and find instead sanctuary harm. Such exposure is likely to be a significant contributor to the workforce crisis that faces the human service delivery system as a whole. Events that cause sanctuary trauma or sanctuary harm in the clients do not just affect them, although they are likely to suffer the most direct harm. The staff members directly involved, those who are indirectly involved, and the organization as a whole suffer "collateral damage," that is, they are affected by such events as well.

In this way, trauma becomes collective. In the case of whole organizations, the concept of "collective trauma" is a useful one. Kai Erikson has described collective trauma as *"a blow to the basic tissues of social life that damages the bonds attaching people together and impairs the prevailing sense of communality. The collective trauma works its way slowly and even insidiously into the awareness of those who suffer from it, so it does not have the quality of suddenness normally associated with 'trauma'. But it is a form of shock all the same, a gradual realization that the community no longer exists as an effective source of support and that an important part of the self has disappeared... 'I' continue to exist, though damaged and maybe even permanently changed. 'You' continue to exist, though distant and hard to relate to. But 'we' no longer exist as a connected pair or as linked cells in a larger communal body"* (p. 233) [355].

The impact of dramatic changes in social service and health care financing that we described in Chapters 1 and 2 can be thought of as a collective trauma to the human service system as a whole, directly impacting the organizational culture of every component of the system and the system as a collective. Since every organization has its own culture, each culture can be traumatized. Patient deaths and injuries—from natural causes, accidents, and most particularly suicide and deaths while in restraints; staff deaths or injuries; loss of leaders; lawsuits; downsizing—all may be overwhelming not just for the individuals involved but for overall organizational function. But as we will explore next, the individuals within an organization may not be aware of the ways in which their own and other people's behavior have been affected by events over which they had little control. That is because much of what goes on in groups goes on at an unconscious level.

Social Defense Systems

There is much in our individual and organizational lives that we wish not to be aware of and we find ways of keeping information out of consciousness, usually things that are distressing and laden with conflicts about the basis of life, or the basis of our reality. The point of defense mechanisms, individually and in groups, is to provide us with illusions of certainty and safety that protect us from being overwhelmed by anxiety, terror, and helplessness. The fundamental problem with these defense mechanisms is that they often keep us from taking constructive action that would eliminate the sources of the stress or threat.

Bion and Basic Assumption Groups

Wilfred Bion was one of the first people to focus on the unconscious defenses that a group uses to deal with anxiety and conflict that distract the group from its conscious tasks. Working as a psychiatrist during World War II, he was one of the founders of group dynamics. In working with groups, he noticed that there were interaction patterns that members of the group were largely unaware of, that appeared to emerge not from one person but were a product of the group dynamic, and that interfered with adequate group performance because they tended to lead to more primitive rather than more advanced levels of functioning. He noted what he called "basic assumptions" that were unconscious, a product of the group, and caused groups to derail from their actual tasks. He called these basic assumptions "dependency," "fight-flight," and "pairing." When an ongoing group strays off course from its actual tasks as a group and continues to function in a way that interferes with the achievement of group goals it is said to have created a "collusive culture" [336–337].

In groups in the thrall of "dependency" assumptions, the members of the group are united by common feelings of helplessness, inadequacy, neediness, and fear and are searching for a charismatic leader upon whom they can depend, who will relieve all anxiety, while protecting and guiding them. When this occurs, group members fail to take initiative, use critical judgment, and depend on leadership too much.

Groups who are susceptible to "fight-flight" are characterized by avoidance and attack. These are the two main strategies group members utilize and the group tends to split into camps of friends and enemies. The fight reaction manifests in aggression, jealousy, competition, and sibling rivalry, while the flight reaction includes avoidance, absenteeism, and giving up. Us-vs-them language is commonly heard. When leaders become a part of this split, they unite followers against the "enemy" and all of the group's energy may be diverted to a dangerous or lost cause.

Bion's third basic assumption group is called "pairing." When this unconscious assumption is in play, people come to believe that the best creation will be a result of pairing up in twos, but unfortunately this means splitting up the group and results in increased levels of intra- and intergroup conflict. "Leave it to the two of us" often does not work as an innovative strategy, and fantasizing that if the "CEO and the COO only worked better together everything would be fine" just keeps the group from progressing.

Jung and Shadow Groups

In a similar vein, Carl Jung described the "shadow," which in Jungian terms represents the darker side to our personality which we do not consciously display in public, although other people may recognize our shadow self before we do. What we cannot admit to ourselves we often find in others; it is the part of ourselves that we are ashamed of and will not admit to ourselves [356]. Building on Jungian ideas, organizational theorists have noted that groups as a whole also have a shadow side. The "shadow group" has been defined as the collection of all the shadow parts of the various members of a work group or other group. *"The shadow group is no phantasm, but rather a hidden reality that parallels the normal functioning of work groups and which takes over their interaction when one or more individual members are engulfed by their shadow selves during emotionally-based interpersonal conflict"* (p. 25) [357].

Menzies and Social Defense

Group analyst Isabel Menzies, building on the work of the noted group theorist Eliot Jaques, described the ways in which mental health systems create their own "social defense systems" [347; 358]. She described how systems develop specific and static protective mechanisms to protect against the anxiety that is inevitably associated with change. The defense mechanisms she describes sound uncannily like those that we see in victims of trauma—depersonalization, denial, detachment, denial of feelings, ritualized task performance, redistribution of responsibility and irresponsibility, idealization, and avoidance of change.

Menzies used as an example of a social defense system a conflict in the nursing staff of a hospital that played itself out at every level within an organization. In describing this she said the nursing staff *"develop some form of relationship that locates madness in the patient and sanity in themselves, with a barrier to prevent contamination. Such an arrangement allows the nurses to stay in the situation without feeling that their minds are being damaged. It justifies the use of control by the nurses, entitles patients to care and refuge, and is a virtual guarantee that they will continue to be thought ill and therefore will not be sent outside"* (p. 604) [359].

Over time and as a result of collusive interaction and unconscious agreement between members of an organization, each organization's social defense system becomes a systematized part of reality which new members must deal with as they come into the system. These defensive maneuvers become group norms, similar to the way the same defensive maneuvers become norms in the lives of individual people and then are passed on from one generation of group participants to the next. Upon entering the system each new member must become acculturated to the established norms if he or she is to succeed and belong. In such a way, an original group creates a group reality, which then becomes institutionalized for every subsequent group, firmly lodged in the institutional memory [347]. This aspect of the "groupmind" becomes quite resistant to change, rooted in a past that is forgotten, now simply the "way things are" [360].

Institutional Uncertainty

In every organization there is the level of "what we say we do" and the levels of "what we believe we are doing" and then there is also "what is really going on," and the members of an organization may be completely unaware of this third level [361]. Depending on what institution we are addressing, unconscious motivations vary. In the health care system, the third level can be addressed as "keeping death at bay" and in a variety of ways denying that death will inevitably occur. In the mental health system, this third level shows itself in attempts to reject the enormous complexity of emotional problems and our relative helplessness in affecting cure and "keeping insanity at bay."

The collective result of this natural inclination to contain anxiety becomes a special problem when institutional events occur that produce great uncertainty, particularly those events that are associated with insanity, death, or the fear of death. Under these conditions, containing anxiety may become more important than rationally responding to the situation. But this motivation is likely to be denied and rationalized. As a result, organizations may engage in behavior that may serve to contain anxiety but that is ultimately destructive to organizational purpose [292; 314; 362]. Likewise, large regulatory systems engage in this behavior after a traumatic event occurs in an organization, often swooping in an effort to address the problem, but ending up simply blaming someone in the organization, arousing more automatic social defenses. They may end feeling better that they did something, but what they did may actually have made the situation worse, not better. One of the ways in which this happens is when a group feels threatened and projects the reason for their fear onto an external enemy, who then becomes dehumanized. This is typically what happens in situations that are confusing and complex. This is most likely to happen when our "social defense systems" begin to fail.

Institutional Trauma and Breakthrough Anxiety

When trauma is experienced, the social defense system goes on "high alert." Intense and primitive emotions are precipitated by exposure to trauma and are experienced empathically by all the members of a group. The occurrence of trauma is a reminder to peers that they too are vulnerable and one way to defend against this sense of vulnerability is by projecting anxiety outward. That can be accomplished by finding something peculiar to the therapist or the worker involved in the event rather than perceiving the risks involved in the work itself. When peers experience this they are likely to distance themselves from the traumatized peer and in that way one person may carry the vulnerable feelings for the entire group [363]. Regulatory agencies often practice similarly by stopping all admissions to the involved organization and essentially sending them into "no man's land" where their survival, already threatened by whatever tragic event occurred, is now further jeopardized by the cutoff of funding. Using the ancient practice of "scapegoating," the group wards off shared responsibility by finding someone upon whom the group can transfer blame and badness, thereby "sending into the wilderness" whatever is anxiety provoking and thus getting it away from the group [364]. In describing scapegoating in human groups, one author wrote:

> Institutions that deal with trauma or with trauma survivors will inevitably encounter secondary traumatic stress... In the case of institutions that deal with physical dangers, their members can be traumatized both directly and indirectly; that is, they can be exposed to both primary stressors and secondary stressors...If any personnel are exposed to primary stressors, then all other personnel are in danger of secondary stress (pp. 232–233) [365].

Postulating that traumatic origins lie behind most psychiatric and social dysfunction reconnects all kinds of behavioral disorders to the social context within which these behavioral problems arise. To take seriously the notion of intervention and prevention in the realm of mental illness, a society must take on issues of systemic violence, abuse, child maltreatment, domestic violence, poverty, racism, and gender inequality. At an individual staff level, the implications of trauma theory are bound to raise anxiety within the institutional setting as the staff become less able to use their usual defenses to protect themselves from the contagious emotion surrounding the traumatic past. In addition, many of them will be themselves trauma survivors and may have unresolved issues that have brought them into the field in the first place.

And it may not be a coincidence that just as the mental health field began to seriously address the issue of violence, abuse, and maltreatment—individual and structural—that research, training, innovation, and treatment were vastly cutback or eliminated altogether in many private and public settings. Over the years many socially engaged psychiatrists and other mental health workers have recognized the connection between trauma, emotional disturbance and social disturbance [1; 139; 294; 340; 366]. Many of the children and adults who end up repeatedly or chronically institutionalized are a product of a society that refuses to face up to and both rationally and adequately deal with its chronic problems: racism, sexism, poverty, child maltreatment, community violence, and domestic violence. "The hospital is landed in a situation where it tries to help an individual on behalf of society which really just wants to be rid of him. This is a no-win situation for the hospital and its staff" (p. 27) [367].

This breakdown of barriers between "us" and "them" can cause massive personal, organizational, and systemic anxiety particularly when beginning to address the patients' past traumatic history triggers reminders in the staff of similar things that happened to them. As one author has noted, *"Talking to patients is dangerous because it threatens to puncture the barrier that keeps sanity and madness in their proper places"* (p. 605) [359]. The present woeful state of the mental health system and related social service delivery components cannot be attributed to a lack of knowledge, research, or evidence. In an extensive review that we referred to earlier, Hubble, Duncan, and Miller have pointed out that many varieties of therapy are very effective and for most people who seek help, positive results are evident in a relatively short period of time [3]. Instead, it reflects a lack of political and social will to address the impact of mental illness in all its form—most of which is preventable—on the health and well-being of the nation.

The Social Defense System Operating Today

This social defense system can be seen operating today in psychiatrists who spend more time deciding on the diagnosis that most adequately fits the *DSM-IV-R* and then prescribing the "proper" medication than they spend actually talking to the patient. The social defense system is operating when the staff fail to ask about a client's trauma history or keep forgetting what the client's trauma history was. The social defense system is operating whenever the "silencing response" is occurring or when we collude to create a blame culture (Chapter 5) or when a collective disturbance (Chapter 8) or groupthink arises (Chapter 6). And whenever staff members engage in reenactment behavior, our social defense system is unconsciously operating, as we will comment on many times in this book (Chapter 11). It is also operating in the institution as a whole, when that institution provides services that are called "treatment" but which are more accurately designed to control or "manage" the individual patient on behalf of the society. It is operating when psychiatrists deal with the constraints on care determined by funding and demands for productivity by exclusively focusing on the use of medications and by making diagnoses that accommodate such a focus, and when the rest of the components of the human service delivery system go along with this.

The social defense system is operative in health care when we deny that health care is a right and a responsibility and that damaging some people's health affects us all. We pretend that the social determinants of health and disease are medical problems, not social problems. It's operating when we fail to take into account the long-term, multigenerational impact of poverty, racism, childhood adversity, and neglect. In reality, the allostatic load on children born and raised under these conditions means that many children do not start out with a level playing field. The social defense system is on full volume when we pretend that one human service sector—child welfare—can simultaneously protect the welfare of children and of families while investigating child abuse and neglect.

If we look, we can see the social defense system in action all around us. The conflict between "controlling" the less fortunate among us for the sake of society and actually helping people by empathizing with and empowering them to make positive change is a source of chronic conflict and anxiety in our systems of care. And this conflict is a source of chronic, unspoken, unrealized stress for everyone working within virtually any social service institution. Conflicts over command and control versus therapeutic empathy are at the heart of many social service environments regardless of whether they serve children, adolescents, or adults.

As an example, as long as the mental health system is responsible for the legal and social containment of mental illness, it will be exceedingly difficult and perpetually stressful for the staff of institutions to offer the kind of care sought by many advocates of the recovery movement. This then presents a major barrier to the goals of the consumer recovery movement [368]. In the juvenile justice system, 30 years of punitive, command-and-control environments have led to escalating levels of violence directed at clients and staff, with relatively dismal outcomes, and yet changing those environments to be more empathic and therapeutic toward the needs, and outcomes, of these traumatized children and teenagers is very challenging. Despite the enormity of the trauma these children have experienced, the general population still believes they should be "punished" and persist in the wrong-headed notion that punitive environments will help these children to change in positive ways.

A good example of the way the unconscious group operates is the way a group selects a "troublemaker" who then performs a function on behalf of other members of the group as well as themselves. This is the person who always challenges administration, who constantly argues, who gives off nonverbal signs of frustration in meetings but never does anything positive, who is always tardy, and who bullies other people [315]. *"Many groups and organizations have a 'difficult', 'disturbed', or 'impossible' member whose behavior is regarded as getting in the way of the others' good work. There may be a widely shared belief that if only that person would leave, then everything would be fine. This view is very attractive, hard to resist and tempting to act upon.... As happens very often, no sooner had one troublesome person left, than another one appeared. ... this unconscious suction of individuals into performing a function on behalf of others as well as themselves happens in all institutions"* (pp. 130–131) [315].

In a similar way, the unconscious, covert aspects of the organization grow up informally alongside or, perhaps more accurately, within the overt organization to provide services and benefits not provided by the overt organization. These arrangements can parallel, complement, or even replace formal organizational structures and processes [369]. Of all the explanations of conflict in organizations, it is these shadowy, largely unconscious sources of conflict that are likely to be the most problematic in caregiving organizations. We may be relatively good at solving many task conflicts and even resolving overt interpersonal conflicts and misunderstandings, but we get blindsided by the unconscious group forces of which we are just dimly aware. We often only observe in retrospect the damage that has been left in the wake of these shadow experiences.

When most of the organizational energy is going into social defensive routines, the organization is unable to fully actualize its mission. As organizational scholar Manfred Kets de Vries has pointed out: *"When social defenses no longer target a specific, temporary danger but become the organization's dominant mode of operation—the permanent, accepted way of dealing with the angst and unpredictability of life in organizations—they become dysfunctional for the organization as a whole. Though they may still serve a purpose (albeit not constructively), they have become bureaucratic obstacles, embedded in the organizational structure. Once firmly entrenched, they have cultural implications for the whole organization"* (p. 314) [337].

Parallel Process: A Trauma-Informed Understanding of Social Defensive Structures

Identifying a problem is the first step in solving it. The concept of parallel process is a useful way of offering a coherent framework that can enable organizational leaders and staff to develop a way of thinking "outside the box" about what *has* happened and *is* happening to their treatment and service delivery systems, as well as to the world around them. It is based on an understanding of the ways in which trauma and chronic adversity affect human function [295; 348–351; 370]. Individual and group conscious and unconscious processes can be put into motion beyond an individual's conscious or deliberate control.

In organizations, conflicts that belong at one location are often displaced and enacted elsewhere because of a parallelism between the largely unconscious conflicts at the place of origin and the place of expression [371–372]. The notion of parallel process derives originally from psychoanalytic concepts related to transference and has traditionally been applied to the psychotherapy supervisory relationship in which the supervisory relationship may mirror much of what is going on in the relationship between therapist and client [373]. Parallel processes are not inherently negative or dysfunctional; it depends entirely on what is being "paralleled." But parallel processes evolve unconsciously, outside of awareness, are at work in all human systems, and can stand in as metaphors, if not actual representations, for each other [374].

Negative, destructive parallel processes occur when another person, series of people, or an entire organization is drawn into re-creating destructive scenarios with people they are supposed to be helping. The result of the parallel process nature of human systems is that our organizations and society as a whole frequently recapitulate for individuals the very experiences that have proven so toxic for them in the first place, while individual reenactments tend to shape the structure and function of those institutions. The concept of parallel process was used in studying the dynamics that unfolded between two consulting groups hired by the same client that mirrored what was happening in the client's organization [374–375]. Here is the way they described it:

> When two or more systems—whether these consist of individuals, groups, or organizations—have significant relationships with one another, they tend to develop similar affects, cognition, and behaviors, which are defined as parallel processes .... Parallel processes can be set in motion in many ways, and once initiated leave no one immune from their influence. They can move from one level of a system to another, changing form along the way. For example, two vice presidents competing for resources may suppress their hostility toward each other and agree to collaborate interpersonally, but each may pass directives to her or his subordinates that induce them to fight with those of the other vice president. Thus, what began as a struggle among executives for resources becomes expressed by lower-ranking groups in battles over compliance with cost-cutting measure. (p. 13) [376]

An even older conceptualization of this process derives from the original sociological studies of mental institutions in the 1950s describing "collective disturbance," which we will discuss further in Chapter 8. A collective disturbance occurs when two people in conflict, each feeling blocked by the other, cannot speak directly about the conflict and unconsciously set up substitute channels of communication through other members of the staff or through the patients [377].

We believe that currently parallel processes are at play that interfere significantly with the ability of the human service system and all of its components to address the actual needs of trauma survivors specifically, and people with mental health and substance abuse problems in general. Instead, because of complex interactions between traumatized clients, stressed staff, and pressured organizations, a social and economic environment emerges that is frequently hostile to the aims of recovery.

Just as the lives of people exposed to repetitive and chronic trauma, abuse, and maltreatment become organized around the traumatic experience, so too can entire systems become organized around the recurrent and severe stress of trying to cope with a flawed mental model that is the present underpinning of our helping systems. When this happens, it sets up an interactive dynamic that creates what are sometimes uncannily parallel processes [120; 123].

The clients bring their past history of traumatic experience into the mental health and social service sectors, consciously aware of certain specific goals but unconsciously struggling to recover from the pain and losses of the past. They are greeted by individual service providers, subject to their own personal life experiences, who are more or less deeply embedded in entire systems that are under significant stress. Given what we know about exposure to childhood adversity and other forms of traumatic experience, the majority of service providers have experiences in their background that may be quite similar to the life histories of their clients, and that similarity may be more or less recognized and worked through.

What Is Denied Comes Back to Haunt Us

The destructive parallel processes that we describe later in this volume—collective disturbance, traumatic reenactment, groupthink, the Abilene paradox—all are part of this shadowy world of group interactive dynamics, the "social defense systems" that rarely get discussed in the social service and mental health world of today. That lack of discussion, of course, makes the influence of the unconscious conflicts at the individual and at the group level much more powerful. Because an understanding of unconscious processes has been almost eliminated from our social service systems, the problems that systematically plague our organizations, create enormous stress in the workforce, and undermine performance are largely incomprehensible. Problems in organizations are often attributed to specific troublemakers, and if only we could eliminate the problem people, everything would be ok. It is important to remember that we organize our social institutions to accomplish specific tasks and functions, but we also utilize our institutions to collectively protect us against being overwhelmed with the anxiety that underlies human existence. We are, after all, the only animal that knowingly must anticipate our own death, fear loss, and fear insanity.

When Tragedy Strikes: The Impact of Chronic Stress and Collective Trauma

When an entire group is exposed to a traumatic situation, it is not just the most vulnerable members of the community who are affected. In an organization that experiences a traumatic event, everyone is affected. In this way, trauma becomes collective. It is our contention that the result of collective trauma, including exposure to chronic and unrelenting stressors over which an organization and the individuals within it can exert little control, leads to highly dysfunctional organizational behavior that directly interferes with the recovery of clients, the well-being of staff, and fulfillment of the organizational mission.

For many institutions the end result of this complex, interactive, and largely unconscious process is that the clients—children, adults, and families—enter our systems of care feeling *unsafe* and often engaging in some form of behavior that is dangerous to themselves or others. They are likely to have difficulty managing *anger* and *aggression*. They may feel *hopeless* and act *helpless*, even when they can make choices that will effectively change their situations, while at the same time this chronic *helplessness* may drive them to exert methods of control that become pathological. They are chronically *hyperaroused* and although they try to *control* their bodies and their minds, they are often ineffective. They may have significant *memory problems* and may be chronically dissociating their memories and/or these feelings, even under minor stress. They are likely therefore to have *fragmented* mental functions. The clients are likely never to have learned very good *communication* skills, nor can they easily engage in *conflict management* because they have such problems with emotional management. They feel *overwhelmed, confused,* and *depressed* and have *poor self-esteem.* Their problems have emerged in the context of disrupted attachment, and they do not know how to make and sustain healthy *relationships* nor do they know how to *grieve* for all that has been lost. Instead they tend to be revictimized or victimize others and, in doing so, repetitively *reenact* their past terror and loss. Their ability to imagine anything other than a repetition of the past, including their ability to set goals, consider in advance the consequences of their actions, and plan for a possible and better future may be severely compromised. Data are beginning to come in that this may be not just a psychological problem but might be based on the brain changes associated with chronic stress [378].

Likewise, in chronically stressed organizations, individual staff members have difficulties differentiating between minor and major stressors. Many of them have a past history of exposure to traumatic and abusive experiences and they do not feel particularly safe in the world. This may manifest as a lack of *safety* with their clients, with management, or even with each other. They are chronically frustrated and *angry,* and their feelings may be vented on the clients and emerge as escalations in punitive measures and humiliating confrontations. They feel *helpless* in the face of the enormity of the problems confronting them in the form of their clients, their own individual problems, and the pressures for better performance from management. As they become increasingly stressed, the measures they take to "treat" the clients tend to backfire and they become *hopeless* about the capacity for either the clients or the organization to change. The escalating levels of uncertainty, danger, and threat that seem to originate on the one hand from the clients, and on the other hand from "the system," create in the staff a chronic level of *hyperarousal* as the environment becomes increasingly crisis oriented. Members of the staff who are most disturbed by the hyperarousal and rising levels of anxiety institute more *control* measures, resulting in an increase in aggression, counter-aggression, dependence on both physical and biological restraints, and punitive measures directed at clients and each other. Key team members, colleagues, and friends leave the setting and take with them important aspects of the *memory* of what worked and what did not work, and team learning becomes impaired. *Communication* breaks down between staff members; interpersonal *conflicts* increase and are not resolved. Team functioning becomes increasingly *fragmented*. As this happens, staff members are likely to feel *overwhelmed, confused,* and *depressed,* while emotional exhaustion, cynicism, and a *loss of personal effectiveness* lead to demoralization and burnout.

Conclusion

And how are these parallel processes manifest in organizational culture? In our experience, chronically stressed organizations manifest many characteristics similar to each other and that can be understood as running in parallel with the clients and with the staff. When this occurs we think of the entire system as "trauma organized"—fundamentally and unconsciously organized around the impact of chronic and toxic stress, even when this undermines the essential mission of the system [9]. In the mental health and social service literature, there is very little recognition of the ways in which these forces are playing themselves out across our horizons. Caught in the grip of monumental assaults upon the systems, few people have had the time or energy to step back and begin to look at the system as a whole through a trauma-informed lens. Organizations are not machines, and they are vulnerable to stress and strain. Many organizations are faced with threats to survival, and they react in the same ways as threatened individuals. In the next chapters we will show how our organizations mirror the very problems we are trying to address in our clients. We begin a more detailed exploration of parallel process in Chapter 5 by describing the loss of basic safety that accompanies chronic organizational stress.

Chapter 5

Lack of Safety: Recurrent Stress and Organizational Hyperarousal

SUMMARY: *The human service system and virtually every component of it, including the mental health system, have been and continue to be under conditions of chronic stress, individually and collectively experiencing repetitive trauma. In many helping organizations, neither the staff nor the administrators feel particularly safe with their clients or even with each other. This lack of safety may present as a lack of physical safety, abusive behavior on the part of managers and/or staff, and a pervasive mistrust of the organization. A perceived lack of safety erodes trust, which is the basis for positive social relationships. As a result these organizations are very tightly wrapped and tensions run high. Under such unrelenting stress, helping professionals and the agencies themselves become more highly reactive and are more ready to see threat rather than opportunity, pathology rather than strength, and risk rather than reward.*

Crisis in Human Service Delivery

A crisis is a sudden or rapidly evolving change that results in an urgent problem or problems that must be addressed immediately, while at the same time what makes the situation a crisis is that we have exceeded our ability to immediately know how to deal with the situation. Crisis represents a condition where a system is required or expected to handle a situation for which existing resources, procedures, policies, structures, or mechanisms are inadequate [379]. It describes a situation that threatens high-priority goals and which suddenly occurs with little response time available [380]. In a crisis, the things that people are used to doing and comfortable doing are not working, and the stage is set for the possibility of either disaster or new learning.

For an organization a crisis is an extreme event that threatens its very existence. Crises exact tremendous emotional costs and are emotionally distressing and arousing. Crises demand that we use our minds in the best way possible, which is a significant problem because severe stress so impedes the use of our higher faculties, as we described in Chapter 3. Crises demand high levels of both social and political skills, as well as whatever technical skills are needed to effectively address the problem. And crises tend to shake up the very ground of our being, both personally and professionally [381–382].

An organizational crisis will be sensed by everyone in the sphere of influence of the organization almost instantaneously, regardless of how strenuously leaders attempt to contain the spread of information. Emotional contagion occurs within one-twentieth of a second, and although employees of an organization may not know what the problem is, they will indeed know that there is a problem [383]. Tension literally fills the air. Within minutes or hours of a particularly disturbing piece of gossip, news, or crisis, everyone in an organization will be in an alarm state with all that goes along with that, including compromised thought processes.

The medical director of a psychiatric program recalls a crisis:

I guess what makes a crisis a crisis is that you are not really prepared to deal with it. When my colleagues and I received the calls about the woman who had killed herself, I felt like the floor dropped out from under me. I had no idea what to do except to get back to the program and meet with my colleagues. I remember just feeling so sick and scared. When we arrived, all the other clients were flipping out and we had to immediately prioritize what to do. I had to listen not just to my head but to my heart as well. Obviously, there were some people more acutely distressed than others, so we attended to them first and then began to rank order what we needed to do and divide up the tasks. I was so glad I didn't have to face this thing alone. It was our shared ability to figure out together what to do that enabled me, and the other members of my team, to decide how to prioritize what needed to be done and decide the best way to meet everyone's immediate needs without making the situation even worse. Because we knew how destabilizing a traumatic event is to our capacity to think, we knew we had to depend on each other as well as everyone in the community if we were to help all of us get through it.

Six Stages of Crisis Management

Norman Augustine, no stranger to crises in his work career, described in an important article for the *Harvard Business Review* the six stages of crisis management: avoiding the crisis, preparing to manage the crisis, recognizing the crisis, containing the crisis, resolving the crisis, and profiting from the crisis.

Avoiding a crisis is, of course, the simplest way to control a potential crisis. But that's not so easy to do when every single person who enters your door for help is in a crisis. We have written this book in the hopes that it will help our readers avoid many of the pitfalls that already exist in the human service delivery system, or if not that, then at least that it helps them prepare for the next crisis. As Augustine reminds us, *"when preparing for a crisis, it is instructive to recall that Noah starting building the ark before it began to rain"* (p. 11) [384].

Recognizing that a crisis is a crisis—and that we name the correct crisis—can be life saving so that we respond before the disaster continues to unfold. We have seen the failure to recognize the correct crisis occur repeatedly in mental health settings usually manifesting as a *collective disturbance,* which we will discuss further in Chapter 8. One of our faculty remembers recalls just such an incident:

> *A patient on our inpatient unit had made a suicide attempt, another had tried to elope, and another had convinced her husband to bring marijuana into the hospital. These were seen solely as individual problems of the patients involved, bearing no relationship to the overall health of the therapeutic environment, so that the result was a series of acting-out behaviors that continued to escalate until we started to ask ourselves whether the problem was the patients or our own unresolved conflicts about some unit policies. But while this was unfolding we all had to endure weeks of a crisis-like environment.*

Containing the crisis and resolving the crisis is much of the focus of this book and requires getting as many people on board as possible to creatively problem solve. To profit from the crisis, we need to have systems in place that allow us to stop blaming each other and instead create environments of social learning where we can learn as much from our mistakes as we can. Brian knows only too well how important it is to prepare for crises because another one is always just around the corner:

> *A key objective here is to keep the organization from constantly spiraling into crisis. While we cannot prevent all crises, we can create systems that minimize them. As far as we can tell, systems that share more and more information and ask all staff to assume responsibility for positive outcomes are better able to avert crisis. The challenge is to anticipate what the organizational triggers are for crisis and get as many people watching for those triggers as possible. I suspect ours are not terribly different from other programs—financial losses in a program, consumer complaints, critical incidents, high staff turnover, and reduced referrals, to name a few. If we can respond to these trends early, we can avoid major catastrophes down the line. Building the systems that help us monitor these trends is a real challenge and often takes us back to the issue of trust. Staff need to have faith that these systems will not be used to hurt them but are, in fact, a protection. Consumer complaints and critical incidents may make the staff involved feel vulnerable, but ignoring them or smoothing them over makes the entire organization vulnerable and ultimately has a negative impact on our ability to deliver on our mission.*

Unfortunately, teams under the pressure of fight-flight respond to acute stress with overwhelming emotions and cognitive impairments. The entire team may engage in behavior that actually interferes with client care or safety and begins to compound an existing problem by not collecting data, not reflecting on the problem, failing to discuss goals, failing to search for alternative solutions, suppressing disagreement, diffusing responsibility, failing to coordinate their actions, and deferring to someone else in a leadership position rather than doing what they need to do. Team leaders often feel compelled to do something to demonstrate a sense of competence and to maintain control, while at the same time, the leaders' focus may have become so narrow that he or she is unable to take into consideration the goals and plans for the entire team [263].

Let's turn now to a few examples of the crises that so greatly impact human service delivery environments. Although loss of leaders, sudden natural deaths of key people in the organization, and tragic accidents all may be the cause of organizational crises, programs have the most difficulty dealing with the violence that unfortunately has become a routine part of many human service delivery environments.

Violence in the Human Service Workplace

The exposure to traumatizing events among human service workers—and therefore the lack of basic safety—is extremely high. Despite this, there is relatively little in the mental health or social service literature about the astonishing risk that many workers in the field are subject to, or the impact of recurrent violence on these organizations. Whether the likelihood of violence is denied or not, in crisis environments the "constant state of arousal" may be a special risk for increasing the likelihood of violence [85]. Living with a chronic sense of fear is one of the most disabling conditions a person can experience. As we mentioned in the previous chapters, stress in the workplace is a widespread problem and is a result of a variety of situations, and being a witness to or victim of violence is one of the most overwhelming situations workers encounter. Since the 1980s, violence has been recognized as a leading cause of occupational mortality and morbidity. On average, 1.7 million workers are injured each year (about half of these injuries occur in health care and social services), and more than 800 die as a result of workplace violence [385]. But these numbers only represent physical violence. Brian recalls his own experience:

> I remember my first job as a child care worker. I was 18 and was assigned to work with an apartment of 16 and 17 year olds. I was afraid from the time I walked into the apartment to the time I left. At times I was physically afraid, but more so I was acutely aware that I was way over my head and was way too young, stupid, and naive to be working there. Almost every interaction confirmed my worst fears.

A significant aspect of job stress is level of risk, and it is the high degree of risk and the fear attendant on that risk that has been a significant contributor to why so many individuals and institutions in the mental health system have been reluctant to change established practices of seclusion, restraint, and forced medication, even though these practices are so frequently associated with negative—sometimes disastrous—outcomes in the patients and for the staff. As Brian has experienced this he notes,

> We believe the escalation in coercive interventions in our organization stems from the fear and the sense that things are out of control. If we ever let down our guard, loosen up, even a little, we get totally run over. It is not possible for staff to help clients feel safe when they have no sense of safety themselves. Beginning to create an organization that feels safe for the staff is crucial for creating safety for clients.

Dangerous Professions

Although workplace homicides attract more attention, the vast majority of workplace violence consists of nonfatal assaults. The Bureau of Labor Statistics data shows that in 2000, 48% of all nonfatal injuries from occupational assaults and violent acts occurred in health care and social services. Most of these occurred in hospitals, nursing and personal care facilities, and residential care services. Nurses, aides, orderlies, and attendants suffered the most nonfatal assaults resulting in injury. In 2000, health service workers overall had an incidence rate of 9.3 per 100,000 full-time workers for injuries resulting from assaults and violent acts. The rate for social service workers was 15, and for nursing and personal care facility workers, 25. This compares to an overall private sector injury rate of 2 [386]. The Occupational Safety and Health Administration in their report wrote:

> For many years, health care and social service workers have faced a significant risk of job-related violence. Assaults represent a serious safety and health hazard within these industries.... The average annual rate for non-fatal violent crime for all occupations is 12.6 per 1,000 workers. The average annual rate for physicians is 16.2; for nurses, 21.9; for mental health professionals, 68.2; and for mental health custodial workers, 69. As significant as these numbers are, the actual number of incidents is probably much higher. Incidents of violence are likely to be underreported, perhaps due in part to the persistent perception within the health care industry that assaults are part of the job. Underreporting may reflect a lack of institutional reporting policies, employee beliefs that reporting will not benefit them or employee fears that employers may deem assaults the result of employee negligence or poor job performance [387].

Emergency rooms can be dangerous places to work, according to a number of studies of workplace violence [388]. A survey of staff in 18 emergency departments in Florida found that 72% of respondents had been physically assaulted during their emergency department career, 42% in the prior year [389]. A recent survey of a random sample of Michigan emergency physicians found that 76% of them have experienced at least one violent act in the previous year, 75% experienced verbal threats, and 28% were victims of physical assault [390]. The majority of violent incidents in the emergency department (as in many other social settings) result not simply from individual psychopathology of the perpetrator, but from the interaction of a number of factors related to the environment, the staff member, the perpetrator, and the interaction between them [391].

After law enforcement, persons employed in the mental health sector have the highest rates of all occupations of being victimized while at work or on duty. In fact, between 1993 and 1999 the rates of workplace violence for all occupational categories fell, and all the declines were statistically significant *except* for mental health. Even law enforcement victimization showed a greater decline (55%) than the decline in mental health (28%). In 1999, for every 1000 people employed in law enforcement, 74 were injured, while for every 1000 people employed in mental health, 46 were injured. The next highest rate is retail sales in which the rate was 14 per 1000 people hired, and for teaching the rate was 12 per 1000. Professional (social worker/psychiatrist) and custodial care providers in the mental health care field were victimized while working or on duty at similar rates (68 and 69 per 1000, respectively)—but at rates *more than 3 times* those in the medical field. Workers in the mental health field and teachers were the only occupations more likely to be victimized by someone they knew than by a stranger [392].

The prevalence of aggression is so alarming on psychiatric units treating adults, adolescents, and children that salaries should–but definitely do not–reflect incremental increases dependent on being in high-risk professions. A recent study of staff working in 15 child, adolescent, and adult mental health programs spread out across the United States showed that aggression and violence are highly prevalent in psychiatric treatment settings: of all respondents, 83% reported being verbally threatened, 65% reported physical assault, and 39% reported injury in a work site during the prior 6 months [393]. In mental health facilities, patient aggression and violence are increasingly recognized as major clinical treatment problems. Violence in these facilities is a safety risk for both staff and patients. The occurrence of violence in mental health settings is costly, both in terms of lawsuits and worker's compensation benefits and staff turnover and also in terms of less easily calculable but no less important costs such as low morale, treatment impedance, and the creation of a negative therapeutic environment [394]. The increase in violence has led to practices that are themselves violent and therefore lead to escalation of violence in a setting, not de-escalation. A variety of terms have been used to apply to the impact on professionals of working with people who have experienced traumatic events: vicarious trauma, secondary traumatic stress, burnout, but relatively little has been discussed about the impact of chronic fear and trauma on workgroups or organizations of helping professionals. Brian observes the following:

> *Many of the trainings I have attended on behavioral support talk a lot about anger and managing anger. There is, however very little talk about fear. I believe many of our staff spend a good deal of their work lives afraid—afraid they will get hurt by a client, afraid they will hurt a client, afraid they will make a terrible mistake, afraid they will look stupid. This fear can at times be overwhelming. We believe the escalation in coercive interventions in our organization stems from the fear and the sense that things are out of control. Staff who feel unsafe cannot easily help clients feel safe.*

Workplace Aggression and Bullying

Workplace aggression has been defined as *"any behavior directed by one or more persons in a workplace toward the goal of harming one or more others in that workplace (or the entire organization) in ways that intended targets are motivated to avoid"* (p. 64) [395]. Investigators have recognized that there are many ways that employees can express aggression. The most obvious—and the most feared—is active, violent aggression against clients, coworkers, and managers. In human service organizations, the threat of physical violence is more likely to come from clients than colleagues.

For the most part, policies and procedures are in place in most workplaces to address the issue of physical violence, and much has been written about safety policies in the workplace. In mental health and social service settings, steps are being taken to protect clients from injury at the hands of staff. The recent national emphasis on reducing seclusion and restraint is instrumental in reducing staff-client injury, and unfortunately the impetus for this change has largely come from deaths of patients that have occurred in restraints. But not enough is being done to protect the workers themselves from violence.

Even more employees are stressed by chronic nonphysical aggression, such as verbal aggression and threats that may come from clients or coworkers. And many workers in social services are bullied—by coworkers, supervisors, government regulators and officials, the media, family members, and sometimes clients themselves. Bullying and all forms of violence are well established as having many negative consequences for health and well-being at an individual level, and at a group level bullying behavior creates an organizational culture that supports and encourages violence in a variety of forms [396–397].

Based on several large-scale studies of bullying and harassment, workplace aggression is a significant problem. In research on work harassment, one study indicated that as many as 30% of men and 55% of women had been exposed to some form of work harassment in the previous year. In addition, 32% said they had witnessed others being harassed in their workplace (being subjected to degrading and oppressive activities [398]. In a Michigan statewide labor survey, 27% of respondents reported mistreatment at work during the prior year and 42% indicated mistreatment had occurred at some point during their working career. In a sample of a number of VA facilities in the United States, 36% indicated that they had experienced one or more instances of aggression on a weekly or daily basis over the preceding year, and 58% reported that they had experienced at least one act of aggression in the previous year [395]. In studies of workplace bullying, which we will discuss at greater length in Chapter 9, based on data from 14 Norwegian studies, researchers found that as many as 8.6% of respondents had been bullied at work during the previous 6 months [399]. Later studies put that figure in Europe to be between 1% and 4% of serious bullying (weekly or daily), and between 8% and 10% of workers report occasional bullying episodes [400]. In a comprehensive series of workplace bullying studies in the United Kingdom, 10.5% of respondents from a cross section of business sectors had some experience with bullying [401].

Every episode of violence has a history. Violent physical or sexual assault that occurs in a workplace always emerges within a context and can usually be traced to various forms of less appreciated forms of violence that may occur routinely within an organization. But even if that is not the outcome, many kinds of abusive behaviors can have devastating effects on individuals and the organization as a whole. Investigators believe there are organizational reasons that explain why mental health, health care, and social service environments remain so dangerous: inadequate employee acquisition, supervision, and retention practices; inadequate training on violence prevention at all levels; lack of clearly defined rules of conduct; failure to introduce employees to antiviolence policies and prevention strategies; inability of managers and supervisors to adequately assess threats; a nonexistent or weak mechanism for reporting violent or threatening behavior; failure to take immediate action against those who have threatened or committed acts of violence (p. 120) [402].

There is a profound organizational silence about the system-wide impact of traumatic and tragic events in human service. We must assume that, if anything, the impact on workers in children's programs is generally even more devastating than in adult programs, consistent with experience in the traumatic stress field indicating that adults dealing with traumatized children are even more vulnerable to severe distress than those working with traumatized adults. Most of the available literature, however, is about adult inpatient suicide and the impact of providing services by child welfare workers so let's briefly review some findings.

Adult Psychiatric Inpatient Suicide

Suicides occur on inpatient psychiatric units at a rate of 5–30 times that of the general population. This amounts to as many as 370 suicides per 100,000 patients. This is in comparison to an overall suicide rate of 10–12 per 100,000 in the general population [403–404]. The Joint Commission on Accreditation of Healthcare Organizations (JCAHO) requests that organizations report inpatient suicides as sentinel events—"an unexpected occurrence involving death or serious physical or psychological injury or risk thereof." Inpatient suicides may occur without warning. Most inpatients who commit suicide are not on special precautions, and about half were last judged by the responsible psychiatrist as clinically improved [403].

Patient suicide is a frightening possibility in the professional life of every psychiatrist. Surveys suggest that as many as one-half of all psychiatrists lose a patient to suicide. A study of psychiatrists in Scotland showed an even higher figure in that 68% of psychiatrists had had a patient commit suicide under their care [405]. About one-third of the suicides that occurred while the client was under his or her care happened while the psychiatrist was still a resident in training [406–407]. Residents may be especially at risk during the first 2 years of training, which typically place residents on inpatient and emergency services, where they are most likely to be confronted with severely disturbed, suicidal patients. It is during these early rotations that they are least prepared, in knowledge, skills, and experience, to deal with such patients or the emotional impact of a death by suicide [408].

The effects of a patient's suicide can last a lifetime. Following interviews with psychiatrists, Brown reported that client suicide had a major effect on their development and *"the details and names remained vivid even after 20 or 30 years"* (p. 107) [409]. Almost 700 mental health social workers were surveyed—all members of the National Association of Social Workers (NASW)—and over half reported that they had experienced either an incident of fatal or of nonfatal client suicidal behavior. Thirty-three percent had experienced a fatal outcome [410]. Not surprisingly, surveys have established that mental health practitioners in general view suicide as their leading source of work-related stress, leading some to view it as an "occupational hazard" [408].

Although psychiatry perceives itself as—and sometimes is perceived by others as—a branch of medicine, there is a certain explicit expectation that once someone is delivered to a psychiatric setting, he or she is no longer in any real danger. This of course denies the reality that there is considerable morbidity and mortality associated with this branch of medicine just like any other branch, but the way that occurs is usually through the individual's own hand.

But unlike many other medical or surgical programs, for people working in psychiatric settings, death is a relatively rare occurrence, even while the threat of death is constantly present in virtually every inpatient case, or they wouldn't get admitted to the hospital in the first place. This can create an illusion on the part of the hospital staff, the clients, the families of the clients, and the general public that all suicide can be prevented and that if a hospital staff has failed to prevent death, then they are morally and legally responsible for the person's death [403].

This is, however, a dangerous and unjust social delusion. In truth, the only way we can keep a person from harming himself or herself—or others—is by using increasing levels of coercion and force, resulting in the nightmare incarcerations within abusive institutions of earlier centuries. If you chain someone to the wall or dose someone with drugs that paralyze their muscles, you can indeed entirely prevent that person from self-harm. Otherwise, people who are mobile can always find some way to exert their will and without force or coercion, we cannot stop them.

The reactions of caregivers to a patient's suicide are in many cases severe and long lasting, as has been showed by a number of studies. Mental health practitioners who are closely involved in the care of a patient who successfully commits suicide are likely to have feelings and reactions not unlike the patient's family members. They are likely to experience shock, guilt, and grief accompanied by a profound sense of self-doubt and loss of confidence. Some will develop symptoms of posttraumatic stress disorder and/or depression that may last a long time. Many will question whether they should keep doing the work they are doing. They are likely to fear administrative censure and litigation. Many times, in an effort to distance themselves from the distressing feelings, colleagues will pull away and not offer the support that is so necessary after a traumatic event [405] [411]. The recognition of the terrible toll exposure to sudden death can take is especially critical for people who are still in training when such a loss occurs.

Following patient suicide, human service workers often have to help other patients who have been traumatized, while at the same time privately coping with their own reactions. Their coping may be delayed because they have had little opportunity to process the incident. After the event, staff members also may be reluctant to discuss a suicide with their own personal support network for fear of violating patient confidentiality or because of a perception that personal reactions should be avoided or minimized—an attitude that may be more common in professions such as medicine and nursing. Many clinicians describe these experiences as the most profoundly disturbing events of their professional careers. Innumerable therapists remain haunted by the deaths, experiencing troubling emotions of grief, anger, guilt. and fear of blame in gripping dreams and fantasies. When asked about the impact of the suicides on their practice, many clinicians report a continuing apprehension about it happening again and several admit to being reluctant to accept suicidal patients into their practice. The intensity of the therapist's emotional response was independent of the therapist's age, years of experience, or practice setting [407].

Working With Traumatized Children: Child Protection Workers

Kendra has been a child protective investigator for the state for the past 3 years. During that time she has interviewed children who have been hit, burned, neglected, and sexually abused by their caretakers. She has written and read reports that include overwhelming details about these experiences, as well as taken and viewed photographs that document the maltreatment. Her caseload has continued to grow, and as she becomes more experienced, new workers talk to her about their cases because they value her opinion and advice. Although she does not mind helping her coworkers, it has become difficult to do so lately because she has been extremely tired. For the past 2 months, Kendra has been waking up at 3:00 each morning unable to breath (p. 39) [412]

Child protection workers are exposed to so much danger that it has been suggested that these workers should be trained in self-defense, should buddy up when they have to go into dangerous situations, and should always have cell phones with them to call for backup. The authors of a study of child protective services (CPS) workers recommended the creation of a supportive work environment where "*supervisors are trained to recognize and acknowledge the effects of being exposed to trauma on a daily basis. Allowing workers a safe place to release emotions and talk about the specific trauma, their fears, and regrets could help minimize the symptoms they experience. Having peer support groups in place, in which workers can engage in group discussion, exchange information, and provide support, can also help in minimizing the likelihood of severe secondary traumatic stress symptoms*" (p. 52). The authors also recommend limiting work hours, since there was such a clear association between level of distress and hours spent per week working [412].

Of course, this fails to take into account the reality that because of relatively low wages, the workers may be working these hours to take home enough money to survive. According to the National Association of Social Workers, the average annual salary for public child protection agency workers is $33,000, while the average annual salary for private agency staff is $27,000. This is a serious problem since according to the University of Washington analysis of salaries that a family needs just to survive, termed the Self-Sufficiency Standard. For Philadelphia, as an example, a family of four with two adults, one preschooler and one school-age child have to take in $60,000, up $7000 just in the last two years. A family of four is considered poor if it makes $22,050 a year - the federal poverty level [413]. In a study of more than 200 mostly female, college-educated CPS workers in a large southern state, Meyers and Cornille found that on the Brief Symptom Inventory, the workers were more symptomatic than the general population but less symptomatic than a population of people receiving services in outpatient psychotherapy. Those who had been employed for a longer period of time in the CPS field, and thus exposed to longer durations of traumatic material, suffered more severe secondary traumatic stress symptoms than those with fewer years. Those who worked more than 40 hours per week were more angry, irritable, jumpy, and hypervigilant, and they suffered a more exaggerated startle response and had more trouble concentrating, more nightmares, and more intrusive thoughts than those who worked fewer hours. Most of them (82%) reported that they had a prior experience of trauma before they entered the field, and 77% reported having been assaulted or threatened while on the job [412]. In their Child Welfare Trauma Training Toolkit, the National Child Traumatic Stress Network assert that:

> Child welfare is a high-risk profession and child welfare workers are confronted every day—both directly and indirectly—with danger and trauma. Threats may come in from violent or angry family members. On top of this, hearing about the victimization and abuse of children can be very disturbing for the empathic child welfare worker and can result in feelings of helplessness, anger, and hopelessness. Those who are parents themselves or who have their own histories of childhood trauma might be at particular risk for the negative effects of secondary traumatic stress. Some professionals struggle with maintaining appropriate boundaries and with a sense of overwhelming personal responsibility. These challenges can be intensified in resource-strapped agencies, where there is little professional or personal support available. It is critical to address professional or personal stress because, if left unaddressed, it can result in burnout and undermine work performance, to the detriment of the children and families served. Signs of burnout might include avoidance of certain clients, missed appointments, tardiness, and lack of motivation [414].

Chronic Crisis Equals Chronic Hyperarousal

These are just two examples of the many kinds of situations that any experienced health or human service worker can expect to be exposed to at some point in his or her career. When the worker fails to recover from a traumatic incident, or when those incidents are compounded, then he or she may become chronically hyperaroused with all the attendant problems we discussed in Chapter 3.

In similar ways, significant problems arise in organizations when the crisis state is prolonged or repetitive, problems not dissimilar to those we witness in individuals under chronic stress. Organizations can become chronically hyperaroused. Organizational hyperarousal may manifest itself in different ways.

The organization may function in crisis mode all the time, unable to process one difficult experience before another crisis has emerged, misinterpreting routine problems as crises when they are not. Alternately, there may be a head-in-the-sand kind of approach, where organizational leaders deny that a crisis is building right in front of them. The chronic nature of a stressed atmosphere tends to produce a generalized increased level of tension, irritability, short tempers, and even abusive behavior. Workers may develop significant mistrust in their managers and managers may fail to understand the chronic hyperarousal of their employees. The urgency to act in order to relieve this tension is likely to impair decision making because we are unable to weigh and balance multiple options, arrive at compromises, and consider long-term consequences of our actions under stress.

One of our faculty consultants told us this story as an example of chronic hyperarousal in a medical hospital:

Hospital beds around the country have been so decreased that many hospitals are under significant community pressure to admit anyone who requires hospitalization, even if they must exceed their normal bed capacity. One hospital began using a crisis code—an amber alert—indicating that the hospital has exceeded its capacity, are now taking on more than they can manage, and that the "no divert" system is in effect. When this occurs, everyone's computer screen flashes orange and announcements are made, causing a repetitive sense of crisis, even though there is nothing anyone can do about it. Nonetheless, everyone's stress response is activated and reinforced, doing continuing damage to physiological and psychological systems. In reality, when the "amber alert" goes off, the staff are already managing the overload, the patients are fine, and order is present even when they have to add extra beds to the rooms or the hallways.

Organizations respond to crisis in observable ways. When a crisis hits, most managers want to do the right thing. But one of the things that makes a crisis a crisis is that no one really knows what to do for certain, yet everyone expects the people in charge to know what to do. Different leaders will respond in different ways, but this is often the time when a charismatic leader exerts the most influence either by creating a different frame of meaning for followers, by linking followers' needs to important values and purposes, through articulation of vision and goals, or by taking actions to deal with the crisis and then moving to new interpretive schemes or theories of action to justify the actions [379].

At such a time, every person throughout the system is under stress, so everyone's ability to think complexly will be relatively compromised. Stress increases a person's vigilance toward gathering information, but it can also overly simplify and perceptively distort what we see or hear. Negative cues are usually magnified and positive cues are diminished or ignored altogether. Furthermore, the stress of an event is determined by the amount and degrees of change involved, not whether this change is good or bad [415]. Under these conditions, command and control hierarchies usually become reinforced and serve to contain some of the collective anxiety generated by the crisis. Command hierarchies can respond more rapidly and mobilize action to defend against further damage. As we discussed in Chapter 3, in times of danger, powerful group forces are marshaled and attachment to the group radically increases. Everyone in the organization is vulnerable to the risks the organization faces as a whole; everyone feels vulnerable [416].

Decision making in such organizations tends to deteriorate with increased numbers of poor and impulsive decisions, compromised problem-solving mechanisms, and overly rigid and dichotomous thinking and behavior. Being in a state of chronic crisis may make it more difficult to discern what is and is not a true crisis. If everything is an emergency, then eventually the emergency response wears out, people become numb, develop avoidant responses, and are no longer able to respond and properly mobilize resources when a true emergency occurs. Whenever we have described this sequence, people in social service settings *immediately* recognize this and inevitably launch into a description of how they have seen this exact thing happen in their organization. One example came from a director of a large social service agency in an urban area:

I have a great example of organizational hyperarousal in a traumatized organization. I was in charge of a large social service agency which had come under serious scrutiny after incidents occurred that resulted in some deaths. As the director, I had replaced the previous director and deputies after they were cast out of their positions due to condemnatory newspaper reports. I knew I was entering a traumatized organization but what that meant did not really hit me until a specific incident occurred. One day, a package arrived at one of the offices. It is not uncommon for people to be threatened in the positions that they hold in our organization, and the package was thought to be suspicious since no one knew who it came from and the recipient was not expecting anything. So a call was put into the police to come check it out. The bomb squad vehicle showed up and parked in the front of the building, although there were no sirens, no one running around looking alarmed. Within a few minutes, I was alerted and went upstairs to check out the situation. When I arrived, the police assured me that they would handle things and there didn't really appear to be anything to worry about so I returned to my office, relieved and ready to get back to work. But before I did, I happened to look out the window. Several hundred workers were already gathered out the doors of our building and across the street. Now, in our building there are other organizations and agencies, not just ours. When I investigated, this is what I found out. In less than 10 minutes, workers in our organization had taken it upon themselves to go floor to floor to alert people that there was a bomb in the building, that management couldn't be counted on to inform them, and that they had better clear out, and so they were doing so.

At first I was furious, and then I realized that this was a sign of how chronically frightened my people were in contrast to the agencies in the same building who were still working at their desks, assuming correctly that the problem was being handled.

But when crisis unrelentingly piles upon crisis—frequently because leaders leave, burn out, are fired, or fail—an organizational adjustment to chronic crisis occurs. As we have discussed, chronic fear states in the individual often have a decidedly negative impact on the quality of cognitive processes, decision-making abilities, and emotional management capacities of the person. Impaired thought processes tend to escalate rather than reduce existing problems so that crisis compounds crisis without the individual recognizing the patterns of repetition that are now determining his or her work and life decisions. The same thing occurs in organizations exposed to chronic stress, a situation that seriously and negatively impacts organizational performance.

Loss of Social Immunity

When we shift our focus away from individual outbursts of violence and instead look at all episodes of any kind of violence as a breach of our social defenses that occurs in a context that is likely to involve everyone in the group, then we begin thinking in a different way about the entire issue. A useful way to think about this interaction between individual and group is through the metaphor of our own immune system, building on what we discussed earlier as the "germ theory of trauma." The idea is that we are each surrounded by potentially harmful bacteria and viruses all the time, and yet we usually stay well. What keeps our immune system healthy?

As long as you are healthy, your immune system is steadily working to keep infectious agents away from your vital organs and as a result, you don't get sick. But if you are overtired, stressed, or depleted, or if the infectious agent is overwhelmingly powerful, then your defenses are breached and you get sick. Once our immune system is vulnerable, all kinds of things can snowball.

We can think of the social body in a similar way. Every group has an invisible protective envelope—what we call its "social immunity"—that keeps its members safe from harm. As complex adaptive systems, groups of whatever size are constantly interacting and exchanging with the individuals that comprise the group. But chronic hyperarousal is damaging to the health of individuals and to the groups of which they are a part. When we are in a poor state of social health, when there are unconscious interpersonal conflicts, when there are secrets being held, when there is a great deal of stress, the usual defenses of the social body are breached and that is when violence is most likely to emerge. Individuals within a group are not safe if they cannot get their basic needs met, if their trust is betrayed, if they are individually blamed for systemic issues, if their normal need to discuss and work through traumatic events is suppressed, if they are unaware of the role they are playing in reenacting traumatic events with others, if they are put in morally compromising positions. All of these factors negatively impact the safety that individuals rely on within a group and therefore erode social immunity that is maintained by a healthy group until no one is safe in the environment.

Thwarting Basic Needs

It is clear from a large research base that employees need to have their basic psychological needs met in order to feel satisfied and safe at work. These include autonomy, which involves having choice, voice, and initiative; competence, being seen as effective and challenged; and relatedness, being connected to others and belonging to the group. When these conditions are met, workers are likely to have greater self-motivation and better adjustment [417]. These necessary elements for job satisfaction run in parallel to the necessary elements for therapeutic change as well [3]. Any work environment that thwarts satisfaction of any of these needs undermines self-motivation, performance, and wellness for staff [418].

Triggering Mistrust

In surveys, a quarter of Americans say that they trust no one at all with their intimate secrets. The proportion of people with no close friends or family members tripled between 1985 and 2004. The result is a notable reduction in social trust. In 1960, 58% of American endorsed the idea that "most people can be trusted"—but by 1998—and continuing through 2008, this number was down to 33% [238]. These trends do not bode well for workplace environments.

It has been clear to organizational development investigators that trust in the workplace is key to productivity and ultimately to the life span of the organization [6]. The fundamental problem with creating atmospheres of threat and mistrust is that such environments directly counter what is needed for effective problem solving. The more complex the work demands, the greater the necessity for collaboration and integration and therefore the more likely that a system of teamwork must evolve to address complexity. In fact, in the business world, "Fortune's 100 Best Companies to Work For" are more likely to have cultures in which trust flourishes, and have half the turnover rate (12.6% vs. 26%) and nearly twice the applications for employment of companies not on the list [419].

Threat does not just arrive in the form of physical intimidation but can come from a number of sources and in a variety of forms. Fear can be conveyed through the actual experience of people in an organization—what has happened directly to a person or what the person has directly observed in the present or the past. Then there are the stories about other people's experiences that rapidly circulate within any organization; these are especially likely to be taken seriously if the person conveying the experience is liked or trusted and when the trustworthiness of the organization is already in question. Threat may also be conveyed via the negative assumptions about other people's behavior and intentions about what has happened that reside within the company and fuel many self-fulfilling prophecies. And then all change is potentially threatening, but externally imposed change is the most threatening, and it has been largely externally imposed change that has characterized the human service delivery system [109].

The list of behaviors that can trigger mistrust in staff is a long one and includes both verbal and nonverbal behavior and is similar to the list of behaviors that also trigger violence. Silence, glaring eye contact, abruptness, snubbing, insults, public humiliation, blaming, discrediting, aggressive and controlling behavior, sexually harassing behavior or suggestions, overtly threatening behavior, public humiliation, angry outbursts, secretive decision making, indirect communication, lack of responsiveness to input, mixed messages, aloofness, and unethical conduct all can be experienced as abusive managerial or supervisory behavior [109]. Dirty looks, defacing property, stealing, hiding needed resources, interrupting others, obscene gestures, cursing, yelling, threats, sarcasm, the silent treatment, "damning with faint praise," arbitrary and capricious decisions, ignoring input, unfair performance evaluations, showing up late for meetings, causing others to delay actions, spreading rumors, backstabbing, belittling, failing to transmit information, failing to deny false rumors, failing to warn of potential danger—all of these actions on the part of management, staff, and clients are forms of aggression which can terminate in the emergence of violence [420]. Some of these behaviors may be subtle but are still violent. They tend to undermine autonomy, competence, and relatedness in interactive and complex ways.

According to Bill Wilkerson, CEO of Global Business and Economic Roundtable on Addiction and Mental Health, mistrust, unfairness, and vicious office politics are among the top 10 workplace stressors [151]. Brian knows what this relationship between trust and power in leadership positions is like:

It is difficult for people in leadership positions to acknowledge just how powerful they are in the lives of people they supervise. We like to think of ourselves as "just folks" or "one of the guys" but we are not. Staff people are very plugged in to what we do and how we behave. Losing your temper, rolling your eyes, sighing, interrupting, talking over people are all picked up by staff and help to shape or damage the atmosphere of trust. Many of us have grown up to believe that the boss does not have to account to others and does not have to play by the rules. The opposite is actually the truth. The more power you have in an organization, the better behaved you must be. The statement "with great power comes great responsibility" is very true and leadership bears enormous responsibility for shaping and reshaping the organizational culture. An organization cannot possibly be a safe place if leaders misuse and abuse their power and authority or permit others to do so.

The Betrayal of Trust

Betrayal of trust is the common denominator for people who have been exposed to abuse and neglect as children [282]. Betrayal of trust in the workplace is disturbingly similar because we tend to replicate our childhood relationship expectations unconsciously, particularly in very hierarchically driven systems where management are "parents" and staff are the "children" in the organizational family. (As Brian points out, in our sector this unfortunate metaphor seems to leave the clients as pets.)

Organizational development theorists have made some observations about betrayal that are worth considering, since trust is such a key aspect of creating environments to serve people who have fundamental issues with trust. The first is that the lower a person's satisfaction is with where he or she works, the higher is the person's motivation to betray trust. The lower the penalty is for betraying trust, the more likely under those circumstances that the person will betray trust. Similarly, the more the person expects to benefit from the betrayal, the more likely it is that the dissatisfied person will betray a trust. People find it easier to rationalize their betrayal when there is inequity in the relationship, when the relationship is not a long-standing one. When people don't feel like "all their eggs are in one basket," when they are not totally dependent on the good feelings of the other person, the more likely betrayal is. The lower the perceived seriousness of the violation, the more likely it is to happen, so an employee who wouldn't considered taking money from petty cash may not think twice about taking some extra supplies from the office [421].

Organizational consultant Ian Mitroff has intensively studied a wide range of organizations who have experienced major crises and traumatic events, and he notes that crises are virtually always experienced as major acts of betrayal because we need someone to blame for how we feel. He defines betrayal as *"the failure of a person, an organization, an institution, or a society to act and to behave in accordance with ways that they have promised or they have led us to believe that they will. Betrayal is the violation of the trust that we have placed in another person, organization, institution, and/or society. Thus, betrayal is profoundly rooted in our basic feelings of trust and goodness with regard to others"* (p. 40) [382].

Brian describes how he and his organization experienced one major betrayal:

Some time back we were confronted with several anonymous allegations of wrongdoing. Because these allegations were anonymous, we were not sure where they were coming from or who was responsible. We knew they were false, but we were at a loss for how to defend ourselves and the organization. For many weeks we held the information to ourselves and did not share it with our staff. Frankly, we did not know who we could trust. We became completely absorbed by the situation. As leaders we became more isolated, withdrawn, and disengaged from the day-to-day events. Important details were ignored and little if any joy was derived from the work. It was an awful time. We finally decided we needed to share this information honestly and directly with the staff, and we conducted a series of staff meetings in which we reviewed what had been alleged. We described our take on the situation and the steps we had taken to investigate what had been alleged. Although we held three meetings with some trepidation, we walked away from them feeling liberated. We had taken a risk, we had decided to trust our staff and take a gamble that they fundamentally trusted us. We received feedback and positive support. We did not only feel relieved we also felt rejuvenated.

The more troubled, difficult, and dysfunctional the organizational culture, the more likely it is that betrayal incidents will occur. Trust in an organization is often far more fragile than people like to believe, and the larger the organization the more likely this is to be the case. Some of the breakdowns in trust that can easily occur and provoke retaliatory mistrust include inconsistent messages, inconsistent standards, misplaced benevolence (tolerating misbehavior rather than dealing with it, false feedback), inaccurate performance reviews, the undiscussables or "elephants" that are in the organizational room (see Chapter 8) [422].

Workplaces that are experienced as fundamentally unsafe—physically and emotionally dangerous, untrustworthy environments—are experienced collectively as dangerous as well. When a large number of people collectively experience fear, difficult-to-resolve and even dangerous strategic dilemmas arise that contain within them the potential for violence [423]. The tendency of a staff to escalate coercive control measures in institutional settings is likely to occur whenever they fear for their own safety or the safety of their colleagues, and when they do not trust the organizational structures and norms to contain potential or real violence. Brian discusses the ways in which his leadership aroused mistrust and a sense of betrayal during a key period of change:

Several years ago we had a leadership change in our education program. The education director, who had led the program for over 20 years, was retiring and it was clear there would be a lot of changes. Although we shared many common values and beliefs and genuinely liked each other, we often disagreed in issues around staff management and supervision. When he decided to retire, I felt I could remake the program the way I wanted it to be. I constructed a brilliant plan in the privacy of my office and then rolled it out to the school staff, a staff still reeling from the loss of a longtime leader. Although I consider myself relatively smart, it was one of the dumbest things I have ever done. My grand plan reinforced the staff's worst fears, that we would totally up-end the program. It also reinforced a sense that the staff needed to be protected from senior administration. While it was quite clear things needed to change in the program, my strategy for change was a complete and utter failure. While this change would not have been easy in any circumstances, my ill-conceived plan knocked us way off course and it took us almost 3 years to recover. My failure to engage staff in the process and my fundamental misunderstanding of what they needed from me cut at their trust in me and ultimately their trust in the organization.

So how did a relatively smart guy make such a huge mistake? This all happened at a point in my life when I was under a considerable amount of stress myself. I was still relatively new to the COO position and was struggling to find my way in our newly acquired mental health clinics. I was on a very steep learning curve in the clinics and frankly was getting knocked around pretty badly. I knew I understood the campus programs, and I knew what needed to happen to make them successful. What was missing, however, was the time and patience to work with the staff to find a new way to operate. Simply announcing we would just go a different direction was a major miscalculation and a colossal error in judgment.

Feelings of betrayal are particularly likely to emerge as a result of a crisis because in a crisis people tend to regress to a more primitive state. This should come as no surprise since as we have discussed in Chapter 3, our fight-flight response is based on our primitive psychobiology. In a crisis, we turn to leaders for safety, as we once turned to our parents, and when they let us down—often by turning out to be no more able to know what to do in a crisis than we are—some very basic assumptions may be challenged or shattered about our ability to be safe, stable, and secure in the organization [382].

The Blame Culture

After a traumatic incident in a social service environment what has been shown to be particularly damaging is the blaming, condemning attitude of officials who came to "investigate" the deaths or injuries with meetings that felt more like tribunals or inquests. This is even more overwhelming when trainees are involved and feel blamed. Because of our primitive responses in times of crisis, the world splits into "friend" and "enemy" and someone must be demonized. An example of this is the suicide review conference that has been found to be especially unhelpful, and even harmful, if performed immediately following the suicide [23]. Brian speaks about the destructive aspects of this "blame game" that are so common in social service environments:

The feelings of fear, anger, worry, and frustration can become daunting. It is common for us to lash out at each other because of the way we feel. "You keep making the same mistake." "You don't raise enough money." "You never hit your billable targets." "You keep changing the systems and the processes—no one can keep up." Over time, the objective becomes more "who can we blame" rather than "how do we fix things." If it is all about blame and shame, then the less powerful people become far more vulnerable and far more scared. They circle the wagons further, and good information and a true understanding of the problem becomes harder and harder to tease out. We spend the better part of our day tearing each other apart rather than figuring out how we can help and support each other. The organization becomes a terrible place to work, and this cannot ever be seen as a good thing for kids or families. Who wants to work in this kind of environment?

In the early stages of the aftermath those most affected by the loss are in a vulnerable state in which normal coping mechanisms are flooded and they may say and do things that are more a reflection of shock and guilt than actual culpability. A formal incident review after a tragic occurrence should be performed after there has been time for a reestablishment of equilibrium, with the resolution of initial phases of shock and recoil. This will vary depending on the staff dynamics and may require a period of at least several weeks [403]. But this is not usually what happens. As the society has become increasingly litigious, the culture has become increasingly a "blame culture" with blaming and scapegoating substituting for complex problem analysis, especially in health and social services. This is especially distressing for health, mental health, and social service teams who come into the profession because they want to assist people and find themselves being blamed for harming them [424]. This is a particularly pernicious reaction when we realize how easy it is for any of us to make errors of omission or commission when under the influence of a crisis event, more often because of our biological vulnerability than because of malice.

The Silencing Response

If you work in a health, mental health or social service setting, you are likely to experience an event you will define as traumatic at some point in your work life. For some, the personal experience of exposure to violence, injury, and sudden death are events that are unfortunately common. Sometimes you may be the person injured; other times you may be responsible for someone who is injured, a witness to the event, a colleague of the person(s) most affected, a supervisor, or administrator in charge. When a violent, traumatic event occurs in an organizational setting like a clinic, hospital, day treatment program, or residential facility, every member of the organization is affected by the events because of our fundamental group nature, our vulnerability to emotional contagion and to dynamic group effects. Trauma is collective. If the event is sufficiently tragic or scandalous, it is likely to be covered by the newspapers but far less likely to be thoroughly addressed at an organizational level because of what has become known as "organizational silence" or the "silencing response" [425–427].

This tendency to unconsciously deny or actively suppress knowledge about a disturbing event and thereby hopefully decrease the disturbing emotions that go along with that knowledge has been described in terms of both the ways in which therapists may silence their clients and disturbing information is suppressed in organizations [425]. Here we are applying it to traumatic events that occur in the workplace that are often silenced as well. After a traumatic event, when people need to debrief, give and get mutual support, and instead have experiences that exacerbate the shame, blame, and guilt already being felt, there is often a mandated silence, insisted upon by administrators, legal advisors, and regulatory agencies. Lawyers often come in and tell you not to speak about an event to anyone; they never come back to announce that "now" you can talk about it. Even long after the event, and long after any legal action could be affected by talking about the event, the silence often remains as a "skeleton in the organization closet" that continues to profoundly haunt the organization even while the actual memories of the details of events have faded.

The results of such silencing and incomplete processing can be extremely detrimental to program function. In one study, staff believed that incidents that had occurred had created a "split" among staff and a general increase in anxiety and tension among team members. Staff splitting was perceived as occurring in two specific spheres. The first area of splitting was related to staff members blaming each other or criticizing how their colleagues had managed the incidents. Participants mentioned they felt scapegoated, ostracized by their peers, excluded from invitations to join others on breaks, or that they were given the "silent treatment." This resulted in a "divided camp" atmosphere, with staff feeling they had to defend one peer over another. No formal investigations related to the actions of the hospital staff found fault; nonetheless, the fear of legal action and criticism of each other was intense. Another area of splitting was related to different opinions as to what should occur after the event. Some staff members wanted to forget it all as quickly as possible and move on, while others felt a need to revisit the events and talk about them. A number of the staff expressed changes in their practice, including an increased vigilance, decreased trust in their patients, and increased rigidity about policy with less room for clinical judgment and significant changes in routines, even though none of these areas were found to be a cause of the patient suicide. The overall tone of the environment became one of fear, anger, and blame [428]. One of our Sanctuary Institute faculty members shared this experience with us:

We were talking to a group of staff members of a psychiatric unit. One woman was notably withdrawn and silent, contributing nothing to the group discussion, sitting herself behind and away from the other members of the group. We had already learned that the program had experienced a suicide on the unit

2 years before, and the date of this meeting had happened to fall on the 2-year anniversary of the death. If the date had been arranged deliberately, it was an unconscious move on the part of the administrative assistant who had arranged that date with us and who was surprised later to learn of the coincidence. Years before, at the time of the patient's death, on the advice of hospital attorneys, little was said about the suicide to anyone but the immediate staff who had been involved and the entire issue was kept closely under wraps, largely because of legal concerns. But despite the fact that these concerns were ultimately unfounded, the staff had never been debriefed about the death, and it was immediately clear that it was a living memory for the staff members present in the room with us—and a puzzle for those who were hired after the incident. We each shared our own experience with a suicide on a psychiatric unit—always an extremely traumatic occurrence—and when we had finished, for the first time the withdrawn staff member tearfully spoke up, "I now know more about your patient and the circumstances surrounding it than I know about the person who died here, even though I was here that night." We were later told that this was the first time the staff member had revealed any emotion about the incident and the first time she had been willing to emotionally engage with her colleagues at all since the suicide.

Moral Distress

The term "moral distress" has been attributed to Andrew Jameton, who wrote about ethical dilemmas in nursing care. He wanted to distinguish between moral dilemmas—situations of not knowing what the right thing is to do—from what is experienced when people believe they do know what the right thing is but are constrained from doing it. He described moral distress as *"the pain or anguish affecting the mind, body or relationships in response to a situation in which the person is aware of a moral problem, acknowledges moral responsibility, and makes a moral judgment about the correct action; yet, as a result of real or perceived constraints, participates in perceived moral wrong-doing"* (p. 5) [429]. The results of moral distress may be physical reactions such as sweating, headache, nausea and diarrhea, and crying. The emotional components include anger, frustration, depression, shame, grief, misery, sadness, and emotional pain [430].

The literature on moral distress has been accumulating at least in nursing references, but most of it refers to medical and surgical nursing. Among nurses, moral distress has been associated high staff turnover, burnout, reduced staff morale/satisfaction, decreased quality of patient care, and increased financial costs [431].

But little has been written about the moral distress experienced by social service and mental health workers under the influence of funding changes, a managed care environment, and increasing levels of social need, uninsured people, and poverty. From what we have perceived in our training institute, in many consultations to a wide variety of settings, in academic teaching situations, and in clinical settings, moral distress—although most people are not familiar with the term—is widespread in our social service settings. It may be a fundamental cause of the crisis in the workforce that we spoke of earlier, even if not identified.

Unrelenting Systemic Stress

Just as individuals respond to acute stress and chronic stress in variable ways, so too can organizations experience the effects of both acute and chronic stressors as a whole. Unrelenting systemic stress producing chronic hyperarousal has become a fundamental characteristic of health care, mental health care, and all human services and has negatively affected the health of organizational cultures. The focus of this book is more on the impact of chronic and unrelenting stress and repetitive crisis than on the reactions of organizations to acute incidents. As we mentioned in the Introduction, one of the terms applied to this difference when speaking of individuals is the use of terminology like "complex posttraumatic stress" in an attempt to emphasize the very complicated outcomes that can derive from recurrent severely stressful situations over time. Similarly, the problems that organizations manifest are also extremely complex and interconnected.

Organizational culture arises out of the history, memory, experiences and formal structures and personnel of the organization and helps to determine the health and well-being of the individual worker. As organizational research has demonstrated, uncertainty is a main contributor to the perception of stress, and there is nothing so uncertain in corporate life as organizational change. As one author from the world of business has noted:

> The combination of economic scarcity, the recession of the late 1980s and early 1990s, the widening gap between demand and resources in public services such as health and education, and the rampant influence of technological change has produced a deeply uncertain organizational world which affects not just organizations in their entirety but groups and individuals at all levels of the organizational matrix. (p. 253) [195]

The literature clearly demonstrates that the combination of uncertainty and the likelihood of change, both favorable and unfavorable change, produces stress and, ultimately, affects perceptions and judgments, interpersonal relationships, and the dynamics of the business itself [193]. In the health care and mental health field for the last two decades, change has been steady and certain only in its tendency to be unfavorable to the practice of the health and social service professions. There are serious consequences to working in such environments, "chronic work stress in a healthcare setting can ultimately lead to *a maladaptive response pattern with a strong impact on a person's emotional health and attitude toward life: the burnout syndrome"* (p. 117) [263].

Social work professor Mimi Abramovitz did a study of senior staff in 107 social service agencies providing a wide variety of services in New York after "welfare reform" was in place. The adverse impact of welfare reform fell heavily on women and children who are the prime users of public assistance and non-profit agency services, all of whom were hard hit by the constraints, sanctions, and penalties exacted by the Personal Responsibility and Work Opportunity Reconciliation Act of 1996. As Dr. Abramovitz wrote,

Rising dissatisfaction, demoralization, and burnout among workers is not unique to New York agencies. A study of 47 of Louisiana's nonprofit social agencies also found increased burnout in more than 46 percent of the organizations surveyed since welfare reform. These outcomes linked to welfare reform do not bode well for workers or for clients who turn to the human services system for support, treatment, and advocacy. Burned out workers often withdraw psychologically, lose their compassion for clients, and reduce their work effort. As the executive director of a child care agency explained: "If they [workers] don't feel good about the job, it is going to be hard for them to really help our clients." When these reactions sweep through the nonprofit human service sector the quality of services surely suffers. (p. 184) [49]

Staff concerns about ethical issues increased in 49.5% of those interviewed. Concerns about protecting client confidentiality, maximizing client self-determination, promoting the general welfare, and supporting advocacy for social justice loomed especially large, troubling individual workers and impeding effective service delivery. Paperwork had increased by 86% and workers were feeling far less effective in their work. They expressed disappointment and great distress at not being able to fulfill the desire that brought them into the work, which was to "help others." Combined with a much greater lack of job satisfaction was a profound sense of demoralization. Although representatives from two-thirds of the agencies (69%) reported that their staff members felt equipped to do their job, the reality of never-ending emergencies, work over-loads, and ethical dilemmas took such a toll that an astounding 83% of the agencies reported higher burnout and stress among their workers once welfare reform was in place. Sick leave requests and higher turnover rates were affecting the entire system.

The effects of stress in organizations and within whole systems are cumulative. A series of small, unrelated, stress-inducing incidents can add up to a mountain of stress in the eyes of people that work there and receive services within these settings. Minor stressors can multiply into often irresolvable dilemmas [415]. Like a client who has been repeatedly abused by his or her family, the mental health system had never achieved parity with the physical health system before the onslaught of managed care and federal and state cutbacks radically changed the face of health care delivery, rapidly bringing the system to the point of crisis that has been ably described in a number of national reports. In observing the fact that spending for mental health care had declined as a percentage of overall health spending throughout the 1990s, former Surgeon General Satcher noted that although some of the decline in resources for mental health relative to total health care could have been due to improvements in efficiency, he concluded that it also could reflect increasing reliance on other (non-mental health) public human services and increased barriers to service access, a conclusion which has been borne out by subsequent reports [432].

As we discussed in Chapter 1, the response has been the closure of psychiatric inpatient units, service cutbacks at clinics, and an inability of psychiatrists and other mental health professionals to support their practice with insurance payments. The existing problems have been vastly compounded by the utilization-review practices of the managed care industry and taken together, the result is "a critical inability of patients to access needed psychiatric care" [90]. Adding to the burden is that current incentives both within and outside managed care generally do not encourage an emphasis on quality of care [432]. As a concrete example of all this Brian observes,

> *The entire system is pretty crazy. As an example, it is built on a fantasy that psychiatrists are providing oversight on clinic cases, but the sheer volume suggests otherwise. Although this is still handled as if it is a high priority in the various regulations, there is inadequate financial support for carrying a psychiatrist on staff. It is a losing proposition. Essentially agencies are paid way too little to have psychiatrists on staff who have way too much to do to actually be effective.*

Conclusion

Our human service system and all of its components are in a state of chronic crisis. As a result, organizations can become overly attentive to threat both from within and from outside the organization. When this happens, all change is approached with fear and suspicion, and feelings of basic safety can become an elusive commodity. Organizational hyperarousal is likely to adversely impact relationships at every level and make recognition of mistakes and subsequent learning from those mistakes more difficult. The bottom line is that chronically hyperaroused organizations have as much difficulty adapting to changing circumstances as do chronically hyperaroused individuals. In Chapter 6 we focus on one of the main results of exposure to chronic hyperarousal: the loss of emotional management. We will try to put words to what is, by now, the experience of so many people who work in human services.

Chapter 6

Loss of Emotional Management

SUMMARY: *A core difficulty for clients served by human services is the ability to manage distressing emotions, while at the same time being able to extend empathy to their clients and not become emotionally anesthetized. Emotions are contagious and under any conditions, human service delivery environments demand the highest levels of emotional labor from workers. Stress and trauma exacerbate those demands. Atmospheres of recurrent or constant crisis severely constrain the ability of staff to manage their own emotions, and this makes it difficult to provide healing environments for their clients. Atmospheres of chronic crisis and fear contribute to poor services. Under these circumstances, conflict escalates and both relationships and problem-solving suffer.*

Emotional Intelligence and Trauma

Emotions provide us with important survival information, most importantly, information about how to get along with other people who are important in our lives. Learning to manage our emotions—modulating and containing them—is dependent on the interaction we have with others throughout our lives. When we are young, caregivers play a vital role in "training" the central nervous system how to respond, and our relationships with other people have a great deal to do with the way in which our brain actually develops [299]. Emotional experience profoundly influences thought, alerting us to contradictions in what we know or perceive and keeping us focused on this discrepancy until we have resolved whatever conflict exists [345]. Our bodies respond to every emotional experience that we have. That is why there are so many language expressions that refer to the connection between the mind and the body, such as "I have a lump in my throat," or "My heart is broken," or "My hair stood on end." The development of emotional intelligence is a prolonged developmental process not dissimilar to the development of cognitive intelligence and may be radically affected by disrupted attachment in early childhood as well as exposure to adversity and trauma.

Emotional intelligence has been defined as *"the ability to perceive accurately, appraise, and express emotions; to access and/or generate feelings when they facilitate thought; the ability to understand emotions and emotional knowledge; and the ability to regulate emotions so as to promote emotional and intellectual growth"* (p. 5) [433]. According to this definition, emotion makes thinking more intelligent and that we need to be intelligent about our thinking. In research findings, emotional intelligence has been associated with success at work, career advancement, superior leadership behavior, effective team leadership and team performance, better physical and psychological well-being, and higher job performance. The dimensions of emotional intelligence most related to the workplace environment have been defined as four clusters of social competencies: self-awareness, self-management, social awareness, and social skills [434].

Emotional Resonance and Contagion

Because we are a social species, dependent for our survival on other people from the time we are born, evolution designed us to resonate with the emotions of others. Such resonance has high survival value. It is life saving for a mother to have a special and specific reaction to the cry of her child, and it is very useful for the entire tribe when one individual scout, spotting danger on the horizon, is able to convey an immediate sense of that danger to his fellows by expressing his emotions through voice and gesture.

This resonance is conveyed in a number of ways. Every emotion evokes a different pattern of response in the nervous system, affecting not just our internal organs but our facial and bodily expression as well. Every emotion also triggers a tendency to act in a certain way [435], and each emotion triggers a response in other people as well called "emotional contagion." Emotional contagion is defined as *"the tendency to automatically mimic and synchronize facial expressions, vocalizations, postures, and movements with those of another person, and consequently, to converge emotionally"* (p. 5) [436]. We are profoundly influenced by other people's emotional states from the time we are born. We respond to another person's emotional state within one-twentieth of a second, and in that time our physiology is changed and our bodies become synchronized to the emotional state of the other. This happens outside of our conscious awareness and is beyond our ability to control.

Many of the core issues surrounding human service delivery are related to difficulties in managing emotions, particularly the distressing emotions of sadness, shame, guilt, anger, and fear. Clients bring their own emotional management problems into every health, mental health, and social service setting and encounter staff members who may be having emotional management issues themselves. What can be a steamy cauldron of emotions is further heated up by the impact of stress on individuals and groups. As Brian points out,

We know that working with our clients provides ample opportunity for our staff to get triggered; in fact it can happen every minute of every day. To create the best possible environment for trauma survivors they need to be around people who are not easily triggered, people who can manage their own emotions successfully and not overreact to events in the environment. If everyone in the environment is crisis driven and staff have relatively little control over their own emotions, things can quickly spiral out of control and become increasingly unsafe. In effect, the treatment environment can begin to look and feel very much like the environment in which our clients were so terribly injured. It certainly does not help to put dysregulated children into dysregulated environments with adults who cannot manage their own feelings.

In many cases the most important work that mental health providers and other social service workers offer to our clients is helping them to manage distressful feelings. Emotional contagion is one of the factors in making human service delivery work so difficult and it is an important component of the most demanding component of caring for other people. It is called *emotional labor.*

Emotional Labor

The concept of emotional labor was first developed by organizational sociologist Arlie Hochschild [437]. She described the work performed by any service employee who is required, as part of his or her job, to display specific sets of emotions (both verbal and nonverbal) with the aim of inducing particular feelings and responses among those for whom the service is being provided. In this respect, employees are being required to control and use their own emotions in order to influence the emotional state of others [438]. Occupations considered to be high in demand for emotional labor include nurses, physicians, therapists, protective service workers, and health service workers [439].

The concept of emotional labor has frequently referred to a deliberate disconnect between felt and performed emotion, "surface acting" that is explicitly a part of the job and is encouraged and supported in performance evaluations. For example, an employee handbook at a deli explicitly stated, *"Under no circumstances should a customer ever wonder if you are having a bad day. Your troubles should be masked with a smile"* (p. 587) [440]. One of the difficulties for people in professional roles such as doctors, nurses, therapists, and other service professionals is that emotional labor is just part of the job, a fundamental part of the job—always glaringly obvious when that labor is carried poorly—but inculcated into the work itself. Emotional labor then becomes part of an each individual's identity and is not separated out as "surface acting" or part of a job [440].

In the human service field, emotional labor happens when you have to induce feelings you may not have or suppress feelings that you do have. It is the everyday work of virtually every therapeutic encounter and constitutes what can go radically wrong in an encounter that is nontherapeutic. Expressing calm and supportive emotions when face to face and voice to voice with a client who may be enraged, attacking, frustrated, shamed, sad, or grief stricken is emotionally demanding. Keeping your voice down and containing your own normal threat responses, and not emotionally escalating on the inside, even when a child or adult is cursing at you, spitting at you, or threatening you with bodily harm requires an extraordinary level of self-control and emotional management. And yet that is what human service workers do every day, often every hour of the day. Brian has spent years watching children and staff interact. But on this day, he thought more about what he was seeing unfold:

> *Recently, I watched several of our youngest children playing on our campus. Two were riding bikes around in an enclosed play area, while three others played basketball. They all seemed fine. There was no fighting or arguing. They were all seemingly content. There was no whiff of trouble. In the corner of the play area sat one of our staff people, a staff person we think highly of, not someone we worry about, talking on her cell phone. My initial reaction was to walk over to her, tell her to get off the phone, and instruct her to do her job. I have learned over the years that it generally not advisable for me to assume my initial reaction is ever the most appropriate or productive course of action. I decided instead to let it go, at least in terms of confronting the staff, but I could not let it go. I spent the better part of the day thinking about what I had seen and how it relates to lots of other sins of omission I have seen and committed throughout my many years in the field.*
>
> *The children I watched playing that day were among our most traumatized children. They are all children in the child welfare system who have been removed from their families as a result of abuse and neglect. Here they were in a program that is supposed to be helping them rewrite the scripts of their lives and what are they getting? More of the same—a morning with an adult who is too caught up in her own stuff to sufficiently attend to their stuff. This is really not what should be happening in a treatment program. It is supposed to be all about recovery and new possibilities.*
>
> *I think I know what was happening. Many of our children are difficult to engage. They push us away and rebuff our efforts to help them. They invite us in and then slam the door in our face when we try to enter. It is all very confusing and disheartening for young staff, and it is not much better for older*

staff either. In many cases, staff check out, but often they do not do it maliciously; they mean no harm. They may convince themselves that this is what the child wants or needs. "They just need some space, they don't need me hanging all over them. I'll just sit over here and make a call and leave them alone." What the staff miss is that they are replaying what has been an all-too-common play for the children we work with: caregivers who are either too overwhelmed with their own lives or their children's behavior to be adequately attuned to the child's needs. It is subtle, but it is powerful, and it is almost always missed in programs like ours.

The idea of emotional labor and the demands of working in mental health and social service environments also help explain why so many people doing this work do not resent their clients as much as they resent unsupportive coworkers, supervisors, administrators, and licensing agency representatives when they add to the burden of the work by creating a "blame culture." When the blaming and shaming happens, usually under conditions of adversity where the worker's defensive ability to deal with the emotional load has already been overwhelmed, the emotional workload automatically doubles and the worker feels he or she is being attacked from all sides. Each of us only has so much emotional energy. If we are spending it on our supervisors or auditors or licensing bodies, we have that much less for our clients. Good managers do not let staff burn up a precious commodity foolishly. We need to be careful what kind of emotional upsets we insert into the life of a worker if we want that worker to be effective with the clients. As one researcher in this field points out, *"Emotional exhaustion results when an imbalance occurs between the emotional demands of work and the personal psychological resources available to fuel the energy to meet such demands"* [441].

Under such circumstances, it is likely that an already compromised emotional management system will collapse. When this happens repeatedly, the reactions will vary from individual to individual. But this process is a prescription for high turnover rates, low morale, counter-aggressive behavior, passive-aggressive behavior, and disengagement or emotional shutdown. In other words, some people will leave and try to find a more supportive environment; others will become chronic grumblers and complainers; some will take out their frustration on the children or adults in their care; others will take it out on their colleagues; and some will just withdraw and in job after job protect themselves from becoming emotionally aroused by simply not engaging enough with their clients to be disturbed.

In her original work, Hochschild suggested that emotional labor does have exchange value and that wages should be commensurate with the amount of emotional labor an individual must extend to do a good job and workers emotional labor should be seen as a form of social capital. In research looking at emotional labor and wages the top five occupations with the highest demands for emotional labor include: 1) police and sheriff's patrol officers, 2) child, family, and school social workers, 3) psychiatrists, 4) first-line supervisors–managers of police and detectives, 5) registered nurses. As we might expect, this research shows that higher levels of emotional labor demands are not uniformly rewarded with higher wages. Occupations with high cognitive demands show that wages improve with increasing emotional labor demands; while occupations low in cognitive demands show decreasing wages as the levels of emotional labor increase. Interesting in this research is the fact that child care workers were considered to have low cognitive demands, although high demands for emotional labor [442]. Herein lies one of the gross misunderstandings that exist system-wide about the requirements for frontline workers in childcare settings, particularly in residential treatment and juvenile justice settings. It is little wonder that there would be such high turnover rates among these key personnel, much to the detriment of childcare organizations and to the children in their care. The workers who spend the most time with the children have the greatest emotional labor requirements but the cognitive demands on them are inaccurately perceived and as a result, their wages are too low for them to adequately serve the needs of the organizations.

Economic Invisibility and the Legacy of Gender Discrimination

Emotional labor and "caring" labor are terms used to pull together concepts from both sides of the institutional divide between home and work. Traditionally, caring for the needs of the young, the old, the disabled, and the ill was "women's work" and was outside of paid labor and outside of the economic system. As a result, all that goes into homemaking is not considered part of the GNP—Gross National Product. Physical and cognitive labor is done for extrinsic reward, but traditionally caring—a form of emotional labor—is not rewarded in any explicit way.

In general terms, jobs are determined by the characteristics of the work required along a scale of increasing work complexity. The work dimensions are usually organized by sets of skills, effort demanded, responsibilities, and undesirable working conditions. Generally speaking, the more complex the work, the higher the wage or salary. But the emotional labor involved in a job is rarely taken into account and those who do that work get little for it. In the social service sector, this just does not make sense, since *"not paying employees for the performance of work that is critical to the accomplishment of organizational objectives and even the survival of the organization is wage discrimination. The invisibility of emotional labor as a compensable job requirement contributes to the gap in wages by gender"* (p. 144) [443].

Depending on occupation, there continues to be a serious gap between men's wages and women's wages for the same jobs. But gender discrimination in mental health and social services may not be the biggest problem for organizations today. Rather, discrimination against traditional "women's work"—caring for others—regardless of whether you are male or female is a more pervasive issue. There is a long background to this. Historically, employers developed separate pay scales by the gender of the job, embedding in the compensation practices cultural assumptions about gender-based roles. These informal practices and cultural assumptions about women's work were then routinely embedded in job evaluation systems that have not necessarily changed very much in the past century. As a result, skills, demands, and responsibilities associated with historically male managerial jobs and with engineering, finance, law, and medicine (with the exceptions of psychiatry, pediatrics, and family practice!) were regarded as complex, while jobs considered historically women's work continued to be low paying: *"Emotional labor remains invisible. It is not viewed as complex. It is not treated as valuable"* (p. 145) [443].

Although caring for others has traditionally been women's work, generally attached to kinship relationships, unpaid, and therefore invisible in the marketplace, much of it is no longer kinship or unpaid. Over the last century, an increasing number of children are in day care, the sick are in hospitals and rehabilitation centers, the elderly cared for in non-family situations, troubled children are institutionalized or put in paid foster homes, mentally ill people are in hospitals, group homes, boarding homes, and outpatient clinics, and a large number of people are in the juvenile and adult criminal justice system. Together they comprise a significant part of the population and other people are paid to care for them as their employment, although not necessarily to care about them. Yet the emotional labor involved in caring for others is not generally considered in evaluating performance and tying the job category to income.

In her original work, Hochschild suggested that emotional labor does have exchange value and that wages should be commensurate with the amount of emotional labor an individual must extend to do a good job and workers emotional labor should be seen as a form of social capital. In research looking at emotional labor and wages the top five occupations with the highest demands for emotional labor include: 1) police and sheriff's patrol officers, 2) child, family, and school social workers, 3) psychiatrists, 4) first-line supervisors—managers of police and detectives, 5) registered nurses. As we might expect, this research shows that higher levels of emotional labor demands are not uniformly rewarded with higher wages. Occupations with high cognitive demands show that wages improve with increasing emotional labor demands; while occupations low in cognitive demands show decreasing wages as the levels of emotional labor increase. Interesting in this research is the fact that child care workers were considered to have low cognitive demands, although high demands for emotional labor [442].

Herein lies one of the gross misunderstandings that exist system-wide about the requirements for frontline workers in childcare settings, particularly in residential treatment and juvenile justice settings. It is little wonder that there would be such high turnover rates among these key personnel, much to the detriment of childcare organizations and to the children in their care. The workers who spend the most time with the children have the greatest emotional labor requirements but the cognitive demands on them are inaccurately perceived and as a result, their wages are too low for them to adequately serve the needs of the organizations.

Emotional Labor and Job Requirements

A gender-neutral job evaluation system (GNJES) has been designed that describes the level of complexity in human relations skills. With every increase in level, there is an increase in complexity and in the demand for emotional labor. Thus, the jobs demanding the greatest amount of emotional intelligence and social skills are jobs that *"require the employee to exercise interpersonal skills in combination, creating a climate for and establishing a commitment to the welfare of clients or the public, coaching and guiding clients through difficult emotional, attitudinal and developmental change around issues that are sensitive, controversial, and about which there is individual resistance as well as providing comfort where people are in considerable pain, dying or gravely ill, angry, distraught, are in drug-induced states, or otherwise unpredictable, physically violent or emotional and may include crowd control when crowd gets out of hand"* (p. 151) [443].

Service jobs have heavy emotional demands and the highest level is applied to *"employees [who] deal regularly with highly physically dangerous and unpredictably hostile or violent people or groups. They may also work directly to meet the needs of people (including family members) who are facing death, through caring for or discussing this or other comparable, extremely sensitive topics with them"* (p. 153) [443]. But in human services, increased complexity in terms of emotional labor does not equal any increase in economic value.

Training for Emotional Numbing

> *He is bothered by the aesthetics of the sick, Walker mused, by the way flesh distorts itself and accommodates instruments of metal and glass. He gives in to the stirrings of distress. He lets the details of suffering and dying overwhelm him. He has failed to accomplish the main thing required of a doctor. He has not become numb.*

> Philip Harper, *Final Fear*

The medical model sets the tone for the whole human service delivery system, just as psychiatrists determine what diagnosis everyone in human services must use when a patient presents with any kind of behavioral health problem. But the training of physicians has within it endorsement and support for emotional numbing, and emotional numbing is both a prime symptom of posttraumatic stress and a poor prognosticator for the ability to engage in the emotional labor required of the caring relationship.

About 50 years ago, Dr. Bertram Lewin, past president of the American Psychoanalytic Association, wondered how the education of a young medical student was affected by having a dead person for his first "patient." This question has never been adequately answered. More recently, Dr. Wolf, from the Louisiana State University School, said, *"Medical education can be a health hazard for many students, and far-reaching reforms are needed to improve it"* [444]. If we dare to gaze critically and humanely at the process of medical education, it becomes possible to understand how a medical professional could become gradually and insidiously dehumanized as a result of his or her experiences. Adverse reactions to cadavers—even in medical school—are hardly unusual. About 5%–10% of students experience some sort of disturbance to their sleeping or eating habits as reactions to dissecting a body. The researcher said their reactions bore a strong resemblance to posttraumatic stress disorder. The experience of training in and practicing medicine is astonishingly stressful and the exposure to traumatic experience is enormous. A study of third-year medical students found clinical levels of depression in 23% of the students, and 57% endorsed high levels of somatic distress [445]. Health care professionals are repeatedly confronted with death and dying, often under horrendous circumstances, are faced with their own shortcomings and failures in fending off death, and are held responsible and accountable for those shortcomings by patients, their families, and their lawyers.

Emotional numbing is one of those good news/bad news issues. It helps physicians, soldiers, emergency medical technicians, emergency room nurses, child welfare workers, disaster workers, firefighters, intensive care unit personnel, police officers, and all those who work under emergency conditions deal with whatever situation confronts them without emotionally falling apart and being unable to think clearly. The bad news is that once we have become emotionally numb, which we do largely through a process of dissociating emotion, those emotions do not necessarily ever become available to us again. And that lack of emotional availability can affect people's personal and professional relationships—sometimes for a lifetime—and lead to the dehumanization of caregiving relationships.

Dehumanizing Caregiving

The word "caring" carries the weight of two meanings: caring *about*—the motivation that activates the caring behavior—and caring *for*—catering to another person's physical and/or emotional needs [446]. If you are an employer, you may be able to hire someone to cater to another person's needs by giving clear instructions about what to do, but you cannot make someone feel the emotions that must accompany "caring about" another person. This issue is particularly pressing in the human service delivery professions because although organizations and licensing bodies can regulate providing food, shelter, clothing, and other basic material needs, the manner in which these material needs are met has been far less amenable to any kind of evaluation much less regulation. Caring about another person is far less tangible while at the same time it is arguably infinitely important to the person being cared for. All too often caring for people without caring about them actually dehumanizes the person being cared for. We saw this happen in many institutional settings in the past, and unfortunately, it occurs in the present as well. Brian sees this firsthand as he travels around various settings:

> I see this in my travels far too often. I see workers who are watching the kids but not really interacting with them. They are making sure the kids do not kill each other but doing little to make sure that they create a different experience for the child. It is the difference between keeping you safe by externally controlling the environment and taking the time to teach you to be safe and caring about you enough to want to take that time.

All You Do Is Talk to People

When we look over the job demands for everyone we know that is in education, health care, mental health care, or social services, they fall into categories denoting the highest demands on emotional intelligence and social learning. But all too often instead of demanding (and having the funding to pay for) that level of skill, we just hire the least problematic and most available "body" to fill a job slot. We are so accustomed to thinking that emotional labor, the work of caring, and exposure to violence, abuse, and physical danger are just a part of the work that we accept the broader social definitions of the relative worth of the work that we do. We can recall many times as clinicians that lay people and other health care professionals would say, "You don't do real work—you just talk to people." It was infuriating but lacking a shared perspective on the value of emotional labor, it was difficult to know how to respond. Brian actually encountered a state official years ago, who said, "Being a child care worker is such an easy job; you get paid to play with kids all day. What's so hard about that?"

Most discussions of emotional labor recognize the skills and effort involved in managing one's own and others' emotions. Less often recognized are the responsibilities inherent in emotional labor. In traditional job evaluation, responsibility factors are given heavy weight in determining compensation, especially responsibility for money or equipment, or for the supervision of a large number of subordinates. But consider the consequences for an alcohol and drug treatment center or a hospital or a residential program for emotionally disturbed children when staff members fail to exhibit the necessary human relations skills or to expend the energy required to perform emotionally demanding tasks effectively. Treatment failure may be the result, not because the client cannot be helped but because the emotional labor necessary to help them is not available. The competent performance of emotional labor has significant consequences, not only for the bottom line but also for the clients who are affected by displays of inappropriate emotional labor [443].

Managers and Emotional Labor

People in management positions are, by definition, emotional managers while they manage everything else. It is one of the most important, challenging, and neglected aspects of any management position. Although we may be trained in certain managerial skill sets, like budgeting, accounting, corporate compliance regulations, policies and procedures, even human resources, rarely do managers routinely get trained in skill sets around emotional management—their own and the people they are supervising—at least not in social service settings. As we mentioned earlier, there is an implicit expectation that if you are *in* these settings, if you have been trained as a psychiatrist, psychologist, social worker, counselor, that ipso facto, you already know how to manage people. This is an entirely false assumption and actually puts social service workers and the organizations they work in, at an extreme disadvantage. The following is a description of an effective manager:

> *Engaged in the development of collective goals and objectives, instilling in others an appreciation of the importance of work activities, generating and maintaining enthusiasm, confidence, optimism, cooperation, and trust, encouraging flexibility in decision-making and change and establishing and maintaining a meaningful identity for the organization* (p. 1027) [447]

This means, of course, that managers must role model effective emotional management themselves. Anyone that is in a leadership position will have to deal with employees' negative emotions aroused as a part of the routine intermingling of a wide variety of people, frustrations secondary to the work environment, frustrations secondary to larger system bureaucratic demands, and the more dire, frightening, and sometimes life-threatening situations that health, mental health, and social service workers must deal with a great deal of the time.

A manager's emotions are contagious and profoundly affect the work environment, as we would expect from the neurobiology of the mirror neuron system and extensive studies of emotional contagion. Negative emotions on the part of managers tend to result in poor outcomes in terms of employee interactions, decision making, and overall organizational performance [448].

Brian describes the emotional contagion that can affect workers and managers alike:

> *It is fascinating that the level of hyperarousal on the part of leadership can serve to actually make things far more dangerous in the long run. While it is important for leaders to have a good sense of the external and internal threats to organizational existence, it is essential that we not become overly reactive to these threats. Ultimately we cannot hope to control all the potential threats. We need to get good enough at recognizing them early and responding quickly. The only way an organization can do this effectively, however, is to have all its members on the case and the only way to have all members on the case is to create an environment that is not on everyone's case. What gets us off course is when leaders think staff are out to get them or are disinterested. Leaders then can become hypervigilant. Staff begin to feel they are not trusted and react accordingly. We really do want everyone paying attention to the people in front of them and not to be overly distracted by what or who might be sneaking up behind them. In an environment where trust is lacking, staff and leadership become adversaries. When problems are uncovered, they are not dealt with as our problems but your problems. We do not talk about what we can do together but what you must do for me.*

If managers are to effectively and consistently do this difficult emotional labor, then they must be taught the skills to do that, even when the emotions are very problematic and/or very intense. To do this, managers need a supportive relationship with whomever they report to, particularly during times of the most distressing emotions. Unfortunately, the unenviable position of managers is that because our systems remain so dysfunctional, it is likely that many managers, all of whom are in the middle of some hierarchy or other, will have to bear the brunt of the negative emotional experiences of their subordinates and the negative emotions of the people above them when a crisis or a trauma occurs. If we want to understand why there is such a rapid turnover of managers, particularly middle managers and directors, we have to look at the incredible demands of emotional labor.

Organizational Emotions

The idea of organizational emotional life is not a comfortable one in most of the literature, largely because there has been a "myth of rationality," a generally held belief that organizational behavior can best be explained entirely in rational cognitive terms [85]. But stress models are fundamentally about emotional reactions and so the emotional nature of organizational behavior can no longer be ignored. In fact, one group of investigators has argued that *"emotions are among the primary determinants of behavior at work .... And profoundly influence both the social climate and the productivity of companies and organizations"* (p. 154) [449].

How does an organization "manage" emotional states? It does so through the normal problem-solving, decision-making, and conflict resolution methods that must exist for any organization to operate effectively. The more complex the work demands, the greater the necessity for collaboration and integration and therefore the more likely that a system of teamwork will evolve. Although most organizations within our society function in a fundamentally hierarchical, top-down manner, in a calm, healthy, well-functioning system there is a certain amount of natural democratic process that occurs in the day-to-day operations of solving group problems, making decisions in teams, and resolving conflict among members of the organization. In fact, research has demonstrated that self-managed teams with decentralized decision-making abilities are among the most important practices for high performance in the current business climate [450].

Unfortunately, in today's human service environment, unreasonable demands on time have reached such an extreme point that time to meet to actually discuss problems, cases, interpersonal anxieties, and build the trusting relationships that are necessary for teamwork has virtually disappeared. Under managed care regimes, it is often only face-to-face time with clients that receives any reimbursement at all and that has resulted in the radical decrease in time for professionals to interact with each other, share information, and get the social support they need to supply the caring labor that we have been discussing. Over time, this has resulted in a loss of emotional management throughout care giving organizations, a crisis-like environment that creates even more stress than is warranted by the immediate demands of the day-to-day work. When we do have time to meet, managers may not know best how to use this time and may actually avoid the tough issues because they are unpleasant and hard to deal with and because they have to do so much with so little time. This is very possibly the main reason why there has been so much reluctance to actually deal with the traumatic backgrounds of our clients—the emotions aroused can be truly overwhelming for everyone and in a system that already has compromised emotional management, simply too much to bear.

Emotions and Organizational Crisis

In organizations under stress, the emotional workload is acutely intensified and if under chronic stress, the emotional workload may easily become overwhelming. Healthy function is likely to be sacrificed in service of facing an emergency. As we discussed in Chapter 4, organizations under stress can manifest traits similar to stressed individuals. As anyone knows who has worked in a setting facing some kind of threat, everyone's attention becomes riveted on the latest rumor and little productive work is accomplished. Because human beings are "hardwired" for social interaction, a threat to our social group can be experienced as a dangerous threat to our individual survival and can evoke powerful responses.

Recall that these responses are called "social defenses" against anxiety (see Chapter 4). Our social institutions are designed to accomplish specific tasks and functions, but we also utilize our institutions to collectively protect us against being overwhelmed with the anxiety that underlies human existence. Despite the fact that tragic loss in human service environments is not an entirely uncommon event, most organizations do not prepare for a crisis, other than for fire or natural disaster. Since the mission of health care, mental health, and social service environments is to care for and about the people they serve, the idea of injury, death, and betrayal is unacceptable, overwhelmingly threatening, and therefore evokes a panoply of social defense maneuvers. The rationalizations internal to the system take on a typical form: "We are so good that nothing like that will ever happen here" because "bad things don't happen to good people."

The collective result of this natural inclination to contain anxiety becomes a problem when institutional events occur that produce great uncertainty, particularly those events that are associated with death or the fear of death, as in the tragic examples we mentioned in Chapter 5. Under such conditions, containing anxiety and distress may become more important than rationally responding to the crisis, although because of our relative ignorance and denial about our unconscious collective lives, this defensive strategy is itself likely to be denied and rationalized. As a result, organizations may engage in group unconscious thought processes and actions that may serve to contain anxiety but that are ultimately destructive to organizational purpose and that create unsafe conditions for staff and clients [292; 314; 362].

Organizational theorist Ian Mitroff has raised a question entirely pertinent to our services: "*How paranoid do we need to be in order to anticipate, plan for, and cope effectively with major crises, and even acts of evil themselves, without in the process becoming totally deranged or evil ourselves?*" (p. 15) [382]. These days the answer, as Brian discusses, is *pretty paranoid*, even in care giving organizations:

> We do fire drills and recently we have done lock-down drills. Lock-down drills are far more emotionally provocative. I think fire is faceless and nameless and, above all, not human. The idea of a client or a former staff person coming in with a gun is more than a little upsetting. We have talked about drilling on the scenario of a child's death, but the idea of it even happening is so overwhelming and horrific that we have not yet gotten up the courage to do it.

This denial that terrible things could happen at any moment is actually considered a sign of health. In his extensive review psychologist John Schumaker reminds us that "*a considerable amount of insanity, in the sense of being out of touch with reality, is requisite to optimal mental health*" (p. 21) [262]. According to one researcher who has extensively studied "positive illusions", our ability to redefine our reality results in an increase in productive work, improves aspects of our intellectual function, improves our memory, inhibits disturbing memories, increases motivation, improves performance, improves coping, and gives us better physical health (Taylor, 1989). It should come as no surprise then, that the terrible events that do occur in many different mental health and social service environments remain unexplored as possibilities before the events and denied after the events, even while they continue to haunt organizational function.

Rarely is an episode of violence in a community a singular and unconnected event. Violence emerges out of a context, but the elements contributing to that emergence are likely to be unconscious, and without a thoroughgoing analysis of each violent episode, the problems are likely to become compounded until the organization is living in a state of chronic crisis and is chronically hyper-aroused. Unfortunately, rather than reviewing the full complexity and deep understanding of emergent violent episodes, it is quite likely that the only thing that will happen is a lot of finger-pointing and development of an entire blame culture as we discussed in Chapter 5. As Mitroff points out, "*Unless we learn from past crises we are doomed to experience those crises over and over again*" (p. 23) [382].

Getting to the heart of violence requires change, and rather than change we substitute scapegoating for real problem identification and solution in far too many cases. The result is a loss in the social immunity to more violence that otherwise is present among groups of people who trust and feel safe with each other. "*Crises exacerbate the splits that are already present in people, organizations, and societies. They increase whatever fears we had before a crisis. Organizations, no less than individuals, are subject to such splits in their personalities. These splits affect not only their financial performance but also the number of crises they experience, and in many cases, the crises they cause. In turn, the number of crises an organization causes affects the financial and emotional well-being of not only those who work in the organization but the larger society as well*" (p. 130) [382].

Let's look at several of the group processes that arise out of unconscious efforts on the part of the group to contain distress, anxiety, shame, and guilt, but that end up creating more distress. In avoiding conflict and failing to engage with each other over the real issues, we make situations far worse than they could be. Here we will focus on groupthink, conformity, and the Abilene paradox.

Groupthink

Organizations under stress may engage in a problematic emotional management process that interferes with the exercise of good cognitive skills, known as "groupthink." The social psychologist Janis looked at how groups make decisions, particularly under conditions of stress. He reviewed studies of infantry platoons, air crews, and disaster control teams and felt that this work confirmed what social psychologists had shown on experiments in normal college students: that stress produces a heightened need for affiliation, leading to increased dependency on one's group.

The increase in group cohesiveness, though good for morale and stress tolerance, can produce a process he saw as a disease that could infect otherwise healthy groups rendering them inefficient, unproductive, and sometimes disastrous. He observed that certain conditions give rise to a shared phenomenon in which the members try so hard to agree with each other that they commit serious errors that could easily have been avoided. An assumed consensus emerges while all members hurry to converge and ignore important divergences. Counterarguments are rationalized away and dissent is seen as unnecessary. As this convergence occurs, all group members share in the sense of invulnerability and strength conveyed by the group, while the decisions made are often actually disastrous. At least temporarily, the group experiences a reduction in anxiety, an increase in self-satisfaction, and a sense of assured purpose. But in the long run, this kind of thinking leads to decisions that spell disaster. Later, the individual members of the group find it difficult to accept that their individual wills were so affected by the group [264]. Here, Brian describes his own experience with this group process:

> Groupthink is complex. In a crisis, people are generally scared or anxious. Conflict in the group may serve only to increase these feelings. The fear people feel can also take a variety of forms. If staff dissent, will they be seen as part of the problem and as a result be frowned upon? At the same time, if they dissent, and as a result the group changes its response, are they then on the hook for the decision and its success or failure? It is very easy to line up behind the leader in a crisis, even if you think that person is wrong. The leader is often seen as the most bulletproof person in the room (although this may not truly be the case) and the leader has ultimate responsibility for whatever course of action is chosen. We have found it useful for leaders to frame the problem but hold off on stating their position until others have weighed in. It is very difficult for staff to oppose the will of the leader and if the leader weighs in first that may be the end of the conversation. If the group goes way off course, the leader can always pull things back on track, but it is best to let others give voice to their thoughts, opinions, and feelings.

In a crisis unit or an acute care inpatient setting, groupthink is easily observable. Staff members are under stress to admit patients, diagnose them, stabilize them, and get them out on the streets again. Typically there is a "mind guard," an individual(s) who encourages others to toe the company line, discouraging all forms of disagreement and dissent. Under such conditions, the staff is likely to develop a high level of cohesiveness, which helps them handle the stress more adequately. However, the result may be that the group is so intent on supporting each other that the group members never engage in meaningful, task-related conflict surrounding the diagnosis or the treatment of the patients. Later, if groupthink has occurred and something terrible has happened, then there will be extreme pressure on all group members from other group members to remain loyal to the group and the group decision. This will effectively silence dissent and arrest all useful conflict, with the group learning little from the experience.

Conformity

Another significant group emotional management technique that is particularly important under conditions of chronic stress is conformity. Social psychologist Solomon Ash demonstrated that when pressure to conform is at work, a person changes his or her opinion not because he or she actually believes something different but because it's less stressful to change one's opinion than to challenge the group. In his experiments, subjects said what they really thought most of the time, but 70% of subjects changed their real opinions at least once, and 33% went along with the group half the time [240].

If a social service or mental health setting is dominated by norms that, for instance, assert that biological treatments are the only "real" medicine that a patient needs, or that the only way to deal with aggressive patients is to put them into four-point restraints, or that "bad" children just need more discipline, then many staff members will conform to these norms even if they do not agree because they are reluctant to challenge the group norms. If a patient becomes a problem and powerful members of the team are insisting that the patient be discharged, others may go along with this decision not because they agree clinically, but because they are conforming to the group expectations. The power differentials in the group can contribute significantly to pressures for conformity. Title, training, degree, authority, years of service, and how strongly someone feels about the issue all can lead us to lining up behind each other more quickly than we should.

The Abilene Paradox

Thirty years ago, organizational theorist Jerry Harvey told a parable as a way of demonstrating an issue that he perceived affected organizational functioning. In the story, four adults are sitting on a front porch in Coleman, Texas (some 53 miles from Abilene), on a very hot summer day. While everyone appears content drinking lemonade and playing dominoes, someone in the group suggests taking a drive to Abilene to eat lunch. Privately, each of the four participants thinks this suggestion is without merit because the only available car has no air conditioner. But each one goes along, so as not to be perceived as a "spoiler" of the group. Upon returning exhausted and disgruntled, the friends recognize that not a single one of them wanted to make the trip. They are unable to justify their original decision to take a 106-mile drive in a dust storm merely to eat a mediocre lunch in such hot weather.

Dr. Harvey believed that something like this happens repeatedly in organizations when there is a false consensus, and it is one of the inherent dangers of focusing on a consensus form of decision making when real conflict is discouraged. There are some warning signs that an organization is in danger of "riding the road to Abilene". There is risk when managers publicly do not fear the unknown and are overconfident to the point of arrogance, when there is an organization with little to no conflict or debate on critical issues, when there is a dominating organizational culture or a dominating leader, when there is a lack of diversity, when there is an indifference to employees in the organization, and when there is a "spiral of silence" in the organization [451].

Chronically Fear-Based Organizations

Specialists in the corporate world have looked at the impact of chronic fear on an organization. As one corporate expert pointed out, *"Fear can make people lash out and transform normally reasonable people into bullies and tyrants... Fear spreads like a virus and encourages corporate abuse to thrive in the policies, structures and operations of a business"* (p. 7) [452]. Just as exposure to chronic fear undermines the ability of individuals to deal with their emotional states and to cognitively perform at peak levels, chronic fear disables organizations as well. Lawsuits, labor unrest, the formation of unions, and strikes are typical signs of a high-fear environment. A lack of innovation, turf battles, social splitting, irresponsibility, bad decisions, low morale, absenteeism, widespread dissatisfaction, and high turnover are all symptoms of chronic fear-based workplaces [109]. *"In all these instances, the hidden factor may be an absence of group cohesion and commitment and the presence of unbearable tensions which create particular stresses for the individual. In these circumstances, the workplace is experienced as unsupportive, threatening to the emotional and physical well-being of the employee. At its worst, the workplace becomes a paranoid-schizoid environment, a nightmare existence"* (p. 250) [195]. Here Brian gives an example of how we often ignore how frightened people often are in the workplace:

> *In our facility we talk a lot about anger and staff being able to manage the anger and frustrations associated with caring for really troubled kids. We talk very little about the issue of fear and sometimes these kids scare the hell out of us. They can be wildly impulsive, extremely provocative, hopelessly depressed, profoundly unreasonable, and on any given day almost anything can happen.*

It does not mean anything will happen, but it can happen. When you're scared, you generally take one of two courses of action. You over control things so nothing gets out of control, or you avoid things so you do not become the target of anyone's wrath. Neither of these is a useful strategy and both lead to eventual conflict. We need to do a better job of acknowledging that fear is a major issue in our organizations and is constantly being managed by the staff. Leaders and managers need to do a better job helping people acknowledge this emotion and manage it more effectively in day-to-day operations. Many managers are cued by their staff to step in and rescue them from these unsettling feelings. This might be acceptable in the early stages of a worker's tenure with the organization, but if it continues to happen it is dysfunctional. Some managers feel affirmed by their ability to dive in and help staff people with this issue, but over time it is crippling to the worker and stunts his or her growth. Managers need to help staff gradually face the fears associated with the work. If the worker cannot do this, the worker is obviously working at the wrong place. If a manager cannot help the worker to grow or help the worker to leave, then the manager is not much of a manager.

Fear-based organizations have great difficulty in adapting to changing organizational demands. Since all of our social service systems are in the business of change, then we should have a clear idea of how individuals and families change but that is an area fraught with controversy, many competing theories, and an overall lack of emphasis on change as the purpose for all treatment. It should not come as a surprise then that our fields are only dimly aware of how to create and sustain organizational change. This is a particularly pressing problem because in the modern world the rate of change has greatly accelerated, demanding almost constant adaptation to changing conditions.

The term currently being used in human services to describe the need for large-scale change is "system transformation". In truth, the need for transformation is so great because we have been operating under the wrong assumptions for a very long time, mainly that are organizations are machines, not living systems, as we discussed in Chapter 1. Living systems, on the other hand, must constantly adapt to changing environments in order to survive. Those that cannot adapt, die. And yet, what is it that produces the "resistance to change" that is such a frequent experience of anyone who sets out to change their organization? We believe much of the resistance is due to chronic fear. Let's look at the typical fears of change that keep our organizations stuck and therefore unable to appropriately adapt.

First of all, animals, babies, and human beings in general have a fear of the unknown. Uncertainty means potential threats to survival are out there. We are a conservative species in that our criteria for whether or not to change is based at least as much on staying put as it is on moving on. We have a deeply embedded notion that if we are currently alive, doing whatever we are doing, it's best to just keep on doing it. In other words in our shared group psyche, "things could always get worse" so we are likely to alter patterns of behavior only when potential disaster is staring us in the face and there really is little alternative to change if we want to survive. Fortunately, we are also driven by curiosity, a desire to explore, and dislike of boredom. These two contradictory motive forces always are at play in our decisions about whether or not to change. But the more fear-provoking, life-threatening situations a person has encountered, the more threatening uncertainty is and therefore the less likely the internal balance will shift toward exploration of new options. Some people avoid circumstances that evoke fear while others try to control their sense of fear by diving into it, but regardless of what defensive strategy we employ, it pretty much comes from the same place: life is scary and fear rules.

Anything that threatens our ability to control ourselves and the people we depend upon threatens this basic primal need to guarantee certainty. So we fear change because change could mean some alteration in the patterns of power and control that we have so far achieved. We adopt specific roles in our relationships with people upon whom we depend and anything that threatens a change in those stable roles makes us fear change. In fact, anything that threatens those relationships, like conflicts of any sort, may make us terrified of changing anything. Change can mean new responsibilities and therefore a change in what we are and are not accountable for and to whom we are accountable, and this may also provoke a fear of change.

All change involves loss and human beings naturally resist giving up what is known in order to risk finding something better in the future. This relationship between loss and change is so important that whenever there is resistance to change in a patient, staff, manager, or organization understanding the losses involved in the change are critically important. Any significant change is associated with emotions and we may fear the distress associated with a change, including confronting unresolved feelings from the past, as well as confronting whatever losses occur concurrently with the change that is happening.

And these are just the fairly routine fears that can be expected when there is change in any of our routines. But there are other significant, meaning level changes that give people reason to fear trauma-informed change particularly. Trauma-informed change challenges us to change the mental models we discussed in Chapter 1. To successfully treat survivors of trauma and adversity requires us to significantly expand our knowledge base, explore our own capacity for violence and difficulties in displaying emotionally intelligent behavior. It requires us to learn from having the foundation of much of our established knowledge shaken. We need to question our own failures of communication, lack of fair play, unwillingness to endure loss, and inadequacy in using our imaginations. The more fear-driven we are, the less likely we are to adapt to the kinds of internal changes that trauma-informed change requires. As a result of all this, it is quite likely that normal conflict will escalate with any system of care.

Conflict in the Workplace

The presences of tension and conflict seem to be essential characteristics of the learning organization. The tension and conflict will be evidenced by questioning, inquiry, disequilibrium, and a challenging of the status quo. (p. 30) [425]

Luthans, Rubach, and Marsnik, *Going Beyond Total Quality*

Ah, conflict—can't live with it, can't live without it. As sociologist Randall Collins has pointed out, human beings are both sociable and conflict prone [453]. Conflict provides us with the drama of life. A movie, television drama, or novel without conflict is boring and life without conflict, even organizational life, is dull, flat, and stagnant.

But conflict in the workplace can be, as one author put it, "good, bad, or ugly" and in part, good or bad or ugly will be determined by the impact of stress [454]. Under conditions of acute stress, conflicts will be submerged as individuals, groups, and the organization as a whole struggle to cope with the emergency, rallying strong group pressure to produce unified group action. But under conditions of chronic and repetitive stress, old conflicts are likely to emerge again—with a vengeance—and new conflicts can be expected to develop as time constraints make it difficult for the normal mechanisms of conflict management to be utilized.

The mental health and social service literature is notable for its apparent lack of interest in the issue of conflict management in our workplace settings, though perhaps no other settings could be more prone to conflict, nor could successful conflict management be more important, since conflict is at the heart of emotional and relational difficulties. And yet, as one social worker in a children's residential treatment program pointed out, *"How can we possibly expect the children to resolve their conflicts when we cannot resolve the conflicts among us—and they see that every day."* The ways in which staff conflict affects service delivery are rarely mentioned, nor do most programs appear to have formal conflict management strategies that work consistently and effectively among and between various components of the organizations. So it is necessary, once again, to turn to the business literature to find a framework for understanding the issue of workplace conflict. In this section we will look at the nature of conflict, the different kinds of conflict, the relationship between conflict and emotional intelligence, the impact of conflict, and what happens to conflicting parties under the impact of chronic stress.

The Nature of Conflict

Conflict or disagreement is characterized by discord of action, feeling, or effect. A simple way of understanding conflict is that it arises when two or more individuals view a situation from different frames of reference and demand mutually exclusive outcomes [455]. Another simple definition is that conflict is a process in which one party perceives that its interests are being opposed or negatively affected by another party [456]. For many people the word *conflict* immediately generates a "mental collision," a perception that a quarrel, a fight, a battle, a competition, or a struggle is occurring. Under these circumstances, people's reaction to this conflict usually reflects their feelings of stress and creates both cognitive and physiological effects [457].

Because conflict is always with us, conflict has been a topic of enormous interest in the world of business and finance. Conflict, of course, is the bedrock of all forms of therapy, and yet relatively little has been written about conflict and conflict management in the human service system itself. This is despite the fact that virtually every mental health and social service setting is rife with conflict in part because we are human beings and human beings engage in conflict routinely. But also because there are fundamental aspects of these settings that breed conflict: differences in personality traits, race, age, gender, ethnicity—the various forms of diversity that affect every setting—but also differences in professional background, ideological framework, values, goals, and basic underlying beliefs about the clients and the role staff members are to play in the clients' lives. These sources of conflict, largely unexamined, have always been with us but have been exacerbated by the influence of the enormous changes that have impacted all of our caregiving systems. Brian describes the very diverse workplace that he helps to manage:

> *The interpersonal conflicts between staff in our organization are frequent and complex as are the sources. Our teams are made up of very diverse staff of different ages, ethnicities, races, genders, sexual orientations, educational levels, disciplines, religions, and all the various personal experiences that accompany these differences. It is extremely difficult to establish the communication necessary on a team that allows people to speak openly and honestly without attacking each other or feeling attacked. Milieu staff are supposed to be patient and supportive with the children in their care, but maintain some level of control. Clinical staff are supposed to understand why clients do the truly inexplicable things they do and suggest effective ways for others to intervene in situations that are dangerous, scary, and chaotic. Teachers are supposed to help children achieve academically, even as the child runs crying from the room every time he or she fails to understand a new concept. We all feel the weight of these expectations even if our coworkers couch their questions in the most gentle language imaginable. When we challenge each other, it is difficult to sort out whether this*

challenge is legitimate or because you think you are smarter than me or better than me.

Conflict is an interactive process manifested in incompatibility, disagreement, or dissonance within or between social entities, that is, between and among individuals, groups, and organizations. Conflict is most likely to occur when any of the following conditions are in play: *(1)* someone is required to engage in an activity that is incongruent with his or her needs or interests; *(2)* one person wants to take a course of action that is incompatible with another person's or the group's preferences; *(3)* there is competition for resources that are in short supply; *(4)* a person possesses attitudes, values, skills, goals, beliefs that strongly influence his or her behavior but are perceived to be contradictory to the attitudes, values, skills, goals, or beliefs of someone else; *(5)* two people (or more) disagree partially or totally about a joint action; and *(6)* people who disagree with each other are interdependent so they must come to some resolution [458]. Then there is the potential for conflicts that exists in five different levels when teams are working together: *(1)* between individual group members; *(2)* around the content of the issue; *(3)* the psychosocial context of the situation; *(4)* the method employed; *(5)* and how what they do or do not do affects others [459]. We would add to this list the enormity of conflicts that exist at the level of theory and mental models that may be completely unconscious assumptions among and between team members.

At the level of the individual group members, people experience a variety of psychological tensions and conflicts and are likely to express them within interpersonal work contexts. These tensions, colored by an individual's past experiences, beliefs, and values, may alter the person's perceptions, feelings, and behavior. The Adverse Childhood Experiences Study and a growing body of research indicate that regardless of the setting, a majority of workers within that setting are likely to have experienced childhood adversity themselves (Chapter 2). Unlike other less emotionally stimulating workplaces, mental health and social service settings are likely to trigger whatever unresolved memories or emotions are leftover from the workers' past lives and may lead to a variety of interpersonal conflicts with clients, their families, other staff members, and management. These effects are likely to be particularly potent whenever someone's safety is jeopardized. The more unsafe the treatment or service delivery environment is, the more likely that these intrapsychic and individual conflicts will play themselves out in the environment, often with detrimental results.

Methods chosen for decision making, problem solving, and simply getting work done may also be a source of conflict. The more complex and interdependent a system is, the more likely it is that a change in one area will produce reverberating changes throughout the system, and change creates conflict.

Leaders, pressured by time and demands for decisions from above, may use methods of problem solving that are not participatory, even though their decision may be the right decision to make and the one that would have come from a participatory process anyhow. But the method chosen—autocratic decision making—may end up creating more conflict, and therefore more problems, than a more participatory process would have created.

And then, always, there is the issue of conflict between one component of a system, like a team, and other teams or components within the organization and conflicts between the organization as a whole and other components of the wider system. It is not unusual in institutional settings to have conflicts between different shifts and different professional groups. And there are usually conflicts between institutions, state regulatory agencies, and funding sources.

But these very rational definitions of conflict leave out the most troubling aspect of all conflict situations: distressing emotions. To be in conflict is to be emotionally activated. In fact, human conflict does not exist in the absence of emotions, and dealing successfully with conflict requires the development of both individual and organizational emotional intelligence [460].

Conflict and Emotional Intelligence

Most importantly, conflict generates high levels of distressing emotion, endangering emotional management on an individual and group level, and dependent on the levels of emotional intelligence that every member of the community is able to achieve. Because conflict evokes emotion, conflict in the workplace has largely been seen as bad or dysfunctional and an interference with the smooth running of any operation, similar to the ways in which emotions at work have tended to be downplayed, considered irrational and counterproductive. To be in conflict is to be in an emotionally charged situation. There probably is no such thing as a purely intellectual conflict. Human emotions and thought are too hardwired together. Effectively managing conflict in the workplace requires the development of emotional intelligence in individuals within the organization and in the organization as a whole.

When people or groups are in conflict, it is never a purely intellectual affair. Our cognitive processes are always being affected by our emotions and when we are in conflict situations, levels of emotional arousal rise significantly for a variety of reasons, some of which are individual and some of which, like emotional contagion, are a product of the group [383]. When conflicts are resolved in a group, the emotion of the group converges. Fear in a group appears to be associated with negative emotions, and in terms of task performance, there is empirical evidence that at least some fear is an essential ingredient that prods us toward change, while high levels of fear lead to impaired decision making [461].

So emotion and conflict go hand in hand and are complexly interrelated. Emotional arousal can cause conflict, can be the product of conflict, and can result from the resolution of conflict [461]. In fact, emotional arousal is what keeps conflicts in play, and it is conflict that propels change. Research has shown that the higher the level of emotional intelligence, the better able employees are to manage stress and conflict and the higher their organizational commitment [462].

Different Kinds of Conflict

If organizations are viewed as machines, then conflict is viewed as an evil that must be eliminated because it creates disorder in an otherwise supposedly orderly world. When this kind of philosophical position is in play, conflict is viewed as a problem of poor design or inadequate structure that must be corrected through more elaborate job descriptions, greater exercise of authority, or through the active suppression of or passive avoidance of conflict. But organizations that must respond creatively to complex problems and that must change rapidly to accommodate changing circumstances must have the ability to successfully manage and even promote conflict or they will stagnate. Conflict creates opportunities for organizational and individual learning and must be harnessed in service of the collective goals. But not all conflict is the same [454].

Research evidence indicates that interpersonal conflict impedes group performance by limiting the ability of individuals and groups to process information and to think well [463–466]. It also diminishes group loyalty, team commitment, intent to stay at the organization, and job satisfaction because of escalation in levels of stress and anxiety [458; 463–465; 467]. High levels of personal conflict are associated with bad performance; if people are fighting because of personal animus, they are less likely to accomplish their tasks. It is also true that group members should neither like each other too much, if too much liking squelches dissent, and they should not like each other too little, if too little liking creates personal tension [468]. As one researcher states it, *"relationship conflicts interfere with task-related effort because members focus on reducing threats, increasing power, and attempting to build cohesion rather than working on task.... The conflict causes members to be negative, irritable, suspicious, and resentful"* (pp. 531–532) [467]. Conflict over process is generally harmful as well—a finding that makes sense in light of the risk that if people argue over process, they will spend less time doing what they are supposed to do [469]. The bottom line is that if people in a group do not like each other and as a result spend their time in personal conflict, the group as a whole will perform badly.

However, "substantive conflict" also known as "task-related conflict" happens when two or more organizational members disagree on their task or disagree on the recognition and solution to a particular problem. Research indicates that a moderate level of substantive conflict is good for an organization or a team because it stimulates discussion and debate and urges a group on to a higher level of performance [548; 470]. Groups that report task-oriented conflict generally have higher performance because there is more likely to be the sharing of various viewpoints and alternative solutions [464–465; 470–472]. This is particularly true for groups performing tasks that were not routine and that require complex problem solutions. Groups that report substantive conflict are also able to make better decisions than those that do not because substantive conflict encourages greater understanding of the issues and that leads to better decisions [463; 473–476].

However, in real life situations, interpersonal conflict and task conflict often occur simultaneously. Conflict over the content of task-related issues can be very useful, but emotion inevitably accompanies conflict and the "heat" of a conflict over tasks can spill over into interpersonal conflict rather easily. Without good conflict management skills in the group, task-related conflict can lead to misunderstanding, miscommunication, and increased team dysfunction. In many teams that have been working together for some time, roles are clearly delineated: one person is the arguer, one person is the creative one, and another individual is passive, while still another tries to settle disputes. Psychosocial conflict arises when a group member feels pressure from the group to assume a role which they do not want or for which they do not feel prepared or when the group constrains someone from changing his or her assigned role when he or she wishes to do so. In many mental health settings, role is determined by professional training and the rigid hierarchy so typical of the medical model. Psychosocial conflicts may arise when changes are suggested that encourage greater participation in decision making of staff members who are lower in the command hierarchy, and especially when structures are created that encourage more participation of clients. The bottom line is that interpersonal conflict and task conflict are inversely related. The more interpersonal conflict there is, the less people will feel safe having healthy disagreements over how to complete a task or solve a problem, and that is bad for organizational well-being.

Conflict Management Strategies

There is a difference between *conflict resolution* and *conflict management*. Similar to the idea of emotional management, conflict management does not imply that conflicts should be avoided, reduced, or even terminated. Instead, it suggests that conflicts must be properly managed so that the dysfunctional impact of conflict is minimized while the constructive functions of conflict are maximized to produce greater organizational effectiveness [458]. But different people have different strategies for handling conflict. Some people face conflict directly and focus on problem solving, collaborating, and integrating various points of view. Others tend to be "peace makers" who try to minimize conflict, smooth the waters, and will yield to others. A third group of people try to maximize their own outcomes at the expense of others through domination, control, competing, and forcing. A fourth group try to avoid conflict altogether by withdrawing, refusing to engage, or not taking action [477]. Different people use different strategies at different times, and part of emotional intelligence is being able to be flexible and apply the right strategy at the most appropriate moment.

There are signs that indicate whether conflict management strategies are adequate to the needs of the organization. Some indicators that conflict management strategies are insufficient include organizational conflicts that run on for years without really changing; a general attitude that conflict-laden problems will never be resolved or even addressed; a predominance of private complaining with little attempt to fix the problem; staff who show little interest in working on common goals but spend significant time and energy protecting themselves or their own interest or just whining and complaining. These are frequently signs of some pathological organizational strategies that have led to this outcome, including non-action, administrative "orbiting," secrecy, and a "law and order" approach.

In *non-action*, conflict is simply ignored or denied with the end result of a significant escalation of conflict. In *administrative orbiting*, managers put people off by telling them that "we are dealing with the problem" but in reality the problem never gets addressed. Management may in fact produce many stalls, including "we are collecting more data," "we are documenting performance," "we cancelled that meeting," and "we have called in a consultant." Another way of avoiding conflict is through *secrecy* and both managers and employees can utilize this approach. Although secrecy may work in the short term to keep people from knowing what is happening, in group settings secrets have a way of inevitably leaking out through the grapevine and when that happens, conflict is escalated even further. Yet another way of not addressing conflict directly is through invoking a *"law and order"* strategy, by leaning on people to repress the outward manifestation of conflict, which does little except to drive the conflict underground where it can grow in destructive power [454].

Many of the existing conflict resolution strategies such as dispute resolution, negotiation and bargaining, mediation, and arbitration can be very useful in minimizing emotional conflict, but they do not necessitate significant change in the organization. Finding and maintaining the right level of task-related conflict, however, is likely to require shifts in fundamental organizational approaches toward double-loop kinds of learning (see later discussion) [458].

Conflict Management Under Stress

As we discussed in Chapter 4, when stress is acute, as when an organizational crisis occurs, interpersonal conflict is likely to be submerged to serve the interests of the group. Human beings tend to "circle the wagons" under conditions of acute stress and mobilize powerful group forces to deal with the crisis. Individual and group conflict and competitive strivings that normally exist between people are always a threat to rapid, unified action during a crisis. Efforts must be made to minimize the normal tensions, conflicts, and aggressive behaviors that inevitably arise in any group. Leadership emerges within the group, and frequently an external enemy is targeted that helps to mobilize in-group bonds.

It is likely that at this point "defensive routines" will be employed that consist of procedures, policies, practices, and actions that prevent employees from having to experience embarrassment or threat. This *"makes it highly likely that individuals, groups, intergroups, and organizations will not detect and correct errors that are embarrassing and threatening because the fundamental rules are 1) bypass the errors and act as if they were not being done, 2) make the bypass undiscussable, 3) make its undiscussability undiscussable"* (p. 43) [458; 478].

The external enemy becomes the object upon whom the group can project all its own negative emotions and desires in service of group cohesion. Blame for the crisis is sought, and the search commences for an external enemy or scapegoat who will shoulder this blame. The more externalized the blame can be, the more the blaming behavior will increase group cohesion as internal conflict is projected externally. The greater the consistency between this psychosocial need and actual events, the easier it becomes to define friend and foe. The greater the perceived differences between "us" and "them," the greater the ease in labeling the enemy and doing whatever it takes to defend "us"[348–351]. Under these circumstances, in mental health settings, there are times when the patient becomes "the enemy," particularly when the behavior of a patient has resulted in staff injury, or when an individual staff member or the institution itself is threatened with a lawsuit, newspaper exposure, or some other public embarrassment. If this goes on for too long, a "blame culture," as we described in Chapter 5, is likely to emerge and can become a part of the permanent organizational culture.

Chronic stress has other impacts on workers. As work-related stressors increase, employees develop negative perceptions of their coworkers as well as the organization as a whole and this may precipitate serious decreases in job performance. Negative interpersonal relationships and the absence of support from colleagues and superiors is a major stressor for many workers. Social support in the form of group cohesion, interpersonal trust, and liking for a supervisor is associated with decreased levels of perceived job strain and better health. On the other hand, unsupportive or inconsiderate behavior from a supervisor appears to contribute significantly to job strain [479–480]. Although the direct effect of social support on stress has been extensively researched, it is only recently that focus has been directed at examining the interaction of social support with a "buffering effect," which suggests that the relationship between stress and outcomes is dependent upon the amount of social support available. For example, coworker support had a more pervasive buffering effect than did support from either supervisor or from one's non-work context [481].

Chronic Conflict and Organizational Learning

Conflict is a necessary component of a learning environment because conflict is a necessary component of learning. Conflict spurs motivation and the desire for change. When organizations cannot deal directly with conflict using methods that utilize good conflict management skills, the organization cannot learn from its own mistakes and error is likely to become systemic. Employees develop escalating negative feelings about the organization that include loss of trust or pride in the organization, resulting in diminished dedication and commitment; an increase in political or self-protective behavior; contemplated or real job transfers; petty revenge or sabotage; lack of any extra effort; making and hiding mistakes or failing to meet deadlines or budgets; loss of effective problem solving, performing work on the wrong priorities and poor methods; loss of creativity, motivation, and risk taking; negative feelings about oneself, loss of self-esteem, self-criticism; negative emotions of anger, frustration, depression, disappointment, disillusionment, and tension; and deepening cultures of cynicism (pp. 111–116) [109].

When these defensive maneuvers are in place and conflict can be neither overtly surfaced nor resolved, it is highly likely that an organization will engage in the repetition of past strategies, whether they have been a failure or not. An initial error, therefore, becomes compounded and when repeated becomes a systematic error. Under stress, lacking social support, and unable to see the larger system influences that are at work, people become frustrated and angry with their coworkers, supervisors, and managers, whom they can see. As a result, interpersonal conflicts increase and this leads to further decreases in collective efficacy [482]. Hierarchical structures concentrate power, and in these circumstances, power can easily come to be used abusively and in a way that perpetuates rather than attenuates the concentration of power. Under these conditions, transparency disappears and secrecy increases. Communication networks become compromised as those in power become more punishing, and the likelihood of error is increased as a result.

In such a situation, conflicts tend to remain unresolved, and tension and resentment mount under the surface of everyday group functioning. Interpersonal conflicts that were suppressed during the initial crisis return, often with a vengeance, but conflict resolution mechanisms, if ever in place, deteriorate under stress. Helplessness, passivity, and passive-aggressive behaviors on the part of the underlings in the hierarchy increase, while leaders become increasingly controlling and punitive. In this way the organization becomes ever more radically split, with different parts of the organization assuming the role of managing and/or expressing different emotions that are then subsequently suppressed. Such conditions as these make an organization ripe for collective disturbance (Chapter 8) that may go unresolved and unrecognized, while policy changes are made that ensure the underlying conflicts will remain out of conscious group awareness.

Conclusion

Under stress, emotional regulation, which is challenging at the best of times, becomes even more difficult to manage and organizations can become dysregulated and hyperreactive. Emotion builds up, conflicts increase, and tensions mount. Problem solving, communication, and interpersonal relationships become disrupted. If leaders are not mindful of this process, things can go very wrong very fast, and, as we will see in Chapter 7, that profoundly affects the organizational ability to learn, remember, and make good decisions.

Chapter 7

Organizational Learning Disabilities and Organizational Amnesia

SUMMARY: *Under the conditions we have been describing, stress interferes with organizational learning, organizational memory is lost, organizational amnesia affects function, and service delivery becomes increasingly fragmented. Decision making becomes compromised and reactive so that short-sighted policy decisions are made that appear to compound existing problems. Dissent is silenced, leading to simplification of decisions and lowered morale. The organization has become learning disabled.*

Organizational Learning Disabilities

Call it escalation of commitment, organizational defensiveness, learning disability—or even more bluntly—executive blindness. It is a phenomenon of behavior in organizations that has been widely recognized. Organizational members become committed to a pattern of behavior. They escalate their commitment to that pattern out of self-justification. In a desire to avoid embarrassment and threat, few if any challenges are made to the wisdom and viability of these behaviors. They persist even when rapid and fundamental shifts in the competitive environment render these patterns of behavior obsolete and destructive to the well-being of the organization. (p. 642) [483]

Beer and Spector (1993), *Organizational Diagnosis:
Its Role in Organizational Learning*

Organizational learning is mentioned frequently these days, but what exactly is it? The idea is that organizations exist in a constant state of interaction with their external environment, and as the external environment changes, the organization must learn to adapt. The concept implies that organizational learning is both a cognitive and social process; that it involves capturing, storing, and diffusing knowledge within the organization. It is the product of certain organizational arrangements and decisions and it often involves reassessing fundamental assumptions and values. Traditionally, organizational learning begins with learning at the individual level and then involves diffusing the knowledge generated to other parts of the organization. The end result of organizational learning is organizational adaptation and value creation [484].

The pace of change in the world in general has radically increased, and the biggest danger to adaptation is a sense of complacency and contentment with the status quo that is both dangerous and unproductive. What is missing, as organizational consultant John Kotter points out, is a "sense of urgency" which is rare and *"immeasurably important in a rapidly changing world"* (p. 10). It requires leadership up and down the organizational hierarchy; a recognition and appreciation for the hazards involved in change; a powerful desire to move and make a difference; urgent activity that is alert, fast, focused, relentless, and continuously overcoming irrelevant activities so that time for what is important is available and measures are in place to prevent burnout [485].

It is this sense of urgency that we need in all human services. People's lives are at stake. And for the children in our services, their developmental trajectory is at stake. In a very literal way, the composition of their brains is being determined by every moment that these children spend exposed to unbuffered and unrelenting external threat. Every disrupted attachment experience is all too likely to do more harm than good as a result. Childhood and adolescence provide windows of opportunity to help even the most injured of children, but those windows close much faster than our present time schedules for intervention and treatment allow.

Unfortunately chronic stress can produce what Kotter discusses as a "false sense of urgency" and what we call "organizational learning disabilities" when *"organizational members become committed to a pattern of behavior and escalate that commitment even when these patterns are obsolete and destructive to the organization's well-being"* [483]. We make the case that the human service delivery system as a whole has developed learning disabilities as a result of exposure to chronic and unrelenting stress.

Chronic Stress Interferes With Learning and Adaptation

All of the stressors we reviewed earlier, as well as the distressing emotions associated with them, are likely to interfere with the capacity of staff and managers to take in new information and change. As we have discussed, cognitive processes change radically under the impact of chronic stress. This tends to drive individuals and organizations to repeat what is automatic and has worked in the past, thus interfering with adaptation to changing conditions. The "case of the separated garbage" that we described in Chapter 1 is an accurate representation of what is commonly noted in every organization that has been around for awhile. As Brian notes:

> We take things in our organizational evolutionary past and carry them forward, even if they no longer make sense in the present. We do not learn

new tricks because we are too stressed to see the need or even have a conversation about the need. Learning is uneven in an organization, and this may create different struggles. One area of a program takes on a new piece of knowledge and another does not. This can cause misalignment in the organization, and we may not be aware of the source of the discrepancy. The work we do is enormously complicated and requires high levels of team work. But the stress of the work and the reduction of resources have made this collaboration seemingly impossible. There are a variety of issues that undercut knowledge development and retention in an organization. It is not as simple as downsizing, or tightening of budgets. It is the result of the totality of stress in an organization.

What Is the Increase in Value We Are Aiming for?

Let's use mental health as an example of the problem we are addressing. What is the "value creation" in the clinical world? Unlike the business sector, the value in mental health services is not as easy to measure since it relates to changes in human performance over a long trajectory and connects complexly to so many other interrelated problems. But as we discussed in Chapter 1, it is clear that enormous value is lost to a society by the toll of mental illness and social dysfunction. Unfortunately, the value that is presently placed on the human service delivery system is almost purely related to dollars spent and dollars saved in the short term. Public funding streams tend to be influenced by the political climate, which may change every few years. Private funding is based on foundations, which are subject to economic ebbs and flows, or for-profit corporations that are accountable to their stockholders for making a profit over a relatively short term. Programs that work are not brought to scale, and innovation is too financially risky. Programs that are effective are often abruptly terminated because the local, state, or national political climate changed and all programs in the public sector are particularly vulnerable to politics.

Effective human services would also prevent problems, and prevention is notoriously difficult to measure. If we spend $100,000 on a residential placement of a child, how do we know that money was well spent until the child grows up? How do we know what would have happened had the child not had that placement? Would the child have gone to jail? Would the child have committed suicide or killed someone else? These are critical questions but impossible to answer: you cannot prove a negative; you cannot substantiate what would *not have happened.* It is difficult to define the return we are looking for and therefore exceedingly difficult to measure it other than in very short-term and sometimes short-sighted ways. The potential value of having an effective human service delivery system can only be measured in longer time frames than are usually employed and that would extend across political administrations, regardless of political views. With adequate treatment and a trauma-informed approach, we should be able to measure not just individual improvement but intergenerational changes. But unless we adopt a longer term point of view this will never happen. And unless this happens, it is difficult for an organization to learn the best ways to approach complex problems.

No Time for Process—Failure of Integration

A way of understanding how organizations learn is by using a framework that involves four processes of learning: intuiting, interpreting, integrating, and institutionalizing. Intuiting occurs when an individual recognizes a pattern or possibility in a situation and shares this intuition with the organization. Through a process of interpretation, the intuition is discussed and refined through a social activity involving the group, producing a convergence of meaning. Integration involves the development of coherent collective action that helps develop a new understanding of how to adapt so that learning takes place at the group level and is linked to the organizational level. Institutionalizing occurs when the learning becomes embedded in systems, structure, procedures, and organizational culture [486].

Today in many human service environments there is a strong bias against anything that implies the need for "process discussions." The advent of behaviorism and biological reductionism justified the elimination of the kinds of broad-ranging discussions that helped people to learn together about the complex nature of human problems and problem solving, most importantly how to integrate scientific knowledge about the body and brain with treatment planning, behavioral support, family patterns, and intrapsychic needs.

What behaviorism didn't eliminate, managed care has. Time for complex discussions, case conferences, and retreats has been virtually eliminated in many settings that previously provided the opportunity for the individual and organizational learning of new information to take place. In many cases these activities have simply ceased to exist, largely because they are not reimbursed and are seen as interfering with demands for increased productivity. There are no research and development departments nor are there knowledge officers assigned to figure out how to retain important information.

The result of all this is a failure of integration across all institutional levels. It is difficult to find a mental health organization where there is one shared theoretical based—and there may be *no* shared theoretical basis for the work people are doing at all. But the hallmark of higher intelligence is integration. In his brilliant book on the prehistory of the mind, archeologist Steven Mithin described three phases for the evolution of the human mind: the development of the domain of general intelligence, then of specialized intelligences that work in isolation from each other, and then the integration of these specialized intelligences into a cognitively fluid, interactive whole. It is this last phase, the integration of various ideas that cannot be achieved without considerable *process.* We have spent over a century developing specialized intelligences in the human services, but what they largely do is compete with each other for attention—including funding for research and the delivery of services. Our fields of endeavor have not yet achieved the breakthrough step of integrating all that we know into a cohesive whole. The dimly held vision of possibility for this level of integration is what excites so many people when they learn about the impact of trauma, adversity, and disrupted attachment. What emerges is a clear sense that to deal with the complexity of psychological injuries, we will have to draw upon *all* forms of therapeutic engagement. In a study of residential treatment centers for children, there were on average, twenty-one different approaches [487]. But that there were twenty-one different approaches is less the problem than that these approaches are not held together and integrated in any meaningful way. As a result instead of having emerging and higher order, we often end up with chaos.

Wisdom Walks out the Door and Is Not Replaced

Extensive research on corporate knowledge concludes that *"knowledge exists in two forms: explicit knowledge, which is easily codified and shared asynchronously, and tacit knowledge, which is experiential, intuitive, and communicated most effectively in face-to-face encounters."* (p. xxxviii) [488] Explicit knowledge can be articulated with formal language. It is that which can be recorded and stored. But even keeping track of explicit knowledge is tricky. Keeping records in order, grant applications in one place, and organizing policies and procedures and other vital information is challenging in highly stressed environments. Things get lost easily because the person working on a project finishes and moves on. To retain information in ways that make future access possible there must be a plan, resources to hire people and machines to store the information, and methods for later retrieving that data. These are time-consuming and expensive processes, but computer technology has made it far more likely that explicit knowledge might be captured.

It's another story with tacit knowledge which is that knowledge which is used to interpret the information. Tacit knowledge is more difficult to articulate with language and lies in the values, beliefs, and perspectives of the system [484; 488]. From an organizational point of view it is *"collectively enacted knowledge"* (p. 869) [489]. There is a widespread failure to capture tacit knowledge because Western culture has come to value results—the output of the work process—far above the process itself, to emphasize things over relationships, doing over thinking [490]. In the mental health world, tacit knowledge has often been referred to as clinical "wisdom" or "intuition", or the much-maligned "anecdotal experience". Although frequently widely agreed upon, clinical wisdom is difficult to test and is therefore vulnerable to getting lost in the present demand for "evidence-based" practices. In the current environment, information that does not have "evidence," meaning a sufficient number of double-blind, controlled studies, is more likely than ever to be discounted as meaningless and this determines what gets funded. But in the effort to provide methods of helping people that have been shown to be effective, we are in danger of retaining only explicit knowledge and losing the equally valuable tacit knowledge within the mental health and social service system as a whole. And that knowledge constitutes centuries of hard-earned wisdom.

Tacit, intuitive, experiential knowledge about the inner workings of the human mind and human group behavior has historically been interpreted, integrated, and ultimately institutionalized within care giving organizations through the sharing of information among a clinical team and in supervisory sessions. In what were frequently prolonged and extensive discussions focused on the many lenses through which that information could be interpreted, individuals, subgroups within an organization and the organization as a whole, could synthesize explicit and tacit information into a working model of the whole human being. Not only was the biological interpretive lens valued, but so too were the psychodynamic, the family systems, the behavioral, the creative, the sociological, the philosophical, and the spiritual lenses.

But biological hypotheses are easier to test, more likely to get funded with research dollars, encouraged by big pharmaceutical corporations, and viewed as less costly. So for the last several decades, the explicit knowledge that has been generated from biological research has come to dominate the treatment environment to such an extent, that in many environments it is all anyone talks about. There are also profound splits between academic research departments who depend on continual grants for their survival and the vast numbers of clinicians out in the field, engaging with the complex problems of individual children and adults as well as their families and communities. The grant money— and therefore the attainment of "evidence-based" status goes to the researchers who have the resources to obtain and manage the grant moneys to do research only on methods that will fit into the achievement of an evidence-base that will get them more grant money.

As a result, a full understanding of the human being labeled as the patient, a human being living within and interacting with his or her personal, social, political, and economic environment, becomes meaningless. Whatever does not get adequate funding in our society becomes irrelevant simply because it has no funding to support it. Important knowledge—perhaps even knowledge that is vital to human survival—is thereby lost to the system. A colleague shared this vignette with Sandy:

> *Visiting an acute care adult psychiatric inpatient unit one day, a consultant sat in on "rounds." The head psychiatrist, wearing what is now the ever-present symbol of medical authority, the white coat, was clearly in charge of the discussion in the meeting. The conversation about every patient consisted of five*

fundamental questions: the date of admission, the diagnosis (es), the medica-
tions the person was on, recent events (in abbreviated form and mostly about
drug effects), and the proposed date of discharge. When the consultant heard of
the recent suicide attempt and the decision to diagnose a formerly healthy and
high-functioning young woman with major depressive disorder, she broke into
the rapidly moving meeting and asked if anything had happened to the woman
in the past year that could explain this deterioration. Silence broke out in the
room and the obviously irritated psychiatrist looked at the social worker in
charge of the case who, paging through the patient's history, reported that yes,
the young woman had been raped the year before. Not only was the past history
seemingly irrelevant to the clinical team, but upon further probing, the team
was unable to even formulate how the previous rape and the depressive episode
might be related, much less what role the staff could or should be playing in
addressing the past traumatic experience. Without meaningful clinical exchange,
organizational learning had, for the most part, come to a halt and team meet-
ings had deteriorated into relatively meaningless ritualistic behaviors.

Labeling That Prevents the Expansion of Knowledge

Individuals create certain ways of knowing, or schemas, that serve to reduce uncertainty. Organizations, too, are said to create interpretive schemes or frames of reference to filter information that is considered within an organization. These organizational-level schemas may then block, obscure, simplify, or misrepresent some of the information that the organization must process and remember [491]. The diagnostic system created by the American Psychiatric Association is an extremely influential filtering system for the mental health professions. *The Diagnostic and Statistic Manual* has become a method for reducing, or at least trying to reduce, the uncertainty that has always accompanied "madness."

Just consider a simple example. A child is physically and sexually abused and when the abuse is reported to child welfare, the child is taken into custody. Unfortunately, this situation alone does not necessarily warrant therapy in our present system. Once the child fails placement in a series of foster homes, the child's acting out leads to a mental health evaluation and the child is given a diagnosis such as "oppositional defiant disorder" or "conduct disorder." Treatment may or may not be effective, but in all likelihood, this is a child who will end up in a psychiatric hospital, residential treatment center, or juvenile justice facility. But the problem has been subtly relocated. Now from the perspective of the child and everyone else who has to deal with him, the problem is centered in the child. The social context that allows so many children to suffer torture when they are young and then experience multiple disrupted attachments is pushed aside.

Using the ancient method of giving a name to what we most fear, we give madness names and descriptions and believe therefore that it is less frightening and more manageable. However, staff members, particularly line staff who are not trained to understand that these are only oversimplified and reductionistic descriptive labels for which we have no agreed-upon etiology, begin to reduce the patients to the diagnoses they carry. In doing so, the patient, whether a child or adult, is automatically dehumanized and pathologized in ways neither the client nor the staff really understand.

Unless patients are willing to pay out of pocket, the only way they can enter the mental health system is to get a diagnosis. The diagnosis then carefully filters what can and cannot be discussed, understood, and shared. The diagnosis implies expected behavior consistent with that diagnosis. Because our minds are set to see what we expect, the diagnosis cues a staff member to expect certain behaviors, provides an explanatory framework for that behavior, and thus minimizes curiosity about what the behavior may actually mean. Being social creatures, and thus vulnerable to being influenced by other people's expectations, the patients respond with the expected behavior. In this way a diagnosis easily becomes a self-fulfilling prophecy.

The sociologist Thomas Scheff described this labeling process years ago, but his work and the work of those like him is little discussed today because it is inconvenient and because it leads to an increase in uncertainty that cannot be tolerated, particularly in a stressed environment [492–494]. The information that has been most systematically screened out via this mechanism is the impact of previous traumatic experience on the evolution of so many diagnostic categories. The traumatic origins of what is perhaps a majority of behavioral dysfunction is enormously threatening to this hugely embracing categorization system that the mental health profession has adopted to feel more secure in a shifting world.

So powerful are the suggestive effects of diagnosis, in fact, that in the early 1970s David Rosenhan experimentally demonstrated that labeling can create a false reality. In an article originally published in *Science* [495], eight pseudo-patients—a psychology grad student, three psychologists, a pediatrician, a psychiatrist, a painter, and a housewife—agreed to be experimental subjects and gained secret admission to 12 different hospitals. Those who were mental health professionals said they were in other occupations, and they used pseudonyms to hide their identity. The pseudo-patients' single complaint was that they had been "hearing voices" that were unclear, but sounded like "empty," "hollow," and "thud." Beyond alleging the symptoms of hearing voices and falsifying name, vocation, and employment, no further alterations of the pseudo-patients' person, history, or circumstances was made. None of their histories or current behavior, other than the report of hearing voices, was pathological in any way.

Immediately upon admission—and they were all readily admitted—the pseudo-patients ceased simulating any symptoms of abnormality, including hearing voices. In some cases there was some nervousness over being admitted so easily to a psychiatric unit, but other than that they behaved as they would behave normally. Each pseudo-patient was told that there was no foreknowledge of when they would be discharged—that they would have to get out of the hospital by their own devices, essentially by convincing the staff that they were sane. As a result, they were paragons of cooperation and were not disruptive in any way. But despite their show of sanity, the pseudo-patients were never detected. In all but one case they were admitted with a diagnosis of schizophrenia and discharged with a diagnosis of schizophrenia in remission. The average length of stay was 19 days, although the length of hospitalization varied from 7 to 52 days. Visitors and other patients were frequently able to recognize that the pseudo-patient was not ill at all, but the staff could not. *"As far as I can determine, diagnoses were in no way affected by the relative health of the circumstances of a pseudo-patient's life. Rather, the reverse occurred; the perception of his circumstances was shaped entirely by the diagnosis.... Having once been labeled schizophrenic, there is nothing the pseudo-patient can do to overcome the tag. The tag profoundly colors others' perceptions of him and his behavior.... The facts of the case were unintentionally distorted by the staff to achieve consistency with a popular theory of the dynamics of a schizophrenic reaction"* (pp. 60–61) [496].

In another experiment, Temerlin took a normal, healthy man, recorded an interview with him, and then played the audio interview to psychiatrists, clinical psychologists, and graduate students in clinical psychology. Just before listening to the interview, the experimental group heard a professional person with high prestige, who was acting as a confederate in the study, say that the individual to be diagnosed was "a very interesting man because he looked neurotic but actually was quite psychotic." The control group did not hear this suggestion. No control subject ever diagnosed psychosis, while 60% of the psychiatrists, 28% of the psychologists, and 11% of the graduate students diagnosed this normal man as psychotic after hearing the suggestion of the expert [497].

If these studies were replicated today, would the results be the same? We can only speculate, but we suspect that although it would be harder for the pseudo-patients in the first study to be admitted to a hospital, they would still likely be labeled as psychotic, and as their labels accompanied them they would find it extremely difficult to shed the diagnosis. Not only that, but they would probably be prescribed powerful antipsychotic medications. Once the diagnosis is in place and unquestioned—as it rarely is in highly stressed environments—it is likely to become self-fulfilling as each subsequent professional believes the assumed expertise and accuracy reflected in the patient's chart and treats the patient accordingly. If the patient is diagnosed not as psychotic, but as having a personality disorder, the course of treatment is unlikely to be a pretty one. Because personality disorders are so loaded with connotations not of sickness but of badness, people carrying the diagnosis of borderline personality disorder or antisocial personality disorder, for example, are likely to be shunned, seen as "manipulative" and "attention seeking," and repeatedly rejected and avoided regardless of the legitimacy of their complaints. Brian gives a personal experiences with exactly this type of problem:

> *Some years ago I did a site visit at an agency, and in the course of that visit I was reviewing a chart. The boy's picture was in the chart, and I was struck by the picture because he looked just like a friend of mine, only much younger. I guess that kind of jolted me out of my mental set for a few minutes. My friend was a great guy and when I saw the picture, I thought, "Wow, how did this kid, who reminds me so much of my friend, end up here in a program for juvenile offenders?" So I read his chart and from all accounts he had had really bad conflicts with his mom. He threatened her one night and she called the police. He was arrested and ended up being placed in the facility I was visiting. It seemed he ended up there because his home was getting more volatile and someone thought he would be better off in the facility. But he had been placed in a unit with other boys who had a history of much more serious offending than he did. When I noticed this, I asked about the agency admissions and utilization review process, because it seemed to me that this boy was not appropriately placed. But when I asked the staff about this, they became furious with me and insisted that it was inappropriate to base my critique on one kid. I emphasized that, sure, he was just one kid, but he was a kid who had a conflict with his mom, ended up in a program for serious juvenile offenders, had been there already 8 months, and had not been involved in a single problematic incident. I thought maybe that meant he hadn't been properly placed. But the staff did not agree. Basically, their attitude was that if he was there, he should be there. End of discussion.*

Self-Fulfilling Prophecies: Setting the Trap for Reenactment

According to sociologist Robert Merton, who first discussed self-fulfilling prophecies (SFPs) in 1948, an SFP occurs when a false belief leads to its own fulfillment, and he noted that these had the potential to produce significant social problems. Research bearing on his analysis has supported both the existence of SFPs and the impact they can have. It's about expectancy. Being inherently social creatures, once an expectation is set we tend to act in ways that are consistent with those expectations. Our expectations then seem to make it come true. If those expectations expect something good to come from us, then good is more likely to emerge. So, too, the opposite occurs. Self-fulfilling prophecies describe the mechanics of how reenactment behavior unfolds.

In 1971 Robert Rosenthal, a professor of social psychology at Harvard University, described an experiment in which he told a group of students that he had developed a strain of super-intelligent rats that could run mazes quickly. He then passed out perfectly normal rats at random, telling half of the students that they had the new "maze-bright" rats and the other half that they got "maze-dull" rats. The rats believed to be bright improved daily in running the maze. They ran faster and more accurately. The "dull" rats refused to budge from the starting point 29% of the time, while the "bright" rats refused only 11% of the time. According to Rosenthal, *"those experimenters who had been led to expect better performance viewed their animals as brighter, more pleasant, and more likable. These same experimenters felt more relaxed in their contacts with the animals and described their behavior toward them as more pleasant, friendly, and enthusiastic and less talkative. They also stated that they handled their rats more and also more gently than did the experimenters expecting poor performance"* (p. 841) [498]. Robert Rosenthal and Lenore Jacobson, in 1968, gave all the children in 18 classrooms a test and randomly chose 20% of the children from each room and told the teachers they were "intellectual bloomers" (though they were actually average). They came back at the end of the school year and tested the same class. The experimental children showed average IQ gains of two points in verbal ability, seven points in reasoning, and four points in overall IQ [498–499].

Brian describes how he sees these SFPs unfolding, even in a school for kids who already have problems:

Recently we have had a spike in property damage at the school. Kids tear stuff off the bulletin boards and people say, "Why bother decorating the boards when they will just ruin them?" So the bulletin boards are bare, the place looks drab and depressing, and we all feel like we are working in a bad prison movie. The behavior of the kids escalates and a hole gets kicked in the wall. It gets repaired a few times, but the response time for the repair gets slower and slower. So more holes appear. We then come to expect that the walls will be damaged, and people stop trying to do anything about it. Then the same thing starts happening in the classroom. Dysregulated kids cannot function in class and so they are removed. Of course, they come to us with long histories of poor school performance and when they get to us, we expect that they will perform poorly. They end up out of class more than they are in class, so they learn less, so they fall further behind, and their sense of being too stupid to learn is confirmed.

So think about the ways in which we are creating self-fulfilling prophecies all the time without recognizing that is happening. What expectations are we setting when we diagnose a child with oppositional disorder or conduct disorder? Or an adult with borderline personality disorder? What expectation are we setting when the first thing a very disoriented patient encounters when he or she enters an acute care unit is a seclusion room? What message are we giving to people seeking shelter when the facility is dark, dingy, cramped, and falling apart? What expectations are in place when insurance companies do not reimburse for team meetings or treatment discussions and consultations? Look around and listen. What are the expectations at your workplace that are being set without anything at all having to be said?

In the last decade alone there has been a 40-fold increase in children diagnosed with bipolar disorder, which may be due to an amazing amount of under-diagnosis in the past, contaminants in the food or water, or may bear a relationship with new marketable drugs for the treatment of bipolar disorder [500]. But has anyone considered the potential ramifications on psychological health, self-esteem, and social adjustment with labeling even very young children with a diagnosis of a major mental illness? Over 4 million children in the United States alone have been diagnosed with attention-deficit/hyperactivity disorder (ADHD). How many of them were screened for exposure to childhood adversity and chronic hyperarousal as a response to traumatic conditions? Screening for the complexity behind these children's problems takes time and taking time decreases productivity. It is far simpler to prescribe a drug and center the problem in the child.

The nature of self-fulfilling prophecies helps us to understand how someone establishes expectations based on previous life experiences and then unwittingly sets up a retraumatizing scenario. For example, a child is sexually abused by her father. Many other kinds of interactions may occur with that adult, but the behavior that is most frightening will have the most value in terms of riveting attention. The data the child selects are that she is bad, dirty, seductive, and worthless as anything other than a sexual object. She concludes that she is indeed bad and that adult men cannot be trusted. She grows up and becomes an adolescent who begins to experience her own sexual desires, which retroactively confirm that she is seductive and bad. So when she meets a man who could disconfirm her feelings of worthlessness, she does not trust him, misunderstands his intentions, and loses his affections. Then she meets a man who does abuse her sexually, thus confirming that the men cannot be trusted. And so forth. A whole life is built on traumatic reenactment, a subject we will describe in more length in Chapter 11.

Most traumatized people who seek service in any of the human service delivery systems have the experience of having their worst fears confirmed over and over. All too often, people who they come to for help end up reconfirming those fears, unintentionally and unwittingly, because we fail to understand how to avoid the trap of reenactment. In order to successfully change those negative expectations and destructive self-fulfilling prophecies, we need to be constantly creative and innovative, and that is much more likely to happen if we do not have to function as isolated individuals but instead are always backed up by a team of people we trust. A nursing staff member who works on an acute care psychiatric unit for adults asks:

What else can you expect from people when they are treated the way we treat them? We diagnose them in terms that if applied to ourselves would be profoundly insulting. We admit them to dirty, dingy, cramped, and broken physical spaces with seclusion rooms and people in restraints screaming. Sometimes we take their clothes and have them walking around in hospital gowns and paper slippers. We often do not even talk about recovery or what it means or what they should do about their diagnoses. I have watched conversations between mental health workers and staff and have been very embarrassed by the arrogant and condescending attitudes of the staff. I have also been party to conversations when clients were made fun of, and laughed at, behind their backs.

At the management level, examples of setting expectations unwittingly are rampant: placing desks as barriers to set a tone of power; paying more attention to what people do wrong than what they do right; failing to give out important information; ignoring people; not getting back to them; changing the subject; and so forth. How do managers communicate low expectations of employees? Doing or not doing the very same things: paying attention to staff only when they do something wrong; failing to praise; failing to give any feedback at all; and failing to provide staff with the information they need to learn how to do their jobs well. Brian describes this in action:

Just like our kids, our staff come with their scripts for how the world works. Just like the kids and the staff, we come with our scripts as well. The easiest thing to do is to always fall into playing the same script over and over again. I am in the role of the unreasonable, abusive father, you are in the role of the misunderstood victimized child. Let's see if we can play those roles flawlessly. I do or say something that hurts or upsets you (it does not matter whether it is true or whether I have a right to say it). You get triggered by the remark because it touches on your vulnerability or fear. You respond by telling me just how disrespectful you think I am. I respond by telling you are not willing to accept responsibility. We are off to the races, playing our dysfunctional roles perfectly.

Filtering out Trauma

Trauma theory restores context to what has increasingly become a decontextualized meaning framework in mental health, substance abuse, and other social service practice. If the origins of so much dysfunction are to be found in the adverse experiences of childhood that a majority of Americans apparently experience (see Chapter 2), then what exactly is the role of the mental health professional, the substance abuse counselor, the domestic violence advocate? What should social service institutions focus their efforts upon? Can we stay comfortably settled in our offices or is advocacy for fundamental change a moral necessity? What exactly do all the diagnostic categories mean when someone diagnosed with posttraumatic stress disorder is six times more likely to be diagnosed with another psychiatric disorder and eight times more likely to be diagnosed with three or more psychiatric disorders [136; 501–502]?

These are disturbing questions for an institution under the best of circumstances but virtually impossible questions for systems under siege to answer. So, for the most part, the issue of trauma is simply screened out organizationally and systemically. With every new war, disaster, or terrorist act, it bubbles to the surface again. Then with every day that passes since the latest trauma, the knowledge fades away a little more or, within the context of this discussion, is socially dissociated. Lacking the time, energy, or knowledge base to use intuition, reinterpret behavior, or integrate new knowledge, the reality of the traumatic origins of mental illness go unaddressed. And the patient, frequently diagnosed with chronic depression, borderline personality, or some other "axis II" disorder, is labeled, everyone in the system colludes to support the reality and meaningfulness of the label in determining future behavior and outcomes, and the patient's more fundamental—and treatable—trauma conditions go untreated.

This represents an organizational learning disability. Organizational development researchers have defined organizational learning as "detection and correction of error" and have described two types: single-loop learning and double-loop learning [503]. In single-loop learning a problem is recognized, diagnosed, and addressed without changing the underlying policies, assumptions, and goals. In double-loop learning the recognition, diagnosis, and intervention require changes in the underlying policies, assumptions, and goals. Double-loop learning is what is necessary to address the astonishingly complex problems of adults, children, and families who enter treatment environments and present challenging problems for staff members whose goal it is to help them. Trauma-informed learning is double-loop learning. Mental health and social service workers have to change paradigms of thought and behavior in order to meet the goals of recovery that trauma-informed change necessitates. But all too often, this kind of shift in underlying paradigm is inhibited by defensive reasoning on the part of organizational members because they so fear complaints of errors in judgment or incompetence that they will not take the risk of making a mistake and learning from it [458].

Organizational Memory and Organizational Amnesia

If an organization is to learn anything, then the distribution of its memory, the accuracy of that memory, and the conditions under which that memory is treated as a constraint become crucial characteristics of organizing. (p. 206)

Karl E. Weick (1979), *The Social Psychology of Organizing*

Memory is vital to our survival. For learning to occur, organizations must have memory. Some modern philosophers believe that all memories are formed and organized within a collective context. According to them, society provides the framework for beliefs, behaviors, and the recollections of both individual and groups [504]. Later, present circumstances affect what events are remembered as significant. Much of the recording and recalling of memories occurs through social discussion. This shared cohesiveness of memories is part of what defines a culture over time. Shared language also helps a society organize and assimilate memories, and eventually to forget about the events.

Critical events and organizational failure change us and change our organizations, but without memory we lose the context. Similarly, there is reason to believe that maintaining silence about disturbing collective events may have the counter-effect of making the memory even more potent in its continuing influence on the organization or society much as silent traumatic memories continue to haunt individuals [370]. Here is a description of collective community memory from the point of view of a director of a shelter:

> We had had a positive reputation in the distant past. But we went through this period of decline, verging on failure; there were other agencies just waiting for us to fail. We cleaned up the leadership, and the quality of services improved enormously, but other organizations still look at as us as if we were the way we were in the past instead of seeing us as we are now. We still have to prove ourselves more than other organizations have to. Every misstep, every miscommunication—just the stuff that can happen in the course of managing a human service organization—becomes a source of scrutiny and there is a kind of attitude that comes out at meetings and in interagency communications that says, "See, I knew you hadn't really changed." It's been hard coming back from that loss of reputation in the community, hard to once again feel safe in the larger environment.

Organizational memory refers to stored information from an organization's history that can be brought to bear on present decisions. This information is stored as a consequence of implementing previous decisions, through individual recollections, and through shared interpretations [491]. Like individual memory, organizational memory is distributed, not concentrated in one place or domain. Brian, who shared with us the mystery of the two garbage pails earlier, gives yet another example here of the strange aspects of organizational memory:

> The first year I was at Andrus, I remember having a most peculiar experience. We used to have an event called the Penny Carnival. Essentially it was a field day with lots of games and prizes. We would invite all the kids, their families as well as all the staff and their families. This event usually took place the Sunday

after Mother's Day, around the middle of May. As we know the weather can be pretty fickle at that time of the year; sometimes it is very hot, sometimes cool, you never know. This particular Sunday, it was hot, probably in the low 80s. I was the Program Director of Foster Hall, one of the adolescent boys' cottages. All of our boys showed up at the Penny Carnival in shorts and t-shirts, which seemed to be appropriate attire for a carnival on a sunny day in May. Everyone had a nice time.

The following day one of the child care staff at another cottage pulled me aside and said, "I noticed all your boys were wearing shorts yesterday." I nodded. Although I had not really noticed that myself, I was willing to take her word for it. She went on to ask, "Did the memo come out from Dyckman Hall, saying it was OK to wear shorts?" Dyckman Hall is our administration building, where all our important decisions were made, including, apparently, when it is appropriate to wear shorts.

I indicated I had not seen a memo on the issue and was unaware there even was a memo on the issue. The worker asked, "Well, if you didn't get the memo, why were your boys wearing shorts?" "Because it was hot," I replied.

She went on to explain that every year a memo comes out from Dyckman Hall, usually in June, indicating when it is OK to wear shorts, and until that memo comes out, kids really shouldn't be in shorts. When I asked what the logic was for this practice, I was told that in the spring it can be cold or hot, you never know. Some days are just not appropriate for shorts and so rather than break out the shorts too early and have to argue with kids on a non-shorts day, we wait for the memo from Dyckman Hall. Fascinatingly, our staff were apparently not even smart enough to know when it was appropriate to wear shorts. I wondered how such a practice could have been instituted and what kind of shorts-related disaster might have occurred to make this an organizational practice. Interestingly enough, I never saw a memo from Dyckman Hall about shorts in my tenure here. I am betting it happened once or twice and this worker got it in her head this was an annual announcement. It is quite amazing how these things take on their own life in an organization and even more amazing how hard it is to kill them.

Failures in Memory Storage

Research shows that organizations keep repeating their mistakes and blunders for two main reasons: they have either lost their corporate memory and are incapable of recalling their corporate history, also known as "time-based" memory loss; or they are unable to communicate lessons from one part of the organization to another part in a timely manner, a phenomenon known as "space-based" memory loss [484; 505]. Time-based memory loss occurs when learning that has taken place fails to be encoded and documented and thus knowledge is lost over time; while space-based amnesia occurs when learning, even when encoded and documented, fails to be shared or diffused [484].

Organizational amnesia can result from a breakdown in any of the four stages of learning: intuition, interpretation, integration, and institutionalization [484]. There may be no mechanism for intuitive knowledge of the individual to be transferred to the organization, or individual intuition may be looked down on, effectively silencing individuals, resulting in time-based memory loss. Tacit knowledge, often in the form of skills or corporate wisdom, is much more difficult to transfer than explicit knowledge, so that much that goes on at a tacit level may not be transferred to other parts of the organization and this causes "space-based" memory loss. Integration and institutionalization may help the organization retain explicit information gained over time, but the tacit information is more easily lost. When this happens, rules may replace norms as guides for the group. Additionally, presumed causal relationships may be in error but may become institutionalized, while accurate causal relationships are ignored. Selective perception and attribution also come into play, as individuals and groups systematically ignore information that does not fit into established schemas. As Brian describes it:

> *Young clinicians commonly struggle to formulate a theory of the case—of what is really going on with their patients, why they are having the symptoms they are having—so they cannot really formulate a treatment strategy that is complex and takes in all the aspects of the person. They may be able to provide a DSM diagnosis—they just struggle to think critically about a case. I have asked myself how I learned how to think about each person, how to develop my own theory for what was going on and test it out. I realize that I had terrific supervision and a lot of it, from experienced people who had a wide variety of experiences. I had the chance to talk to them, to review my cases, to watch them in action. I don't think that happens in training programs as much as it used to.*

Downsizing Memory

Organizational or "corporate" amnesia becomes a tangible problem to be reckoned with when there is a loss of collective experience and accumulated skills through the trauma of excessive downsizing and layoffs [506]. It is now generally recognized that corporate layoffs can have devastating effects not just on individual but on corporate health as well, even producing what has been termed "survivor sickness" in the business world [507–508].

It is the valuable tacit memory that is profoundly disturbed by the loss of personnel in downsizing. According to investigators in the field, the average length of a U.S. employee's tenure with any given company is approximately

5 years. *"The dramatic shift in the nature of employment toward short-term tenure is among the biggest damaging influences on productivity and competitiveness in companies today. That's because short-term tenure translates into short-term organizational memory. And when a company loses its medium and long-term memory, it repeats its past mistakes, fails to learn from past successes and often forfeits its identity… Hard-won and expensively acquired organizational memory walks out the door every time an employee retires, quits, or is downsized"* (p. 35) [509].

Corporate memory loss at any level in the organization is significant. However, some investigators believe that when it happens at the senior team level, it has the greatest impact. Senior team members hold a strategic place in the organization and hold the vision for the future direction the organization should take. There are fewer members at this level, and they hold more power. Therefore, decisions made have a greater global impact throughout the organization. They are responsible for maintaining the integrity of the organization and that loss of integrity can impact not only the organization but also the community it serves [488].

Organizations must reckon with past failures and the fragmentation of meaning and purpose that accompanies these failures. Organizations can distort or entirely forget the past, or important parts of the past, just like individuals do, and the more traumatic the past the more likely it is that the organization will push some memories out of conscious awareness. Changing leaders, even changing the entire staff, does not erase the organizational memory, nor does it excavate and provide decent burial for the skeletons in the organizational closet. As one author puts it, *"Pain is a fact of organizational life. Companies will merge, bosses will make unrealistic demands, people will lose their jobs. The pain that accompanies events like these isn't in itself toxic; rather, it's how that pain is handled throughout the organization that determines whether its long-term effects are positive or negative"* (p. 12) [510].

Organizational Amnesia and the Mental Health System

Looked at from a developmental point of view, the mental health system represents an example of arrested organizational development attested to by systemic fragmentation, lack of clear purpose, lack of innovation, and a foreshortened vision of the future [511]. This failure of development is most poignantly recognizable within the institutional setting. Since the origins of the state systems in the nineteenth century, the course of institutional psychiatry has been plagued by a seemingly terminal repetition: a positive vision of healing, empowerment, and recovery in all its complexity is washed away by ignorance, greed, and a lack of commitment on the part of society as a whole. The small, treatment-oriented programs with a high staff-to-patient ratio and a rich network of relationships that characterized moral treatment were supplanted by the huge bureaucratic institutions that came to be called "state hospitals," and we have been busy disassembling them for the past three decades. But rather than seeing that many people need and can benefit from 24/7 care when it is done properly, we have substituted once again ignorance, greed, and a social lack of commitment called "managed care." Managed care is slowly strangulating inpatient treatment in all of its forms, while laying all of the blame for systemic shortcomings on the mental health system and then blaming it for its own failures.

Those Who Cannot Remember the Past...

The early-twentieth-century philosopher George Santayana wrote, *"Those who cannot remember the past are condemned to repeat it"* (p. 82) [512]. The mental health system keeps forgetting lessons learned and having to learn them all over again. This cycle of protest-reform-regression has been going on for centuries. Only the times, places, and people have changed; the issues are recurrently and depressingly similar.

The current enthusiasm for "evidence-based practices" as the only form of service delivery that should be permitted is the latest flavor of the month. Indeed, a rigorous concern about outcomes should be the basis of any form of treatment, and as we mentioned in Chapter 1, we would be better served if competition among providers was over improvement in client outcomes. However, the burden of expecting practitioners to only use double-blind, scientifically demonstrated treatment methods is short sighted and absurd for many reasons. A real problem with evidence-based treatments is that they are generally owned by someone, cost money to implement, require rigorous and expensive data collection, and may not really conform with the way funders fund programs. Agencies can spend lots of money on implementation and then within a couple of years that investment can walk out the door in the form of staff turnover.

The reality is that we already know that therapy in a wide variety of forms works as long as certain criteria are inherent in the therapy. According to those who have thoroughly reviewed the existing literature, successful outcomes hinge on four fundamental factors: *(1)* factors related to what the client brings to the situation (accounting for about 40% of outcome); *(2)* the therapeutic relationship (accounting for about 30% of outcome); *(3)* expectancy and placebo factors, also known as "hope" (accounting for about 15% of outcome), and *(4)* an explanatory system that guides healing rituals (accounting for the last 15% of outcome) [3]. This means that 60% of what accounts for whether a person responds to treatment hinges on relationships with the people delivering the treatment. If caregivers develop a positive, warm, supportive, and empathic relationship, support the development of hope that progress can be made, have a clear rationale for what they are doing that outlines a therapeutic map of recovery, and empower the clients to help themselves, there is likely to be improvement. It will be interesting to discover how much we can gain in client improvement once we pay attention to the traumatic origins of mental illness that applies to the 40% of outcome attributable to what the client brings into treatment.

Factors Contributing to Loss of Knowledge

What are factors that repeatedly cause this loss of knowledge in the mental health system? There are several challenges to effective organizational memory that can be addressed:

1. Informal organizational knowledge, being tacit and intuitive like a wild animal, resists capture. Without being able to openly communicate about and discuss this tacit knowledge, we always are in danger of simply repeating what we have done in the past automatically, whether it was useful or not.
2. The usual approach to organizational memory, by keeping files and preserving documents, fails to preserve context. For many reasons, it may cease to provide accurate records of past events.
3. Under some circumstances, knowledge loses its relevance, and thus its value, over time. What may lose its relevance at one point in time may at a later point in time be entirely relevant, but by that time everyone has forgotten what it is or how to do it.
4. The current litigious environment may create an economic incentive for "organizational amnesia" [490].
5. The institution may have experienced a traumatic experience that is organizationally dissociated.
6. The subject matter of memory may demand such major organizational change that it simply must be "forgotten" because it places the institution in conflict with the larger society.

Informal organizational knowledge is lost when individuals, particularly long-time professionals, leave the organization and do not pass on hard-earned knowledge to new employees. Much of the tacit memory in organizations is passed on through the mechanism of organizational culture, "the way we do things around here." Culture is massively affected by layoffs, program closures, and leadership changes. Organizational structure tends to be more lasting, but the structure and function may cease to inform each other so that the structure itself becomes meaningless, repetitive, and hollow because the tacit information formerly embedded in clinical wisdom that has now left the system no longer informs the structure. Even the knowledge that seems embedded "in the walls" of an institution is lost when the physical structures themselves are torn down, or when the entire program moves to a new, and frequently diminished, locale. An experienced administrator describes a cycle that many people in this field can relate to:

> A residential treatment program for children was highly structured around behavior management. Children lost points for an almost infinite variety of infractions and the decisions about consequences remained largely in the hands of childcare workers who were indoctrinated into the system by other childcare workers. The staff members who had previously started the behavior management system as an almost revolutionary way to address difficult problems that had not been responsive to psychodynamic forms of treatment had long since retired or gone on to other positions. Without a guiding and integrated theoretical framework, the behavior management system had come to bear absolutely no relationship to the child's history and was performed as a relatively meaningless ritual. A similar behavior management plan was set out for every child who came into care. If the child continued to be disobedient to the rules, no one on the staff stopped to inquire about the intended consequences of the child's behavioral plan and how it fit into an overall recovery process for the child. There was no discussion about the meaning behind the child's behavior. Childcare workers were taught to believe that their job was to manage behavior through this system and were led to believe that they did not need to know anything about the child's previous experience in order to successfully achieve this. Without a conceptual framework or strategy to fall back upon, staff members frequently simply "dosed" the children with more behavioral consequences that did not work to actually change behavior, or worse because it was so punitive, consequences did bring about behavioral change while the child was in the setting, but after discharge the child's behavior rapidly went back to its baseline of dysfunction.

Organizational memory is kept within the files and records of the institutions. But the actual physical archive of a patient's file becomes essentially meaningless when the record-keeping is based on satisfying the demands of what is frequently seen as an oppressive, arbitrary, and capricious process of justifying admission. As a psychiatrist working in an acute care setting tells us:

> On an acute care inpatient unit, the case manager or psychiatrist may have to call the managed care company every day to get permission to keep a patient in the hospital. Unless they can demonstrate concretely that the patient needs what the insurance company defines as hospital level care—usually requiring an imminent threat to life—the hospital stay is likely to be denied. Although human beings rarely change dramatically overnight, the hospital charts indicated that radical and dramatic change frequently did in fact happen within hours. According to the chart, a patient would continue to be suicidal for days

and then seemingly miraculously be ready for discharge, or a psychotic patient's voices would suddenly disappear. In fact, patients were improving at the pace at which patients have always improved, but reality could not be truthfully explained in the chart without damaging consequences. Additionally, staff were taught never to write anything positive about changes the patient was making until the end of the stay because these comments could be used to justify and mandate discharge, even if the improvement was still quite fragile from the point of view of the clinician. As a result of these and other adaptations to adversity made by hospital staff, over time, even the physical archives of a patient's progress have become corrupted and can no longer be considered an accurate portrayal of what actually happened in the treatment process.

Knowledge loses its relevance when it is no longer valued by the organization as a whole. *"Even though organizations do not have a biological existence, they can still act in ways that suggest they have forgotten key lessons previously learned. Lessons learned and knowledge previously generated are sometimes lost and forgotten"* (p. 273) [484]. If an administrative system is emphatically concerned about reducing costs, or reducing hospital stays, and pays only lip service to clinical care, it is not long before knowledge that relates to clinical care is lost. It is lost because it is no longer considered relevant to what employees perceive as the real organizational mission—and what will get paid for—even if the stated mission says something else.

The loss of organizational memory can be witnessed in many settings where the staff—even the most professionally trained staff—seem unable to formulate anything but the most rudimentary ideas about human motivations, drives, and problems. Losing the history of the patient is a common occurrence in many settings today. As if they were journalists instead of clinicians, staff carefully record the "who," "what," "where," and "when" of their patients' lives but may never get to the "why" because they have no thorough theoretical grasp of causality. The meaning in the message is lost as communication within an organization breaks down and organizational memory becomes increasingly impaired. The patient's history is not conveyed to other members of the treatment team, resulting in space-based memory loss, and the patient's history is not carried through time, a situation particularly applicable now to the longer term treatment of disturbed children, resulting in time-based memory loss. One of our faculty consultants shared this experience with us:

A multidisciplinary team of a residential treatment program was meeting regularly to create significant change within their organization. Children often stayed in this program for several months, and sometimes years. In a discussion about a particularly difficult little girl who had already been in the institution for over 2 years, the social worker mentioned that this was a child who had been sexually abused. A childcare worker who worked in the cottage with this girl piped up indignantly, "How is it possible that I have worked with this child for the last year and a half and no one ever mentioned that she had been sexually abused?" This caused the entire team to step back and look at the many ways in which they repeatedly lose the children's histories in the day-to-day struggle to control behavior.

Similarly, as staff and leaders leave an institution, the memory of organizational events, like the histories of the patients, becomes like a cheesecloth, filled with holes. Parts of the institutional memory are kept in consciousness but because it is only part, the result may be a serious distortion of the past. Another of our faculty consultants shared this story:

An outpatient organization with a variety of different programs decided to work on better integrating their overall system. To serve this goal, the consultant urged the group to review their long history. One of the conflicts that surfaced was a generalized but nonspecific fear and suspicion of the financial department in the organization that seemed to make no sense in terms of present operations. The consultant asked the most long-term members of the organization to form an inner circle to talk about the past, and the other members of the group sat in a wider circle around them. What surfaced was a part of their history that many people in the room knew nothing about; it was part of the tacit memory that was still playing a role, unconnected to any context. Thirty years before there had been a financial crisis that almost caused this venerable institution to shut its doors. Financial specialists, one of whom was still running the department, were called in to attempt to rescue the situation. At the time, everyone felt enormous pressure but particularly the newly hired financial people. The organizational grapevine warned everyone about "staying away from finance" and some personal vignettes about short-tempered responses from the people in finance reinforced this warning. Although the situation had long since righted itself, the "word on the street" was still "stay away from finance." The current leader had known nothing about this piece of the history so had not been able to do anything to correct the misapprehension that targeted one lonely and isolated department until this fragment of organizational memory was retrieved, made conscious, and therefore available for change.

Lawsuits are known to be extremely stressful and, in some cases, traumatic for many of the people involved in the proceedings. There may be an unconscious and conscious bias toward only remembering experiences that support the defense of the suit, and this may encourage organizational amnesia. Instructions given by lawyers at the time a professional or an organization encounters a potential lawsuit may unwittingly encourage forgetting, especially when all talking or writing about the events is discouraged [513]. And it is also likely that events that led to litigation have been traumatic to the staff involved, not just the person who has been in some way injured.

The result of organizational amnesia may be a deafening silence about vital but troubling information, not dissimilar to the deafening silence that surrounds family secrets like incest or domestic violence. Maintaining silence about disturbing collective events may force the memories to go underground, where they have the counter-effect of making the memory even more potent in its continuing influence on the individuals within the organization as well as the organization as a whole, much as silent traumatic memories continue to haunt traumatized individuals and families [346]. Topics that are actually central to organizational function frequently do not get openly discussed: race, sex, power, and fairness. It seems that the agreement not to talk is at times a collective agreement. Silence is reinforced by a groan, an eye roll, or some other unfavorable response so that everyone quickly learns not to bring that subject up again.

Here a faculty consultant shares a story about an organizational "secret"—a secret report—that many years later was still powerfully affecting organizational function:

> A social service organization had endured three leadership changes in 2 years. The internal situation was becoming increasingly chaotic, and the Board of Directors requested an evaluation from an external agency. The report obtained through many personal interviews with the staff was largely negative, probably more to make the point for funding sources that there was great need than that the authors wanted to criticize the staff. Unfortunately, however, the leader at the time, herself just making the transition, chose to keep the findings of the report secret from the staff but based much of her changed policy upon the report. She was an authoritarian leader and the changes she made were perceived as insulting, unfair, and cruel by the staff. She only lasted in her leadership position for 2 years. When the organization again changed directors, a consultant was brought in to help with the reorganization that was obviously needed. In the interim, the level of service delivery had radically slipped, staff morale had plummeted, and the organizational reputation was sliding progressively downward. After a number of meetings with a multidisciplinary team, the issue of this elusive report now 5 years old, finally surfaced. Fortunately, the current director managed to find a copy of the report buried in the organizational files. Once the "secret" report was exposed to the staff, put into context, and emotionally and cognitively worked through, the organization could begin the healing process so necessary for it to recover its former level of function and status in the community.

Previously hard-earned knowledge may be lost and then rediscovered as if new. We are currently in a climate where seclusion and restraint are being actively discouraged and even prohibited, due in part to the activism of mental health consumers and the deaths of patients while in restraints. However, reforms to curb the use of restraint have repeatedly been followed by the escalation of coercion for the last several hundred years, in a pattern dating back at least to the birth of moral treatment in the late eighteenth century. Reformers come in, demonstrate that psychiatric care, even of the most violent people, can be delivered without violence in environments conducive to healing, and as long as the reformers are active, this proves to be largely true. But then the knowledge gradually slips away again. A psychiatrist shared this story with us about how easily old knowledge can be lost:

> A psychiatrist experienced in operating inpatient settings using milieu therapy, assumed leadership of an inpatient unit that had been in existence for decades. Although the level of restraining people was relatively low compared to many current settings, the staff denied any knowledge of ever hearing about anything called "milieu therapy", leaving the psychiatrist curious about how the staff knew how to handle tricky and potentially violent situations. They actively resisted the suggestions of the new psychiatrist to align their current practices with milieu treatment, openly stating that the psychiatrist had herself invented the "milieu" ideas and the staff viewed her suggestions as the impositions of radical new ideas that could never work. And then one day one of the nurses brought in an old nursing book from the 1940s. The staff were shocked to see clear definitions and explanations of "milieu therapy," not as the new psychiatrist's radical ideas, but as previously established and accepted nursing practice. It was clear that at some point in time, milieu therapy knowledge had been embedded in the practice of the unit program since the "footprints" were still visible, hidden in some of the policies on the unit that supported noncoercive treatment. But the theory and practice of those policies had been cut off from the context, much like posttraumatic fragments of experience are cut off from the total context of a person's experience. The psychiatric unit as a whole had become amnestic for entire bodies of previously gained knowledge and experience and was unable to access those memories and incorporate that experience into ongoing practice.

In this way, why we do what we do gets separated from what we do. So for awhile at least, people go on doing what they do even though they don't know why they are doing it. But over time, and particularly under the influence of chronic stress, without understanding or being able to talk about the "why," they stop doing it and eventually have to relearn cycles of understanding and behavior that previously was established knowledge.

Trauma and Organizational Memory

Mental health and social service organizations can be traumatized in many ways: layoffs, closures, and loss of funding, patient deaths, staff deaths, staff injuries, and other acts of violence. And it may not be possible to traumatize

an institution without producing defects in organizational memory. In traumatized individuals, memory problems follow two main, often alternating,
patterns: too little memory or too much. After a traumatic experience, individuals may develop amnesia for the worst aspects of an experience, while at
the same time fragments of the traumatic memory may continue to intrude
into consciousness at inappropriate times. Either way, the trauma may radically
interfere with current information processing, decision making, problem
solving, and life choices.

Historically, the reality of traumatic experience in the lives of psychiatric
patients has been recurrently "unknowable" by the mental health system. As
Judith Herman has pointed out, *"the study of psychological trauma has a
curious history—one of episodic amnesia. Periods of active investigation have
alternated with periods of oblivion. Repeatedly in the past century, similar lines of
inquiry have been taken up and abruptly abandoned, only to be rediscovered much
later. Classic documents of 50 or 100 years ago often read like contemporary works.
Though the field has in fact an abundant and rich tradition, it has been periodically forgotten and must be periodically reclaimed"* (p. 7) [139].

Dr. Herman and others have pointed out that the study of traumatic stress must
occur within political and social contexts that give voice to the disempowered
and the disenfranchised. The reality of traumatic amnesia in individual trauma
survivors has repeatedly left us with a cultural amnesia—a gap in the societal
narrative that could fully round out the reality of those traumatic events. The
reluctance of victims to dredge up memories of a past trauma and thereby
become triggered into states resembling the initial horrors has been paired with
a social reluctance on the part of witnesses to listen to those stories and to bear
witness to the terrors of the past. This is accompanied by an unwillingness on
the part of those in power to take responsibility for the perpetration of acts of
violence or the failure to protect citizens from those acts [514]. This social
amnesia is particularly great when the trauma has occurred to an oppressed or
marginalized social group—women, children, minorities—and the mentally
ill. And importantly, the course of development transiting from traumatic
event through posttraumatic reactions to symptomatic behaviors can span
decades and travel through a variety of intervening variables, each of which can
negatively or positively impact on the ultimate course. As a result, it has been
easy for both survivors and witnesses to lose the thread of cause-and-effect
relationships, and this always serves the interests of the perpetrators, who are
rarely held accountable for their acts [348–349]

Compromised Decision Making

Every day, all day long, people working in human service delivery systems
of every variety must make decisions that affect people's lives. Making good

decisions isn't innate; it is a learned skill necessitating on-the-job, hands-on training and supervision. The best decisions are likely to come out of a process rather than "just happening," which are unfortunately the kinds of decisions we are most likely to make under stress. The process of effective decision making is characterized by thoughtfulness and information informed by emotion, past experience, and intuition. It is careful, methodical, and well reasoned. It is also difficult and demanding and the greater the complexity of the situation or the decision that needs to be made, the greater the demand on the individual. It is for this reason that repetitive and routine decisions are expediently managed by authoritarian systems of control, while complex decisions require a very different approach. And for the same reason, repetitive and often poor decisions are made under stress.

Decision making may be profoundly affected by emotion. Positive emotion increases creative problem solving and facilitates the integration of information, while negative emotion produces a narrowing of attention and a failure to search for new alternatives. People who are in pleasant moods tend to deliberate longer, use more information, and reexamine more information than others. People in aroused or unpleasant moods tend to take more risks, employ simpler decision strategies, and form more polarized judgments [515].

But this analysis of decision making focuses on the individual decision maker. At the workplace, individual decisions certainly must be made very day, but even individual decisions must be made in the context of "the group"— whatever that group happens to be. What do we know then about the process of decision making when many factors must be taken into account, when many people must participate in the decisions, and when decisions that are made may have significant and lasting consequences?

Absence of Participation in Decision Making

In the world of business, there has long been discussion about the advantages and disadvantages of encouraging, creating, and supporting ways in which a larger number of people in the workplace can participate in making decisions about workplace issues that affect them. Lack of participation in the decision-making process, lack of effective consultation and·communication, office politics, and lack of a sense of belonging have all been identified as potential organizational stressors for workers. However, increased opportunity to participate has been repeatedly associated with greater overall job satisfaction, higher levels of emotional commitment to the organization, and an increased sense of well-being [85].

In truth, regardless of the work that people are doing, it has to be organized, and the typical form of organization is that of the hierarchy. For the most part, hierarchies are assumed to be necessarily autocratic: the higher level tells the next lower level what to do and they do it. *"This assumption explains why most of the organizations and institutions, even government agencies, in a democratic society are managed autocratically. It is argued that they need hierarchy to orga- nize work, and that hierarchy is necessarily autocratic. Those who are bothered by the irony of this try to soften hierarchical autocracy by decentralizing some of the decision-making"* (p. 115) [329]. Hierarchy is often also equated with bureau- cracy, defined by sociologist Max Weber as *"a fixed division of labor among participants, a hierarchy of offices, a set of general rules which govern performance, a separation of personal from official property, and rights, selection of personnel on the basis of technical qualifications and employment viewed as a career by participants"* (p. 12) [516].

When lives, not just the bottom line, are at stake, participatory principles become even more important. Given the challenging physical, emotional, social, and ethical problems that confront most helpers and caregivers today, creating more participatory systems is critical. The difficulties our clients have are simply too complex to be addressed by the stagnant, bureaucratic, and autocratic environments that are so typical of the nonprofit world. Furthermore, in the private, for-profit sector of the health care environment, the search for profitability in a financially constrained environment makes it necessary to apply both internal and external pressures that advocate for good patient care. Getting everyone in an organization in alignment is necessarily a democratic process because everyone needs to be able to move their feet, at least a little. But ensuring better participatory systems and therefore relying on less individual decision-making judgment means that we must become aware of the dynamics of group decision making and the forces that can affect those kinds of decisions.

Decision Making Under Stress

Under stress, individual performance changes and problematic group processes will be exacerbated. Stress tends to increase performance quantity while decreasing quality. Attention becomes narrowed to include only the most vital task features. Information processing becomes simplified [517]. Under stressful conditions, decision makers are likely to experience what has been termed *decisional conflict* referring to the simultaneous tendencies within a person to accept and to reject a given course of action. Prominent signs of this are hesita- tion, vacillation, feelings of uncertainty, and signs of psychological distress [280]. All of these are threats to self-esteem and threaten the aura associated with leaders and the centralization of authority that typically occur in a group under stress. As a result, decision makers are likely to display premature closure by terminating a decisional dilemma without generating all the possible alterna- tives and consequences of the decision so as not to be seen as "flip-floppers." To add to the problem, under stress the cognitive function of decision makers is not likely to be at its best but instead is typified by a narrowing of focus, atten- tion only to threat, and increasing cognitive rigidity. These deficiencies result in a premature narrowing of alternatives, overlooking long-term consequences, inefficient searching for information, erroneous assessment of expected outcomes, and oversimplified decision rules that fail to take account of the full range of values implied by the choice being made [264]. In this way the gap between effective decision making and impaired decision making is likely to widen.

Apparently, the best defense against stress is recognizing that stress is likely to affect performance. In a study of flight crew performance, the one item that discriminated most clearly between outstanding performance and average performance among airplane pilots was whether they admitted that their decision-making ability was negatively influenced by stress. Outstanding pilots, contrasted with below-average pilots, realized that their abilities could change under stress; because they realized this, they appeared to be more receptive to inputs from others [518].

What happens to decision makers who later regret their decision? They are likely to suffer from strong and distressing feelings of post-decisional regret, which may further interfere with the ability to curtail losses or to make new decisions that will enable recovery from the setback. Post-decisional regret entails intense emotional distress—anxiety, rage, guilt—which then creates a higher level of stress and can give rise to psychosomatic symptoms as well [264].

Stress and Group Performance

If we look at how groups respond to stress, groups adapt to stress at first and the increase in stress may actually increase performance. But then as stress increases, group performance begins to degrade as does individual performance [517]. Stressful group work conditions tend to increase the "need for closure"—the desire for definite, nonambiguous solutions—within the group. Groups under stress exhibit a strong desire for uniformity of opinion and are likely therefore to exert influence on anyone who diverges from this uniformity. Pressures to conform to the will of the most powerful and persuasive members of the group intensify. As a result, stress tends to result in a "closing of the group mind" described as an aversion to unpopular options and an acceptance of authoritarian leadership and existing group norms [517].

As a result of these pronounced tendencies under stress, one organizational consultant has emphasized that *"given the tendency for communication among equals to turn hierarchical under stress, it would appear necessary that those at the top of the hierarchy explicitly legitimate and model equal participation if they are to override the salience of hierarchy"* (p. 142) [518].

In organizations, as systemic stress increases and authority becomes more centralized, organizational decision-making processes are likely to change as well. We like to believe that important decisions are made rationally and unemotionally, and under normal conditions this may indeed be the case. But under stressful conditions, emotions are likely to play a much more important role in a decision-making process that may already be compromised by inadequate access to all needed information. Stressful conditions do not just originate from actual life threat, particularly within organizations. Instead, stress is generated by feared losses, worrying about unknown consequences that may negatively impact on the work environment, concern about self-esteem, conflicting values, and emotional contagion. As C.O.O., Brian shares the things he worries about when he makes decisions, particularly the ones he must make under stress:

I worry about getting the decision wrong. About hurting somebody as a result of this decision. I worry about failing and looking stupid. I worry that people may not like me because of this decision and some people may think I am being duplicitous.

The Destructive Aspects of Silencing Dissent

Dissent can be defined as expressing disagreement or giving voice to contradictory opinions about organizational practices and policies [519]. Dissent can be triggered by a number of circumstances, but research has shown that the most common causes for dissent were related to perceived unjust treatment, organizational change and the implementation of those changes, decision making, inefficient work practices and processes, roles and responsibilities, use and availability of resources, unethical practices, performance evaluations, and dangerous circumstances involving self, coworkers, or clients [520]. The challenge for leaders is to encourage and allow dissent without compromising on values. It's often a tough line to walk.

Given the pressures within a group that may push for conformity, groupthink, and group polarization, it may take a great deal of courage to dissent, but given these same pressures, it is vital that individuals use their own perceptions when they see something they believe to be problematic within an organization.

Creating environments that support direct and open dissent is important for a number of reasons. Worker satisfaction is increased when employees feel they can freely voice their opinions and be heard. Participation appears to increase satisfaction and commitment. Workers sense whether dissent is acceptable in the organizational culture and then determine their reactions based on their perceptions [519; 521].

But most importantly perhaps, dissent serves as corrective feedback within an organization that can avert disaster. Dissenters serve as the "early warning devices" for systems, sensing impending disaster even before anyone else-including the people in charge-recognize that something is wrong. But to be useful dissent must be direct, unmitigated by fear or distrust, and therefore the conditions that promote dissent within an organizational culture must be conducive to free speech without retaliation.

Group Polarization: Why It Must Be Safe to Dissent

Group polarization has been found in hundreds of studies involving over a dozen countries, including the United States, France, Germany, and Afghanistan. In countless cases, like-minded people, after discussions with their peers, tend to end up thinking a more extreme version of what they thought before they started to talk (p. 112) [468]. When the majority of a group initially leans toward one position—even when that position is extreme—their consensus tends to influence others in the group that hold a more moderate position, and then the whole group moves toward the extreme position [522]. People respond to the arguments made by other people, and when a number of people are predisposed in one direction, the entire group will become skewed toward that predisposition. Those who hold a minority position often silence themselves or otherwise have disproportionately little weight in group deliberations. The result can be *hidden profiles*—important information that is not shared within the group. Group members often have information but do not discuss it. The result is to produce inferior decisions [468]. It is also through this mechanism that rumors are both bred and fed, *"deliberation among like-minded people often entrenches false rumors"* (p. 32) [523]. Because of the effect of this group polarization, a proposal or decision that insists on a strong response is likely to lead to an even stronger response. If that proposal is one that suggests something aggressive, then aggression is likely to increase.

Additionally, people with extreme views tend to have more confidence that they are right, and as people gain confidence they become more extreme in their beliefs. By contrast, those who lack confidence and are unsure what they should think tend to moderate their views. The result is that increased confidence can increase extremism as well. This is particularly likely to happen if the person exuding confidence about his point of view also has high status in the group. Other people keep quiet about their reservations, simply because of their desire not to incur the disfavor of the high-status speaker. Indeed, they might silence themselves simply because they do not want to cause internal tension. Seeing their views corroborated and uncontradicted, the first speaker then becomes even more confident still, and hence more extreme. Groups that are highly bonded through emotional ties may be particularly susceptible to polarization because group polarization tendencies combine with groupthink to produce a very unhealthy stew. All these effects, however, are invisible to the participants, so as other people continue to reinforce the extreme position, confidence grows based on further agreement, not necessarily because evidence has actually been presented that supports the conclusions that are being reached.

It is interesting to consider the influence of biological psychiatry in this light. Faced with the profound uncertainties of human existence and the complex social realities that have such an impact on our patient's lives, how comforting it is to be utterly confident about the function of neurotransmitters and the drugs designed to affect them. How easy it is to become contemptuous of those who minimize or even question the utility of such treatments. Did the virtual takeover of psychiatry by biological psychiatrists and the accompanying displacement of most psychodynamically oriented psychiatrists have everything to do with "truth" and "best practices"? Or could it be a recent example of group polarization in mental health practice?

Over time, group polarization can have very detrimental effects on an organization because those with more moderate opinions stop contributing or leave the group altogether. As a result, extreme positions may come to dominate the organizational climate, and these extreme positions may significantly interfere with healthy organizational adaptation and change.

Dissent Is Rarely Welcomed

As useful as dissent is, however, dissent has rarely been welcomed in the workplace. There is empirical data that employees often feel compelled to remain silent in the face of concerns or problems—a phenomenon that has been termed *organizational silence* [427]. In one study that interviewed employees from 22 organizations throughout the United States, 70% indicated that they felt afraid to speak up about issues or problems that they encountered at work. The "undiscussables" covered a wide range of areas, including decision making, procedures, managerial incompetence, pay inequity, organizational inefficiencies, and poor organizational performance [109].

The silencing of dissent is arguably even less welcome in environments characterized by chronic stress. One investigator who characterized organizational expression as *"an enduring problem of fundamental tension between the individual and the collective"* (p. 127) noted that such tension tends to be resolved in favor of organizational interests [524].

For managers, particularly under stressful conditions, dissent may be seen as a threat to unified action. As a result, escalating control measures are used to suppress any dissent that is felt to be dangerous to the unity of what has become focused organizational purpose, seemingly connected to survival threats. This encourages a narrowing of input from the world outside the organization. It also encourages the development of split-off and competing dissenting subgroups within the organization who may passive-aggressively or openly subvert organizational goals. As group cohesion begins to wane, leaders may experience the relaxing of control measure as a threat to organizational purpose and safety.

They may therefore attempt to mobilize increasing projection onto a designated external enemy who serves a useful purpose in activating increased group cohesion while actively suppressing dissent internally.

But the suppression of the dissenting minority voice has negative consequences. As dissent is silenced, vital information flow is impeded. As a result the quality of problem analysis and decision making deteriorates further. If this cycle is not stopped and the organization allowed the opportunity to recuperate, the result may be an organization that becomes as rigid, repetitious, and ultimately destructive and even suicidal as do so many chronically stressed individuals [348–351].

Conclusion

Organizational stress interferes with the capacity of organizations to learn from their clients, their staff, their mistakes, or from anyone else. Organizational memory and decision making can be negatively affected by stress. In the next chapter we look at the ways in which these impacts of stress negatively affect organizational communication, creating more conflict and greater numbers of events that cannot be discussed, all resulting in "organizational alexithymia" and collective disturbance.

Chapter 8

Miscommunication, Conflict, and Organizational Alexithymia

SUMMARY: *Under conditions of chronic stress, breakdowns in organizational communication networks occur. The feedback loops that are necessary for consistent and timely error correction no longer function. Without adequate networks of communication, the normal conflict that exists in human groups will escalate and increasing amounts of important information become "undiscussable." At the same time, the organization as a whole becomes increasingly alexithymic, unable to talk about the issues that are causing the most problems and that remain, therefore, unsolvable. One of the consequences of this is the emergence of collective disturbances that may turn into chronic unresolved conflict and violence.*

Patterns of Organizational Miscommunication

Organizations are built, maintained, and activated through the medium of communication. If that communication is misunderstood, the existence of the organization itself becomes more tenuous. (p. 136) [518]

K. E. Weick (2001), *Making Sense of the Organization*

In the human body, communication occurs via the circulatory system, which connects every part of your body to every other part of the body and conveys the nutrients we need to stay alive. Communication represents the flow of life in an organization as well. Everyone brings his or her own perceptual lenses to every communication exchange, and the interaction between sender and receiver can be exceedingly complex. Every organizational communication network is multidimensional and complex: formal and informal; vertical (up and down the organizational hierarchy) and horizontal (across levels); emotional and cognitive; verbal and nonverbal; conscious and unconscious.

When the body is conveying information, it self-regulates the flow of information—of nutrients, oxygen, hormones—that is required in each area of the body, and it does this through constant feedback information. Whenever a feedback loop stops working effectively, is cut off, or is blocked, we get sick or, in extreme cases, we die. Similarly, in organizations anything that negatively impacts on communication begins to create dysfunction in the organization that rapidly begins to decrease organizational effectiveness.

Different Lenses, Different Points of View

Organizational miscommunication is a major stumbling block in the human service delivery system. Information is not easily shared among different components of the mental health system, much less with systems that interact with mental health—a phenomenon that is called "silos." There is not a shared conceptual framework or language between components such as mental health, substance abuse, and physical healthcare [171]. It is as if every individual puts on a different "lens" to understand the client. But there is little recognition that everyone is wearing some kind of distorting lens that may be a result of our professional training, our ethnic background, our gender, our class, our race, our age, our previous life experience—virtually anything that separates us as individuals. This diversity of "points of view" is not necessarily a problem *unless* it is ignored and we pretend that it doesn't exist. When there is adequate time to recognize, understand, interpret, and synthesize these different views, it is possible to develop a much more complex idea of who the person is who sits before you. But when this more complex interpretative process does not occur, then everyone in a treatment environment simply works independently, assuming that everyone else sees things the same way they do. As one administrator put it:

> We see this all the time. Children in our state receive services from the State Education Department, Child Welfare, Mental Health, and Juvenile Justice, and often the same child bounces from program to program and system to system depending on what event put the child in the system, not the child's actual need. These systems do not work well with each other and rarely share information. Although there is increasing recognition of this, bureaucracies do not change easily. I am told that there are 100 kids in this county who bounce from system to system, and the cost of services for these 100 kids is greater than the entire budget for mental health services for everyone else in the county. While at the same time, the kids rarely get much better; they just age out of the system.

Different Theories, Different Mental Models

In the human services fields there are many more theories—or lenses—than there are truths. People adopt different theories to explain human behavior, and the theory or theories they adopt become invisible over time because they are so deeply entwined in the way they view the world. They become mental models upon which people tend to base their professional and often personal identities.

This fragmentation of theory, approaches, and services is not unique to children's services. We see it everywhere in the human service delivery system. It has stymied researchers, clinicians, and administrators [487; 525]. It generates both practical and theoretical dilemmas. As another example, if you received training as a psychoanalyst or psychoanalytic psychotherapist, then you have a complex and rich mental schema that helps you understand the patients who come to you for help. You will include certain information and exclude other information and to some extent what you include and what you exclude will be determined by how old you are, your gender, your race, and the thoroughness of your own analytic experience. When you are just learning, this process is intentional, but over time, it becomes so automatic that you are no longer even aware of what you are excluding. So you may avoid getting much training in the use of medications and will talk endlessly to your patients about symptoms that could be relieved by the judicious use of antidepressants. Or you may spend more time paying attention to your patients' intrapsychic dreams and fantasies than their real-life experiences.

If however, you were trained as a biological psychiatrist, then you may have very little interest in knowing about anything other than the person's symptoms, his or her physical status, his or her present stressors, and his or her reactions to the various medications that you use. You may not take the time to find out anything about the person's past history of attachment, childhood development, life course, or traumatic experiences because within the scope of your basic assumptions, it simply isn't relevant. Nor is the person's intrapsychic life relevant to your work together—if it is relevant at all.

As another example that we referred to earlier, in treatment settings for children, more than 17 therapeutic approaches have been found operative at one time in many residential treatment centers around the country. Within any of these approaches, one can find many variations from person to person [487]. Programs try to cobble these approaches together in order to have a coherent program, but given the impact of chronic stress, depletion of resources, and relatively untrained staff, this effort often does not succeed. *"Few centers can now provide a substantive (much less a theory-based) written account of their program,"* and they still lack criteria *"that rationally link diagnosis, etiology, prognosis, and (sic) criteria for specific forms of residential treatment"* (p. 324) [526–527]. Mirroring the disorganization that we find in the lives and the brains of traumatized children, the programs designed to treat them often suffer from a lack of integration of services, even while individually, the approaches may be excellent.

There are too many theories in mental health service delivery to go into all of them here—that could be an entirely separate book, so hopefully you get the point. But it is not just the mental health system. These kinds of automatic assumptions based on mental models can be spotted in virtually all of human services if you look for them.

For example, let's take a domestic violence shelter staff. Most of the staff are women. Some of them have been working in the domestic violence system for decades. These older women have witnessed the development of the field and remember when the interpretation of being a battered woman was that you were a crazy woman who was asking for it or a woman who was lying. Therefore, people in the domestic violence field heartily repel any notion that any of the women who come into the shelter are "crazy" or have mental health problems. People newer to the domestic violence field that join the staff are likely to have heard about the history of the domestic violence movement, but for them it is just that: history. What they see are very traumatized and depressed women who cannot seem to adequately self-protect, who are often using alcohol or drugs and are heavily involved in the underground drug economy, who have great difficulty caring for their children, and who are often far less than grateful for any interventions the staff employ in the shelter. The older women and the younger women share a common commitment to help women who have been battered, but their underlying assumptions are likely to be radically different. Unless these differences are surfaced and worked through, the shelter is quite likely to become an unhealthy place for everyone.

Let's take another example from health care. A program is implemented to help HIV-positive teenagers in an urban pediatric hospital. The staff members of the program are comprised of pediatricians, nurses, social workers, and peer counselors. The teenagers are mostly black and Hispanic children who have been raised in poverty. Many of them were born HIV positive, and some of them are substance abusers and became HIV positive as a result. Others developed the problem as a result of unprotected sexual behavior. Other than the peer counselors, the staff are well educated, and they are from diverse backgrounds. But only the social workers are likely to have had any psychological skills training, although their knowledge base will probably be largely determined by where they trained and when they trained. And none of them is likely to know much about the impact of childhood adversity and trauma on the development and current presentation of the teenagers in their care. Nonetheless, each person will make his or her own assumptions about the children, their parents, and each other automatically and at least partly out of awareness. Without a systematic method for integrating these varying points of view, how likely is it that the needs of these children will be fully addressed?

And to expand that last example further, let's speculate that in the HIV program, it is possible, with some work, to get everyone on the same page. As a result, the teens in the program start to show progress, until they get back into school and one teacher (real incident) tells a young HIV-positive boy that the reason he has AIDS is because his mother slept with a monkey. In another class (another real incident) attended by an HIV positive girl, a teacher divides the class according to who would and who would not have sex with someone who is HIV positive, and then proceeds to encourage the other kids to talk disparagingly about anyone who is HIV positive or has AIDS. The mental model clashes in these examples are so radical that it's hard to know even where to begin. Not surprisingly, in both of these examples, the young people took a turn for the worse in their medical status and compliance with their medication regime.

Inadequate Information Systems

Information systems, if they exist in other than a primitive form, vary between different settings and are not necessarily compatible with each other. Dr. David Satcher, the former Surgeon General commented that:

> *Effective functioning of the mental health service system requires connections and coordination among many sectors (public–private, specialty–general health, health–social welfare, housing, criminal justice, and education). Without coordination, it can readily become organizationally fragmented, creating barriers to access. Adding to the system's complexity is its dependence on many streams of funding, with their sometimes competing incentives. For example, if as part of a Medicaid program reform, financial incentives lead to a reduction in admissions to psychiatric inpatient units in general hospitals and patients are sent to state mental hospitals instead, this cost containment policy conceivably could conflict with a policy directive to reduce the census of state mental hospitals.* [432]

To make matters worse, confidentiality laws and practices for mental health, child welfare, and substance abuse programs are more stringent than for physical health care. A study of three Medicaid behavioral health plans found that information sharing between clinicians in different systems is hindered by differing confidentiality rules. Before records can be shared, individuals must sign a separate release authorizing their mental health or substance abuse care-givers to furnish information to their primary care physician. Some behavioral health clinicians simply do not ask for authorization, nor do they discuss the advantages of sharing information with others who are involved in the consumer's care [528]. Particular problems arise when the client can block the flow of information between systems and the information turns out to be a secret that is vital for the providers to know, such as a history of substance abuse, child abuse, or domestic violence. Additionally, and very importantly, state-of-the-art treatments, based on decades of research, are not being readily transferred from research to community settings [166].

The Ease of Miscommunication

In an organization, communication is going on all the time, but it is going on at many different levels simultaneously. Formal communication occurs in memos and meetings. Informal communication occurs at the water cooler, in the coffee room, over lunch, or in stairwells. We convey what we mean through words and through all of the subtle nonverbal exchanges of our bodies and voice. Where we are in the hierarchy often determines what we do and do not convey and the way we convey it. In any communication we are providing both cognitive and emotional information. And then our communication is determined in part by what we consciously decide to say but is always colored by our unconscious motivations as well.

So even under normal circumstances there are multiple ways for communication to go wrong. Just as an example, let's say that one person, Tommy, needs to convey information to another person, Bill. The message is conveyed by Tommy in a language they both presumably understand, and then Bill decodes the message and puts it into context, that is, he makes sense out of it. But what happens when the way Tommy uses the words does not convey the same information to Bill as was meant? Or what if Tommy's nonverbal information contradicts the verbal message being sent? Or what if Tommy's message does not say precisely what he intends to say? What if Tommy is lower in a hierarchy than Bill and he is fearful about what he has to say? What if Tommy catches Bill and conveys information he believes to be very important when Bill is in a hurry to get to a meeting or to go home?

So Tommy's message has been sent to Bill. When the message arrives, "noise" may interfere with Bill hearing the message accurately. The "noise" may come from the way Tommy is dressed, Bill's previous experience with Tommy, Bill's preoccupation with something else, Bill's present mood, or Bill's disagreement with the last person he talked to. Bill may by nature be very good at interpreting verbal information but is oblivious to the nonverbal aspects of communication. Or Bill might reject the information as not being that important or something he doesn't want to hear. Bill may misinterpret the information. He may have unconscious biases about the information Tommy is conveying. Tommy may have been emotionally upset when he conveyed the information, and Bill tends to shut down whenever he is confronted with distress. Even if all goes well and accurately in the communication between Tommy and Bill, the feedback loop from Bill to Tommy may clear up many of the communication problems or it might just make things worse.

Now, what if the situation changes a bit and Tommy is not a man but a woman? What if Tommy and Bill are from different racial groups? Have different sexual orientations? Have different ethnic backgrounds? Are different ages? What if Tommy comes from the North and Bill is from the South? What if they are from different countries? What if they don't speak the same language? When you look at it this way, it's not so incredible that we have so many communication problems—it's actually amazing that we do as well as we do at communicating with each other [529]. It's one of our human gifts.

Miscommunication in Systems

Tommy and Bill illustrate how easily miscommunication can occur between individuals. Now crank the possibility of confusion up a couple of notches and we get to miscommunication within systems. The multidimensional nature of interpersonal communication does not change; it becomes more complex because now information must flow not just between two individuals but between and among groups of individuals through communication "channels." But these channels may be inadequate for the volume of information that is entering them, or the channels may be too few, too narrow, or too slow [529].

In mental health and social service organizations, clinical communication networks have traditionally been defined by team meeting structures as well as the informal sharing of information that occurs between people in relatively confined spaces. As time pressures have increased, both informal and formal communication systems have been eroded with staff members in acute settings having little time at all to communicate the valuable informal information and team structures being limited to only the most vital and simple information delivery. With little time or incentive to chart data about the context of the patient's life, the patient file may have relatively little value and be too narrow in form to be of much use. Likewise, the time delay of information between various shifts or components of the system may increase the likelihood of miscommunication so that a day later, the staff is just beginning to respond to events that have occurred the day or days before.

Pathologies of information flow can happen when excessive or improper filtering of useful data or the inadequate filtering of useless or erroneous data occurs. For example, when the traumatic roots of mental disorders are ignored and forgotten, and when knowledge of milieu management is lost, then it is likely that information vital to the patients' recovery will be systematically filtered out of the flow of information and judged as irrelevant to the immediate concerns. The loss of psychodynamic and systems perspective means that far-ranging information about context and meaning will be eliminated from discussion and often replaced by or even swamped by erroneous or irrelevant information about details of behavior that do not necessarily lead anyone anywhere.

And Then There Is E-mail, Texting, Cell Phones, Blackberries, Twittering...

Technology has been created—allegedly—to enhance communication. Telegraphs, telephones, and e-mail all represent technological advances, and all have their drawbacks. First, there is a lot of communication that is far too nuanced to be handled by the written word of the average person, and it can easily lose its meaning and impact as it travels along the fiber optic threads that now connect us. Second, e-mail creates the illusion of communication. While it is great for general announcements or for planning a meeting, it is of little help in solving complex problems, resolving conflict, or achieving consensus. Brian discusses his personal experience with communication and technology:

> *On the technology front, while there are clearly gains, there are probably more losses for the work we do. At the end of the day it has become easier for us to disengage from our work, our clients, our coworkers, and our direct reports, while at the same time creating the illusion that we are fully and constantly engaged. "I'm too busy to talk right now, I'll shoot you an e-mail." "I really should discuss this with so and so, I'll leave them a voice mail." We don't sit and chat with our coworkers and our kids because we have to check our e-mail or take that cell call. Although technology is a key driver in how we share, retain, codify, and store knowledge, there are other new challenges as well. Years ago we used to struggle with workers who would sit and read the paper at work, now it is cell phone calls, checking Blackberries, playing handheld games, wearing iPods. All of these distractions, many of which we have introduced into the work to make things better, serve to allow all of us, starved for engagement, to disengage.*

But electronic communication is less than useless and often actually destructive in dealing with issues that have any emotional content. It creates the sense that we are communicating without all that messy eye contact and back and forth. But lack of eye contact, and the other important nonverbal information that is conveyed in face-to-face contact—tone of voice, facial expressions, body posture—makes it possible for us to fire off an angry flurry of messages in a moment of extreme frustration and crankiness. Our intemperance has now been committed to paper and can be shared with countless other people from now until the end of time. It can easily create conflict where no real conflict existed. As Brian points out,

> *The other thing about electronic e-mail is that people send it off when they are charged up. It is so easy to sit alone in your office and fire off an angry e-mail that has the potential to ruin someone's day. It is the communication equivalent to dropping a bomb from a plane. You never have to look into the faces of the people you hurt.*

Third, electronic communication robs us of the integration that is so important in our work. There are just these strands of thoughts thrown out there, usually not terribly refined, that trick us into believing we have sufficiently weighed in on or contributed to the problem-solving effort. It is, however, the integration and synthesis of these ideas that really counts for something and that does not always happen. And it certainly is less likely to happen by electronic means.

Fourth, electronic communication can become a vast wasteland, and separating the chaff from the wheat is no small task. On any given day it is common for a manager to receive 150 e-mails. Perhaps 10 of these e-mails contain some piece of information we can really use. The problem is that it is impossible to know which line of which e-mail contains the gold. If you skim your e-mail, you probably get 5 out of 10 of these nuggets. If you read it all thoroughly, you probably waste a lot of useful time. Another aspect of this glut of information is that many of us take for granted that e-mail is a great communication device and that the receiver agrees with this assumption. The only problem is not everyone reads e-mail and not everyone reads it all the time. It becomes easy to say to yourself, "Hey, I sent you an e-mail on that" and assume your job as communicator is done. Again from Brian:

I personally skim my e-mail looking for words like injury, blood, ambulance, fire, flood, and police. This suggests a certain focus. I rarely look for the words great, happy, successful, and wonderful and if I see these words it is often my cue to stop reading because it suggests there is nothing to worry about here. But in a setting like ours, where people are working directly with kids and not sitting at computer monitors all day, e-mail is hardly instant communication, and the assumption that it is really effective is quite flawed. Problems with technological advancements also apply to cell phones. It causes one to wonder, "How did we ever get by before cell phones?" On the plus side cell phones do allow people to stay connected in a crisis and seek out a second opinion quickly if they are struggling. On some level, however, it robs us of the sense that we can make an independent decision and use our own judgment. "If I have a phone and my boss has a phone, and I make an independent judgment, and did so without calling my boss, who is on my speed dial and says call me anytime, and that decision is a bad one, I'm dead". We have also seen cell phones adversely impact the work by allowing staff to divide their attention between the work at hand and some affairs that are clearly not the affairs of the organization. We can get distracted, lose focus, and become inattentive.

Size Matters: Communication and Group Size

In the early 1990s, anthropologist Robin Dunbar from the University of Liverpool started measuring monkey brains. Well, not just monkeys but all primates, including the great apes, and he noticed that each species tended to have a group size that was proportional to the size of their brains; the bigger the neocortex, the larger the social group. He suggested that for every species there is an upper limit to group size which is set by purely cognitive constraints, determined largely by whether the animal has a large enough brain to maintain the cohesion and integrity of the group. How many relationships can one chimpanzee keep track of? In nonhuman primates, this number is determined by the maximum number of individuals with whom an animal can maintain social relationships through personal contact, also known as social grooming [530].

Dunbar developed an equation relating group size to brain size and found that for humans, the maximum number is about 150. He believes that this represents the maximum number of relationships with whom we can maintain stable relationships, based on our neocortical processing ability. When we go beyond that number, we need a wide variety of more formal structures and methods of enforcement. At this point in group development there is a proliferation of laws and regulations as well as agencies, bureaucracies, and governments to maintain some sort of stable society [531]. As Dunbar points out:

If you belong to a group of five people, you have to keep track of ten separate relationships: your relationships with the four others in your circle and the six other two-way relationships between the others. That's what it means to know everyone in the circle. You have to understand the personal dynamics of the group, juggle different personalities, keep people happy, manage the demands of your own time and attention and so forth. If you belong to a group of twenty people however, there are now 190 two-way relationships to keep track of, 19 involving yourself and 171 involve the rest of the group. That's a fivefold increase in the size of the group, but a twentyfold increase in the amount of information processing needed to "know" the other members of the group. Even a relatively small increase in the size of a group creates a significant additional social and intellectual burden. (pp.178–179) [532]

Now, think of our huge schools, large residential programs for children, bulky bureaucratic child welfare systems, giant insurance companies. The larger the organization and the more people in that organization, the more challenging maintaining healthy communication is likely to be and the more likely we are to fall back on old forms, technology, rules and regulations, and other bureaucratic necessities. The larger the organization the greater the importance of actively promoting new and innovative communication structures but this rarely happens. And all because of the size of our brains! What we need are vertical and horizontal communication structures so that planning is done with a team, horizontally or laterally, and reported up and down the vertical hierarchy.

Communication Under Stress

So as complicated as this is, communication gets even more problematic during crisis and particularly under conditions of chronic stress. Crises are never totally secret: all stakeholders in an organization are likely to feel the anxiety and uncertainty in the environment, even if they know relatively little about what is happening. Informal networks of communication—rumors, gossip— are likely to increase under these conditions as formal networks withhold information. But it is during times of crisis that leaders most need to get feedback, adjust actions accordingly, rather than wall themselves off or "shoot the messengers" who bring bad news. By definition, in a crisis things are out of control and there are no easy and obvious solutions to the problems. Constant feedback becomes more critical because of the high degree of uncertainty about ongoing actions taken to address the crisis. Organizations that already have poor communication structures are more likely to handle crises poorly [533].

It is very difficult to help people, or help people to help people, when you feel you need to be secretive about your processes. If you make a mistake, it is easier to just say "we made a mistake, we'll fix it." The current climate does not make this an easy or desirable position to take. In fact, you need to be incredibly brave to ever say "we dropped the ball." This is not to say there is no forgiveness— there certainly is, and more often than we might think—it is just never clear how badly you will get hurt for your honesty.

As stress increases, perception narrows, more contextual information is lost, and circumstances deteriorate to more extreme levels before they are noticed, all of which leads to more puzzlement, less meaning, and more perceived complexity. Communication is necessary to detect error, and crises tend to emphasize vertical, one-way communication structures where information flow is going from top to bottom but not bottom up. This is problematic since lateral structures are often more appropriate for detection and diagnosis of crisis. In any crisis situation, there is a high probability that false hypotheses will develop and persist. It is largely through open exchange of messages, independent verification, and redundancy of communication channels that the existence of false hypotheses is likely to be detected. Therefore, in a crisis there is a premium on accuracy in interpersonal communication [518].

Research has shown that organizations are exceedingly complex systems that can easily drift toward disaster unless they maintain resources that enable them to learn from unusual events in their routine functioning. When communication breaks down, this learning does not occur [534]. Brian notes the difficulties inherent in trying to be more transparent in an organization:

Transparency is a double-edged sword for everyone. In the old way of operating, senior managers make decisions and then deliver the news to middle managers and so on down the line. On the negative side, obviously staff do not take kindly to being told about a decision that affects their lives that they had no input in making. On the other hand, sharing information on potential changes that are not fully formed can be extremely anxiety provoking. Recently we had a conversation with some of our staff about a potential change in one of our programs. Referrals were way down, and it was clear we needed to make a change in the program. The need for a change was evident to everyone, but initially there was a sense among the line staff and middle managers that there were clandestine meetings taking place at the highest levels in the organization. It seemed there was already some resentment building that staff were not included in these imagined meetings. The only problem was there were no secret meetings. When we met with the staff to discuss the problems of occupancy, staff were appreciative, but had lots of questions. Who would the program now serve? When would the change take place? How would the changes impact the current resident? Part of the problem with transparency is that you begin the conversations before you have the answers, in part, because you want the stakeholders to participate in constructing the answers. Staff members who do not feel particularly powerful, may not grasp the notion of sitting with the anxiety that comes with not knowing and not having all the answers. The anxiety associated with change can get acted out in a variety of ways. It is crucial that middle managers are able to sustain the conversation and help folks contain the emotions associated with change. If staff begin to act out excessively and their emotion spills out all over the place, senior managers get the cue that the staff cannot handle an unformed plan and as a result they may not share information as readily in the future.

Instead of increasing interpersonal communications, people in crisis are likely to resort to the excessive use of one-way forms of communication. Under stress, the supervisory structure tends to focus on the delivery of one-way, top-down information flow largely characterized by new control measures about what staff and clients can and cannot do. Feedback loops erode under such circumstances and morale starts to decline as the measures that are communicated do not alleviate the stress or successfully resolve the crisis. Brian describes the way miscommunication easily becomes an organizational style:

One of the most obvious things that happens in our organization under stress is that people stop meeting and talking with each other. The general sense is there is no time to meet because the workload is way too intense. So meetings get cancelled or certain staff members are allowed to miss meetings repeatedly. We have the sense that meetings are predominately for information sharing and so we convince ourselves that if we keep good notes and circulate them, the folks who missed the meeting can and will keep up. Unfortunately there is no substitute for face-to-face meetings. Gathering together as a group serves two major functions in a team: planning strategically and emotional management—both functions that even the best note taking will not replace.

In chronically stressed organizations, it may be the constant "noise" of interruptions that decreases the efficiency of complex thought processes and effective communication. Text messages flying, cell phones ringing again and again, calls for urgent responses all can provide information or simply be tremendous distractions. According to Mandler's theory of stress, autonomic nervous system activity is triggered by interruption which he defines as "*any event, external or internal to the individual, that prevents completion of some action, thought sequence or processing structure"* (p. 92) [535]. Both actions and thoughts can be interrupted, either when an expected event fails to occur or an unexpected event occurs. Crises, by definition, involve interruptions in actions and thoughts.

Another source of systematic error resides in the hierarchical nature of most organizations that is exacerbated by stress. When people are fearful of the response of the person above them in a hierarchy, they are likely to do things to communicate in ways that will minimize the negative response from their superior but which may significantly distort the message [536]. They do this in a variety of ways: by gatekeeping and thereby filtering some information in and other information out; by summarizing; by changing emphasis within a message; by actually withholding information; and by changing the nature of information [537] .

The way this plays out in the typical social service organization is that as stress increases and communication networks erode, the more complex team organizing strategies to deal with the complicated problems surrounding an emerging crisis with a patient, another staff member, or the organization as a whole are eliminated. The administrators at the top are likely to know the least about solving the problems at the bottom, and yet everyone turns to them, expecting them to solve the problem. As a result, the staff and administrators are likely to resort to simple, punitive, draconian, and restrictive methods of intervention more characteristic of their own childhood experiences than any rational theoretical, psychologically informed complex solutions to complex problems. Since these responses arise from regressive responses, they may not be entirely rationale and are likely to be ineffective. But because of the nature of group regression, it is difficult for the group to admit its own irrational responses, and therefore self-correcting mechanisms are not likely to readily occur and systematic error is likely to be the result.

When some or all of these communication pathologies are already in play, small events can lead to potentially disastrous outcomes. Organizational theorists have observed that when important routines are interrupted, when pressures lead people to fall back on what they learned first and most fully, when coordinated actions break down, and when communication exchanges become confusing, more errors occur, error detection is decreased, and errors pile upon and amplify each other. Complex and collective responses are all more vulnerable to this kind of disruption than are older, simpler, more over learned cultural and individual responses (Weick, 2001).

Poisoning the Grapevine

The notion of "the grapevine" originated during the American Civil War when telegraph lines were strung from tree to tree resembling grapevines, but the messages transmitted often were garbled, and these distorted messages were said to "come from the grapevine." One study contended that 70% of all organizational communication comes through this system of informal communication, and several national surveys found that employees used the grapevine as a communication source more than any other vehicle [538].

The grapevine carries accurate information *and* it carries rumors as well as gossip. Studies have shown that employees are most likely to rely on the grapevine when issues are perceived as important but ambiguous, when they are threatened, stressed, or insecure, when there is impending change, and when they feel that management is not communicating [538]. As one investigator put it, *"Rumor defines a thin line between impression and reality"* (p. 14) [539].

The commonly accepted understanding of rumor is that it is talk that is unsubstantiated by authority or evidence [540]. Rumors represent hypotheses about how the world works and are therefore attempts to make sense out of uncertain situations [539]. Four different types of rumors have been described as follows: *(1)* the pipe dream expressing what those circulating the rumor hope will happen; *(2)* the anxiety rumor, which is driven by fear and unease and often represents the "worst-case scenario"; *(3)* the anticipation rumor, which is usually precipitated by ambiguous situations where people are not sure what to expect; and *(4)* the malicious or aggressive rumor, which is motivated by an intention to harm others [541].

Rumors fill in the gap where facts are absent. Rumors frequently represent at least a kernel of truth. *"Lacking personal knowledge, we tend to think that where there is smoke, there is fire—or that a rumor would not have spread unless it was at least partly true"* (p. 5) [523]. Rumors are most likely to occur when something is happening that is particularly relevant to people's existence but they do not feel they actually have control over events. This is why rumors are likely to escalate when some organizational change is taking place. This is particularly true when the change itself challenges established beliefs or practice, but before the change has actually taken place and demonstrates the nature of the new reality. In contrast to gossip, the primary role of the rumor is to help people cope with uncertainty [540].

In highly stressed organizations, rumors have special influence because people are frequently not receiving enough accurate information to quell their fears and will thus grab onto any source of information, regardless of how ill informed it is, as a means of "knowing." Under these circumstances, rumors, which may not be given any credibility under the calmest of circumstances, spread faster than fire in a paper factory. Once set into motion, the rumor mill is likely to further escalate the sense of mistrust and apprehension that already exists.

The word *gossip* itself derives from the act of spreading the word about a new baby's birth, but that of course is not the way it is used today [541].

Put people together, men or women, old or young, anywhere in the world and we will gossip. Gossip occurs in virtually every group and workplace setting, but in times of uncertainty and chronic stress—usually a time of increased inter-personal conflict—negative gossip is likely to increase. In a work setting, nega-tive gossip enhances the gossiper's coercive power over the recipient of the gossip and the more accurate the gossip, the greater the gossiper's power [542].

The grapevine becomes poisonous as malignant rumors and negative, hurt-ful gossip increases. This is most likely to occur when people are uncertain and frightened. When it occurs it is likely that dysfunctional relational styles learned in a troubled family are brought into and played out in the workplace, as when bosses engage in gossiping and backbiting in order to maintain control, power, and security [543]. Managers may gossip with subordinates about other employees or clients and play one employee against another. The supervisor may make disparaging comments about one employee to another. All of this lends itself to the promotion of a toxic environment.

The Undiscussables and Organizational Alexithymia

Empirical data indicates that employees often feel compelled to remain silent in the face of concerns or problems, the *organizational silence* [544] or silencing response that we discussed in Chapter 5. As you may recall, in one study that interviewed employees from 22 organizations throughout the United States, 70% indicated that they felt afraid to speak up about issues or problems that they encountered at work. Harvard University educator Chris Argyris has dis-cussed the "self-fueling group processes" that group members consider to be potentially or actually embarrassing or threatening and therefore they cannot be discussed [545]. Brian knows his phenomenon only too well:

> You know that fear of speaking up is rolling when even folks who are willing to raise an issue begin the conversations by saying, "I am going to take a risk here…" and then they ask a question like "Why did we stop putting salt shakers on the lunch table?" That doesn't seem all that risky, but it flags that even asking the simplest question of leadership is risky business. It is worth paying attention to this.

The problems that people in organizations are afraid to go near, and that serve as major communication blockages that can lead to figurative—and sometimes literal—death are known as "undiscussables" or more commonly, "the elephants in the room." "*An undiscussable is a problem or issue that someone hesitates to talk about with those who are essential to its resolution*" (p. 78) [109]. The "undiscussables" can cover a wide range of areas, including policies and procedures, coworker performance, pay inequity, organizational inefficiencies, and poor organizational performance. But almost half of the undiscussables are likely to be about management performance, competence, and interpersonal style—most particularly how decisions are made by management; favoritism; management's role in promotions, assignments, and terminations; ethics; managerial motives; and corporate politics [109]. The undiscussables in mental health services often center on these very same issues as well as on past traumas, abuses, and inadequate delivery of services.

Subjects become undiscussable for reasons that have little to do with rational practice and everything to do with emotions. They are designed to keep people in a group from experiencing distress, or at least to keep some key people in a group from experiencing distress. They are the taboos that everyone knows about but can never be put out on the table; therefore, the underlying problems can never be addressed. And the longer these subjects go undiscussed, the harder it is to talk about them and the more they become both a cause and a result of fear [109]. Brian describes this at Andrus:

> *Many of our conflicts, which get played out over and over in program, stem from our inability to identify and clarify our basic assumptions about the work or the way things should operate. Things like the role of punishment, the role of families, the role of leadership, who does what task, how power is exercised, the etiology of the clients' problems. We come to the work with very different ideas about how these issues should play out, and we need to have ongoing clarifying conversations about our assumptions.*

In tracing preventable disasters, as in the *Challenger* spacecraft explosion, the fundamental problem frequently boils down to the "undiscussables"—what can and cannot be talked about, who is allowed to talk and who isn't, and what they are allowed and not allowed to say [546]. Decisions about what is undiscussable are rarely overtly made but are signaled nonverbally and through the organizational norms that exist at a cultural level.

The less of a participatory environment and the more hierarchical the organization is, the more likely that there will be an accumulation of undiscussables. The more authoritarian and punitive the organization is, the more likely it is that this accumulation of undiscussables will include some very nasty, threatening, and disturbing items. The more people in an organization cannot talk about those things that lie under the surface, the organizational secrets and skeletons, the more likely it is that the organizational culture will become dominated by self-fulfilling prophecies and reenactment behavior.

As we described in Chapter 3, the inability to give words to feelings is called "alexithymia," and a significant body of research has accumulated around the connection between alexithymia, somatic disorders, and a history of trauma [289]. We use it here, however, to apply to what happens to an organization as a whole when many important topics become undiscussable. We believe that an accumulation of traumatic experiences that become undiscussable produces an organizational state that resembles alexithymia in traumatized people who must find other ways to express troubling emotions because they cannot directly express these feelings and work them through within a social context.

When this happens, the organization becomes increasingly isolated and is likely to reenact traumatic experiences in a wide variety of ways that are ultimately detrimental to organizational functioning. We believe that the social service system in general and the mental health system in particular are suffering from "organizational alexithymia," unable to fully discuss what has happened in the overall environment, fearful of any sociopolitical analysis, avoiding painful memories and thoughts, and increasingly marginalized from the mainstream community. This makes the reenactment of trauma much more likely. The greater the number of undiscussables, the greater the amount of unresolved conflicts in the organization and the more likely it is that those conflicts are interfering with healthy organizational behavior. The greater the number of undiscussables, the more likely it is that the organization will be helpless to effectively react to the group phenomenon known as "collective disturbance."

Collective Disturbance As Organizational Dissociation

A "collective disturbance" is a common group phenomenon representing a profound disturbance in the communication network, unfolding when conflict higher in a hierarchy is being actually played out lower in the hierarchy, without anyone recognizing that there is a destructive parallel process going on. Extensively described in the first sociological study of a mental hospital and later in descriptions of democratic therapeutic communities in the 1950's and 1960's, it became clear to researchers that individual patients who became the focus of attention on a psychiatric unit were those who were the subject of unexpressed staff conflict [377; 547]. As soon as the staff conflict and communication blockades were surfaced, the individual patients' behavior improved. Similarly, collective disturbances involving several patients or an entire unit could be traced to conflicts originating near the top of the institutional hierarchy. The intensity of emotional interpersonal conflict and the separation of the cognitive and emotional content of information could be traced through the staff and into the patient community, traveling down through the vertical hierarchy largely via nonverbal, unconscious, and informal communication network. The staff/management conflicts usually seemed to revolve around disagreements between the priorities of institutional purposes or incompatibility between a given purpose and some institutional need. The level of immediate stress, collective emotional intelligence, and health of the communication system in an organization is likely to determine how rapidly and effectively a group manages this common but largely unconscious phenomenon.

The Natural History of a Collective Disturbance

When a conflict occurs in a hierarchical group that is felt but undeclared, the emotional and cognitive components of the conflict split, or dissociate outside of anyone's awareness and the emotional information is conveyed downward quickly, because of the rapid nature of emotional contagion, while the cognitive information remains largely unknown, held by authority figures, and sometimes secret. Group tension rises, but the tension is ascribed to other, often inaccurate sources. In such a climate, people withdraw from each other, errors accumulate, and vulnerable members of the staff begin acting out. Rumors abound and everyone tends to look for the source of the conflict in the clients who, by this time, are indeed beginning to respond to the emotional turmoil by acting out in whatever ways are typical for them individually. Formal communication decreases, but informal communication increases.

The signs of an impending collective crisis are abundant and largely non-verbal: errors in technique, doors left unlocked, messages forgotten, increased absenteeism frequently due to functional illness, staff preoccupation with problems of or with other staff, increased withdrawal by key staff members, an increased sense of helplessness, distorted or inaccurate information, increased rumors and gossip, missed or canceled meetings, an inability to make decisions, and finally, a sense that "something bad is going to happen," representing a vague understanding that unconscious factors are in play. If the evolving crisis is not attended to and resolved, violence on the part of several, although not all, patients/clients/students will be the result [377; 547]. If the managers and staff members are able to confront their own unspoken conflicts and restore more integrated communication, they can prevent or at least terminate a collective disturbance and, in doing so, reduce the level of violence within the community.

A collective disturbance often develops over several days. There are typical symptoms of an evolving group crisis that can be experienced by individuals or by everyone in the community. Initially, there is a period of unease, with a rising level of anxiety, irritability, and generalized stress. The usual interventions that a staff uses to reestablish equilibrium do not seem to work. At this point, staff members generally look for an individual cause for the problem, either within themselves or within a particular staff member who is lower in the organizational hierarchy or in a client. One person may be singled out as the "cause" of the problem and steps may be initiated to get the designated person out of the community, but such steps fail to resolve the problem. As the problem evolves, however, the milieu environment becomes more uncomfortable and every individual escalates whatever behavior he or she typically uses to manage stress.

As this spiral continues, everyone in the environment begins to sense a shift in the power balance. The sense of partnership between clients and staff and/or between staff members is supplanted by a growing sense of antagonism. The line staff members are likely to feel increasingly helpless and paralyzed. Everyone seems to be waiting for someone else to fix the problem. There is a reluctance to actively intervene in conflict situations accompanied by a minimization of the problem and even a denial that a problem exists on the part of some of the community members, while others become more loud and insistent that "somebody" needs to do something. *"It is bad enough to hear denial expressed by a single person in an organization. It is quite another to hear it voiced by a majority of the members of an organization. That is truly scary. When this happens, the denial is collective, and for this reason it is much harder to confront and to root out"* (p. 36) [382]. As the milieu heads towards the seemingly inevitable crisis, people feel increasingly attacked, everyone senses that individual and group safety is being threatened, boundaries that are usually respected are violated, rules are broken, until finally, violence erupts demanding a response on the part of the entire community. Here Sandy shares an example of her own experience with a collective disturbance:

An experienced nurse from a therapeutic community in the United Kingdom came to visit the Sanctuary program for two weeks. As we mentioned earlier, this was a program devoted to treating the profound psychiatric effects of childhood trauma. This visit occurred a few months prior to a major and unwanted change that had been announced to the staff the week before. The Sanctuary program was due to move to an entirely new hospital, forcing all of us to adjust to many unwelcome changes, including the loss of important relationships, while also offering more opportunities for growth and the potential for greater safety in an increasingly hostile economic environment. It was the only way the program was going to survive. As the leader, I had met with the staff and announced the move, but I was very angry about the circumstances, felt very guilty that people's lives were about to be so disrupted based on a decision I had to make, and as a consequence I had unwittingly shut down debate or even much conversation about all that went into this decision. I thought I was protecting the staff but really I was protecting myself—it was just too painful to talk about.

Our visiting nurse was initially an outsider to the group, but she rapidly integrated into the staff milieu and provided a unique observer/participant role for the time she was present. The first week, the patient community was unusually obstructive. The patients were not functioning well as a group. There were frequent complaints about the usual things—staff not being attentive enough, poor food, not enough hot water, and the like—all of which consumed an inordinate amount of time in individual and group discussion while serving to allow everyone to avoid the necessity of dealing with their real reasons for being in the hospital. No amount of staff redirection seemed able to get the community back onto its therapeutic tasks. The level of acting out in the form of self-mutilation, suicidal ideation, and minor boundary violations escalated throughout the week. Yet these patients were in no substantive way different from a similar group of patients on any other week. By the end of the week, the staff were bitterly complaining that "this is the worst community we have ever had."

There was a regular staff meeting scheduled for the end of the week, and although the focus of the meeting was supposed to be on individual treatment plans, when she heard the staff complaints about all the patients in the community, our visitor tentatively broached the subject as a question for the group. "Could there be something going on with us that was impacting the community—were we in the grip of a collective disturbance?"

In doing so, she took the valve off the pressure cooker and the staff began voicing their concerns, conflicts, and fears about upcoming changes. Because someone outside the group brought it up, and in doing so temporarily became the informal leader and was not a part of our "social defense" system (whose job it is to protect the leader and the group from too much anxiety), I as the leader was able to hear what she was suggesting and that allowed me to more calmly listen and not get in the way of the conversation. What also came to light was a previously unexpressed recognition that this week signaled the second anniversary of a suicide that had occurred on the unit and that had been a traumatic experience for everyone involved. It is important to recognize that neither the move nor the prior suicide could be changed. There was no decision to be made, only formerly undiscussables to discuss. We did exactly that and then went back to our tasks at the time the meeting was designated to end.

But seemingly miraculously, and through no other intervention, by the next week we had "the best community ever." The patients—the very same patients—were eagerly and wholeheartedly embracing therapy, focusing on their significant issues, and working together with care and compassion as a group. At the level of staff and management, reassociating the emotional and cognitive components of information, making the unconscious conscious, encouraging communication vertically and horizontally, and reading the message in the nonverbal information we were getting from the clients and the staff allowed healthy communication channels to be re-established. The patients, as the most vulnerable members of the community, no longer needed to carry the burden of expressing in behavior what needed to be integrated and assimilated with words by the staff.

Chronic Collective Disturbance

To become more effective at managing these kinds of collective emergent phenomena, management and staff members must realize that such phenomena exist. In our highly individualistic culture, this can be a hard sell. In general, we are not accustomed to perceiving unconscious motivations of individuals, much less those of entire groups. In the case of a collective disturbance, what occurs cannot simply be explained by the usual emotional contagion that occurs in groups. A collective disturbance has a structure that may not always be immediately visible because so much is going on underground, in the "shadow group." But the disturbance is a sign that the social defense system that we discussed in Chapter 4 has been activated and organizational communication is shifting to a defensive mode. If this conflict is not confronted, the result may be a state of chronic collective disturbance.

Without an understanding of how the unconscious minds of individuals and of groups function, organizations may remain in total ignorance of the collective emotional disturbances that begin to repeatedly impact their organizations. New leaders and other new employees may walk into an organization that is in the grip of collective disturbance and be able to recognize it but lack the skills, influence, or opportunity to do anything about it. When this is happening, an organization is becoming "emotionally disturbed" itself.

Dehumanization and Bureacracy

These collective processes and the unconscious social defenses that give rise to them help to explain how distance from suffering people can permit decisions to be made that may be completely lacking in empathy or understanding of their plight, by otherwise caring and committed individuals. When we don't actually *see* the suffering, our own emotions are not mobilized. When we feel a sense of divided loyalty—who should we be loyal to? Our bosses, our organization, the clients? It is then much easier to dehumanize people and dehumanization is a slippery slope. Dehumanization occurs when people begin treating another person or groups of people as less than fully human, inferior and unworthy of respect or equal experience. It occurs whenever some human beings exclude other human beings from the moral order of being a person and is the central process, the beginning first step, of every evil, every atrocity committed by man against man [548].

When we are distanced from another suffering being, it is far simpler to mount intellectual reasons—that often make a great deal of sense from a purely logical point of view—that serve to justify decisions and policies that would otherwise be unacceptable. It becomes simple to propose either-or arguments and turn complex problems into simple ones. It becomes infinitely easier to turn people into economic indicators, or budgetary nuisances, or productivity figures. In this way, layers of bureaucracy allow decision makers to create policies and send them as instructions downward through the layers of a hierarchy without having to experience the consequences of those instructions because the natural human activation of the mirror neuron system does not occur. In doing so, our systems *systematically* eliminate that which makes us the most able to deal with complex problems—integrated thoughts *and* feelings—and we end up creating collective disturbances completely out of conscious awareness.

Without empathy it is easy to suggest apparently "logical" solutions that are actually fundamentally immoral. Processes that dehumanize people can easily be put in place by otherwise caring and concerned people unless there are clear standards of moral safety that actively guide people at every level in communication and decision-making processes. As Brian describes,

This can also be the source of misalignment in organizations. We make a decision at one level in the organization and then when a manager actually has to look someone in the eye at the next level and make this happen, the manager picks up the sad eyes or the irritation and then waffles. The manager makes concessions and changes and often does not come back to his or her own manager and say, "You know when we rolled this out, people really had trouble with it." The manager just allows drift. All of a sudden what we thought was happening was in fact completely derailed and there is no clear explanation for how or when that happened.

Conclusion

Communication is essential to the health of organizations and yet there are multiple interactive barriers to good communication, particularly under conditions of chronic stress when conflicts are not resolved and increasing numbers of undiscussables cloud judgment, perspective, and common sense. The result of broken communication networks is likely to be the emergence of collective disturbances that will lead to violence if they are not resolved. In the next chapter we will explore in more detail the influence of power relationships, authoritarianism, and the helplessness that abuses of power can induce in everyone.

Chapter 9

Authoritarianism, Disempowerment, and Learned Helplessness

SUMMARY: *As communication breaks down, errors compound, and the situation feels increasingly out of control, organizational leaders become more controlling and authoritarian. Under these circumstances, workplace bullying is likely to increase at all levels, and organizations may become vulnerable to petty tyrants. As the organization becomes more hierarchical and autocratic, there is a progressive and simultaneous isolation of leaders and a "dumbing down" of staff, with an accompanying "learned helplessness" and loss of critical thinking skills. The organization and the individuals in it become highly risk avoidant. Efforts to empower workers may pay only lip service to true participatory processes.*

Exerting Control: An Adaptive Evolutionary Response to Fear

At present, most organizations and institutions in our society are more hierarchical and bureaucratic than democratic. Investigators in the field have pointed out the strong tendency within organizations to gravitate toward hierarchical modes of structuring themselves [549]. In the early part of the twentieth century, Michels described "the iron law of oligarchy," which contends that as organizations grow larger and become more complex, increased specialization occurs along with the need for more expert leadership; when this happens, participation in organizational decision making declines. He was pessimistic about the possibility of success for any democratic experiment [550].

A strong tendency toward hierarchical control has been noticed, even in organizations that claim to be democratic. It has been argued that management resists free speech more stubbornly than any other concession to employees [551]. This has been substantiated by a review of court decisions pertaining to freedom of speech in the workplace revealing a general assumption *"that conflict and dissent are always bad and no good can come from them; a concept that flies in the face of modern thought on organizational conflict and free speech"* (p. 260) [552]. Conflict needs to move us, not stall us. As Brian describes:

A major hazard of having power is that people often do not tell you the truth. This is not malicious or mean spirited; it is simply self-preservation. I have found that the story of the Emperor's New Clothes captures a reality that is a very real threat to healthy organizational functioning. If you are in a position of leadership, it is not uncommon for people around you to agree with you and tell you you're brilliant, regardless of what you actually do or say. To be effective as a leader, you need people to tell you that you are naked when you are. You need to trust that people can be honest with you, but to make this possible you need to make sure that at every turn you are willing to listen to contrary points of view. You need to remain open minded and accepting of opposing points of view, or they will stop coming, even when we most need them. The larger the organization, the more difficult it is to establish a participatory kind of work environment so each level needs to have this approach with the next. Since trust is crucial, how do we come to trust people who we have little or no contact with? It is particularly challenging to make this shift in an organization which has historically had a more autocratic style. It may be possible for senior leaders to make this shift, but middle managers need to be able to make the shift as well and their sense of vulnerability may make this very difficult.

Everyone Wants to Be Powerful

Everybody wants to be powerful; after all, what is the choice other than being powerless? But power can be expressed in ways that create and in ways that destroy. One can use power to do something, to prevent or to delay something from being done. Power can be directed inwardly toward oneself or outwardly toward others. Power can be exerted against, over, or with someone else. Inward power can influence people outside oneself. Outwardly expressed power can change people on the inside. Power can be used to exert control or to give over control. Power can be used to coerce and force, or power can be used to free people from oppression. There are overt displays of power and there is the subtle use of power [553]. Power can be enforced or it can simply be assumed. The following story of Brian's is an example of the exercise of assumed power.

About a year ago I was supposed to be speaking at a conference in Maryland. I told the conference organizers that I would bring my own LCD projector, since renting one would cost them several hundred dollars. It was my intention to drive down to the conference, so bringing the projector was not a major inconvenience. I was planning to leave for the conference on Wednesday, so on Monday morning at 9:30 a.m. I called our MIS staff and told them I needed the projector for Wednesday. About 45 minutes later one of our MIS staff appeared at my office door with the projector. I thanked them for dropping it off and told them I would return it on Thursday when I got back from the conference. I put the projector on the floor next to my desk and returned to doing my work.

At 12:00 noon our Training Director, Tito, appeared at the door of my office. I said hello and asked him what I could do for him. He looked a little irritated and the first words out of his mouth were, "What's the deal, what is going on here?" I responded by saying, "huh?" He pointed to the projector sitting on the floor of my office. I said I was doing a presentation on Thursday in Maryland, and I promised I would bring a projector. To which Tito replied, "What's wrong with you?" I didn't think there was anything wrong with me, but I am often the last to know when something is wrong with me, so I replied, "What are you talking about?"

Tito then proceeded to tell me the story of his morning. He had been conducting a training session in the training room on campus that was scheduled to run from 9:00 a.m.-12 noon. He began the training at 9:00 a.m. and at about 10:00 a.m. the door of the training room opened up and our MIS staff members walked in. They announced to Tito that "Brian needs the projector"; they proceeded to unplug and disconnect the projector in the middle of the training and walk out with it.

Tito was left to finish the training without his visual aids. Fortunately he was left with more than enough resentment to finish off his presentation. I can only imagine how pleased he was to see the projector in its carrying case on the floor of my office. I explained I had called and asked for the projector, but had no idea they were going to yank it out of the training. I apologized profusely, and Tito seemed to understand what had happened and accepted my apology.

This was a sobering experience. I have known Tito for over 15 years, and I am pretty sure he does not think I am a jerk. But in that moment he certainly had his doubts. He was, however, grown up enough and brave enough to come and confront me and get to the bottom of what had happened. I wondered how many times that happens and I never find out about it. How often do maintenance guys get pulled out of repairing the broken radiator in a child's bedroom to come over and tighten that screw that is sticking out of my door? You know— the work request I wrote that said, "When you get a chance, could you tighten that screw. No hurry." Yeah, the one that 3 seconds after I wrote it the foreman called the guy on the walkie-talkie while six staff were in earshot working to repair the radiator in a kid's room who was freezing last night and told him to drop everything to take care of my loose screw.

These incidents serve as reminders that there are forces that exist way beyond me, as the leader, that are in play. But even if I don't know what they are, these influences and experiences serve to shape my image in the organization and paint a picture that people in power only care about what they want and need. In this example, no one intended any harm and in fact had the best of intentions, and yet things went off the rails and could have easily snowballed from there. If Tito wasn't Tito, and we didn't trust each other, then he could have held a silent grudge against me for years that could have affected many people over time. If Tito wasn't a trainer but instead was a staff person, the power differential would have been too great for that person to confront me, and instead he or she would be more likely to take out his or her frustration on the kids and tell other staff members that I am obviously a jerk. It is extremely important that people in leadership positions at any level recognize that even if they don't feel they have power, other people believe they do and that perception can change all sorts of things, not necessarily for the better.

Learned Helplessness and the Lust for Power

The fundamental existential reality that all human beings must face is that we will die and that all we work for, dream of, and know will be gone. So incomprehensible and awesome is this knowledge that from the moment of our birth we are struggling to overcome it, to control ourselves, other people, and the world around us, all in service of denying our existential vulnerability. Even before the onslaught of the twentieth century, the English historian Lord Acton wrote in 1887 that *"Power tends to corrupt, and absolute power corrupts absolutely"* [554]. We believe that for the most part this corruption is rooted in fear. The more one develops defenses against the reality of mortality, the more one fears losing those defenses and in this way, power itself becomes addictive because it offers the illusion that somehow "you can take it with you." As in so many traumatized clients who use money, drugs, alcohol, food, and other substances to fend off their terrible despair about what has happened to them, those who seek ever-increasing levels of power do so to satisfy a craving for certainty and control over deep and largely unconscious feelings of existential terror and despair.

When People Become Poison Containers, the Poison Leaks Out

The result is a lust for power that is commensurate with our fear—the more frightened we are, and the more we are compelled to deny our fear, the more we struggle for control. Given that other people and nature are impossible to completely control without violence, it is essential that we learn how to manage the fear in ourselves, our societies, our workplaces, our families, through methods that ensure checks and balances on our desire for power and the basic terror that drives it. At the same time, the enormity of the threats we face are staggering in their ability to arouse fear, and therefore it is astonishingly easy for the most fearful and the most powerful among us to seize control of an organization or even an entire society and manipulate other people into becoming psychological and physical defenses against the fear they feel inside [348–351].

The magnitude of these existential fears is rooted in our experience in childhood. The psychohistorian Lloyd DeMause has written extensively on the ways in which historical and modern parents have used the exercise of power over children as a way of overcoming their own basic helplessness and fear, leftover from their own childhoods, projecting all of their own unruly and unresolved distress onto their children and using children as what he has termed "poison containers" [555]. In this way, the use and abuse of power over others is conveyed across the generations and becomes the family and the social norm. Although applied here to family relationships, it is easy to extend this metaphor more generally. Consider the many ways in which poisonous, toxic feelings are spread around an organization.

When the lust for power in a person is paired with intelligence, a genetic predisposition for psychopathy, and an abusive or neglectful upbringing, the results are likely to be devastating for other human beings. The neurocircuitry of empathy appear to have evolved to serve the social bonds between mother and child and then for pair-bonding. When these neurological connections are examined, the brain circuits that are interconnected are for social behavior, physical pain, and the ability to represent both the self and the other in the mind. As a result, empathy is built into all mammals, and when we see someone else in pain, we feel pain ourselves and will naturally act in some way to alleviate the pain [556]. The latest research information indicates that individuals with high psychopathy scores, at least those who have been studied—all of whom were in prison (which is *not* where the majority of psychopaths reside)— have brain deficits that leave them unable to experience emotions as other people do, including empathy, and bullies appear to enjoy other people's pain [557–559]. However, most people with high psychopathic traits end up working in the same office or the same community as the rest of us, *"among the professions likely to attract psychopaths are law enforcement, the military, politics, and medicine"* (p. 8) [557]. According to one writer on the subject, 4% of the population have these impairments, but they account for only 20% of the prison population [559]. These are the people most likely to bully and terrorize others in the workplace. Conditions of external threat are likely to induce many others to go along with them.

There is no getting away from the exercise of power, but in any organization it is important that people are safe enough to discuss this fundamental aspect of existence that is so central to our personal and professional lives. The human preoccupation with the exercise of power, particularly the tendency to oppress others and abuse power can only be understood by grappling with the universal human experience of helplessness. Repeated experience with helplessness decreases our ability to survive regardless of whether we are chickens or humans [296; 560]. Helplessness is toxic and human beings, unlike other mammals, are only too aware of our utter helplessness in the face of the inevitability of death.

Trauma Is Inescapable Shock: Learned Helplessness

Learned helplessness was first defined as a concept in the early 1960s when Overmier and Seligman began doing experiments on the reaction of animals to inescapable shock. The basic idea was that a perceived lack of control over one's environment leads to future inaction. Seligman suggested that human beings, born in a state of total helplessness, gradually develop a sense of control as the child learns that his intentions direct his voluntary movements and that he or she also has an impact on the people around him [296]. Under the right circumstances a child comes to believe that his or her actions will predictably affect outcomes and increasingly develops a sense of mastery and self-efficacy.

On the other hand, repetitive experiences with a lack of mastery, loss of control, helplessness, and failure teaches people—both children and adults— that regardless of what one does, there will be a negative outcome. Trauma, by definition, represents a devastating experience of helplessness. This engenders an internal experience of what has come to be known as "learned helplessness." *Learned helplessness* is a phenomenon containing three components: contingency, cognition, and behavior. Contingency addresses the relative uncontrollability of the situation. Cognition refers to the attributions that people make regarding their situation or surroundings of which they are a part. Behavior allows individuals to decide whether they will give up or proceed with the obstacle set before them [561]. The less controllable the situation, the more the person attributes the situation to being inevitable or his or her own fault; the more the person has failed to act in a helpful way or acted in a way that did not help, then the more likely the experience is to produce helplessness and therefore be a toxic one.

Learned Helplessness and Blaming Others

Studies of learned helplessness in humans have shown that exposure to recurrent unsolvable problems in the present can undermine performance on a future task. In terms of the original theory, these deficits result from a reduction in a person's expectations of being able to control the outcome. Upon recurrent failure to solve a problem, people may develop the expectation that nothing they do will affect the outcome and may generalize this expectation to other tasks. As a result, they may put less effort into subsequent tasks and consequently show performance deficits. Research has consistently shown that people who attribute failure to internal, stable, or global causes perform worse in a new task than people who make an external, unstable, or specific attribution of causality [562–563]. This is probably the underlying defensive purpose of blaming that we discussed in Chapter 5—attributing failure to something outside of oneself—something that is potentially controllable, feels better than blaming oneself, or what we call "taking responsibility for one's mistakes". Hence, the more helplessness a person has been exposed to, the less likely the person is to take responsibility and will instead find someone or something else to blame to try and in doing so protect his or her already fragile self.

The more uncontrollable existence has been, therefore, the more helpless a person has been in childhood, particularly helpless to self-protect or protect others, the more heightened will be the person's defenses against helplessness and the deep sense of shame that inevitably accompanies helplessness. When people self-protect against the shame of being helpless, a common protective mechanism is to "attack others." It is against this background of early childhood helplessness, abuse, and neglect that Dr. Jim Gilligan understood the criminals that he worked with in a prison for the criminally insane: *"Physical violence, neglect, abandonment, rejection, sexual exploitation and violation occurred on a scale so extreme, to bizarre, and so frequent that one cannot fail to see that the men who occupy the extreme end of the continuum of violent behavior in adulthood occupied an equally extreme end of the continuum of violent child abuse earlier in life"* (p. 45) [300].

When instead that strategy is to "attack self," people are more likely to become depressed and self-destructive. Learned helplessness has been expanded to describe some people's pessimistic explanatory style in which individuals attribute negative events to internal or stable causes over which they believe they have no control, and people with this style are said to be more likely to develop a helpless response in the face of new challenges. Learned helplessness has also been used as an explanation for the ways in which people learn to cope with repetitive trauma and as a model for depression. Dr. Donald Nathanson has written extensively about the importance of shame in understanding the various defensive strategies that people use to protect against the overwhelming nature of shame [435]. Although over the years there has been a great deal of discussion and debate over the exact mechanism of learned helplessness, it has been applied to a wide cross-section of people from test-taking students to disruptive children and their mothers [564].

Our Systems Promote Learned Helplessness

Learned helplessness at work has been defined as a debilitating cognitive state in which individuals often possess the skills and abilities necessary to perform their jobs but exhibit suboptimal or poor performance because they attribute prior failures to causes which they cannot change, even though success may be possible in the current environment [565]. When applied to the mental health system, it is possible to see parallels between the helpless responses of the clients and the helpless responses of the staff and managers who serve them. Historically, our systems of care have not focused on empowering clients to make their own decisions but have instead created "expert" cultures within which the client is chronically dependent for help on a medical model that places expertise solely in the hands of caregivers. Helpless passive or passive-aggressive dependency is likely to be the result. Visit many mental health care, health care, or social service environments today and you will see the same behavior mirrored in the staff.

In a controlling, non-participatory environment exercising top-down management, every subsequent lower level of employee is likely to become progressively disempowered. This organizationally induced helplessness has been described as the antithesis of empowerment [566]. After years, decades, and even generations of controlling management styles, reversing this sense of disempowerment can be extremely difficult, particularly under conditions of chronic, unrelenting organizational stress. To be effective, hiring people with a sense of self-efficacy is really crucial, but if you are running an autocratic shop you will avoid these folks like the plague. So instead, the autocratic institution keeps reenacting failed strategies: hiring or retaining people who will support the notion that they have to be told what to do and will not take responsibility for their own decisions, creating a self-fulfilling prophecy.

All workers bring to the workplace environment various personal dispositional factors such as optimism or pessimism—seeing the glass as half full or as half empty. The big five personality factors that have been shown to positively influence performance include extroversion, emotional stability, agreeableness, conscientiousness, and openness to experience. These factors are likely to influence the way workers do their job and the results they get. Individuals then attribute cause for the outcomes they get. When the cause is obvious, this factor plays less of a role but when the cause is ambiguous, people tend to fall into their own habitual way of explaining bad events that befall them.

Learned helplessness is associated with a style that is stable—happens all the time—and internal—"it's because there is something wrong with me"[567]. This style is likely to lead to one where the person is always in the victim role. In other research this "external locus of control"—believing that you are a pawn at the mercy of external forces—contrasts with an "internal locus of control" where you believe you are in control of your own behavior [565]. When people develop an external locus of control, they are reluctant to take any responsibility for their own behavior and attribute all problems to external causes over which they have no control.

As we discussed in Chapter 2, there are significant situational factors that may influence performance level. People regularly subjected to role conflict, role overload, and role ambiguity accompanied by a pervasive sense of helplessness may feel prevented from asking for help, getting clarification, and receiving support. Tasks may be ambiguous or poorly defined. Feedback may be nonexistent or be so distant from the actual behavior that it is meaningless. Success may be very difficult to assess and may be only distantly related to day-to-day actions on the part of the worker [567].

In many mental health situations, roles are very ambiguous, particularly for institutional front-line workers, and their tasks are frequently ill-defined.

Although they are supposed to help clients "recover," what this means is unclear, while they are likely to be punished if they fail to "control" the clients and punished if they are excessively punitive or controlling. Feedback for the ways in which they convey empathic regard for the clients may be minimal, while feedback for the ways in which they do not make the clients follow the rules may be rapid, punishing, and pervasive. And in virtually all mental health and social service environments, there are great distances between what individuals do on a day-to-day basis and long-term outcomes. In this way, providing these services bears a closer similarity to parenting than to most other kinds of jobs.

Staff members in juvenile justice settings are expected to help these troubled young people become more accountable and responsible for the problematic behavior they have directed at others. Unfortunately, however, they have been asked to do this in what is often a largely nontherapeutic context and instead have to try somehow to bring about change in these children through punitive command and control measures. To try and control the children's behavior, the environments tend to become increasingly rigid and rule bound and in doing so inadvertently promote more helplessness rather than more mastery.

This is exacerbated by the abuse that can happen while they are in a facility. According to recent figures released by the Department of Justice, an estimated 12% of youth in state juvenile facilities and large non-state facilities (representing 3220 youth nationwide) reported experiencing one or more incidents of sexual victimization by another youth or facility staff in the past 12 months or since admission, if less than 12 months. Over 10% (2730) reported an incident of sexual victimization involving facility staff [568]. The problem is that given the background of abuse and neglect that these children are known to have experienced, unless the environment can help young people deal with locus of control, and the helplessness and shame that underlies it, it is impossible for these young people to become more accountable and responsible citizens.

In other social service settings, clients are only occasionally consulted in how they are to solve their own problems. Collaborative problem solving has become increasingly rare in residential placements, child protective services, shelters, and health care programs as stress on these programs increases. Adults have little enough say in the way care is delivered to them, while children get virtually no say at all. On November 20, 1989, the United Nations adopted the Convention on the Rights of the Child, a landmark for human rights. Here for the first time was a treaty that sought to address the particular human rights of children and to set minimum standards for the protection of their rights. The Convention on the Rights of the Child is the first legally binding international instrument to incorporate the full range of human rights—civil, cultural, economic, political, and social. It sets forth basic standards which individual nations agree to pursue on behalf of children. With 193 nations having ratified it, the Convention is the most widely adopted human rights treaty in history.

The United States is the only nation that has not ratified the Convention, other than the failed state of Somalia [569]. What does this tell us? Perhaps that in the United States, people see their kids as possessions, and the state has no right to tell us what to do with our property.

The Parallel Process of Organizationally Induced Helplessness

So the clients who routinely require services in human service systems are people who are likely to have experienced situations, often traumatic ones, over which they have had little control. This lack of control has been repetitive and has profoundly influenced their view of themselves and other people. They come to be "fixed" or to get their problems "solved." But their problems are not readily fixed by anyone else. Sure, there are some things we can do, prescribe, suggest, and even implement. But for the most part, people who need help must rouse themselves to take mastery over the chronic problems that plague them.

Our diagnostic system encourages helplessness. For example, when someone comes into a setting with a diagnosis of a personality disorder, the typical response is that there is nothing that can be done to change that person and the best thing to do is to get them out of the setting, or at least away from you. Children diagnosed with conduct disorder may be perceived as unchangeable, bound for a life of imprisonment. Under such conditions, the least trained people—who are usually those who spend the most time with the clients—are likely to be the most profoundly influenced by what ends up many times being the kind of self-fulfilling prophecy we described in Chapter 7.

In an organization, employees may engage in specific behaviors that contribute to organizational helplessness. They may stop striving for high levels of achievement because they harbor a fundamental belief that no matter what they do, they will not make a significant difference. Other people become passive, failing to seek out any new or innovative ways of approaching a problem and resisting anyone else's suggestions as impossible. Some become passive-aggressive, sticking to the letter of the rules and doing nothing above and beyond following the rules. Many will not make decisions, even when urged to do so, because they are afraid of negative consequences [570].

Research has demonstrated that employees of centralized, bureaucratic organizations that rely on formal rules and policies often experience feelings of alienation, frustration, and helplessness [571]. Not being able to control work methods, performance evaluations, and decision making all contribute to the sense of helplessness within an organization. The less participation an employee has, the more this is likely to be the case. As one investigator stated, "*Aspects of the organizational environment such as traditional appraisal systems, flawed reward systems, poor leadership, counterproductive personnel policies, and inappropriate organizational structure are all said to lead to feelings of helplessness on the part of organizational members. If organizationally induced helplessness results in lowered feelings of performance efficacy, both for new tasks and those currently being performed by these members, strategies to decrease and even reverse these feelings are critical"* (p. 408) [572].

Learned helplessness is visible everywhere in the human service system. In the mental health system, the systematic takeover by managed care, the pressures of deinstitutionalization, the devaluation of the sacred nature of psychotherapeutic healing, along with the increased medicalization of service delivery have represented an uncontrollable series of events to everyone within the system [573]. Individual personality differences not withstanding, it appears that the system as a whole has responded with an inability to protect itself, suffering blow after blow with little if any protest. Culture is important because it acts as a buffer and supportive system for its members and provides members with a stock of knowledge about the way things work and a set of meanings that makes sense of that work. Collective trauma tests that stock of knowledge, and if the organizational culture cannot answer the test of explanation to its members, then the members are left disempowered, helpless, and unable to make sense out of their experience [574]. This is an apt description, applicable to all of the social service professions who have rallied little organized protest to the devastating impacts of the changes that have occurred, whether those changes have resulted in significantly diminished services to their clients or significantly diminished incomes and job satisfaction for themselves.

Many human service organizations promote further helplessness in their workers through fundamental flaws in structure and process. Then the staff of these organizations encounter the complex problems presented by their clients as insolvable problems that simply frustrate them further. Helpless to protect themselves, feeling embattled, hopeless, and helpless, the staff and management often engage in risky risk avoidance—risk management policies that may virtually prevent therapeutic change.

Risky Risk Avoidance

The notion of risk comes from the French word *risqué*, which at the turn of the nineteenth century referred to a wager between individuals taking account of the probability of losses and gains [575]. In its present usage, risk has been defined as *"the projection of a degree of uncertainty about the future on to the external world"* (p. 5) [576]. Between 1967 and 1991, the number of articles published about "risk" went from 1000 article in the first 5-year period, to 80,000 in the last 5-year period reviewed, suggesting to the investigator that medical practice specifically and Western society in general have become preoccupied with minimizing risk, just at a point in time when the risk of so many major threats to human health are lower than at any other point in history. One author calls this a "risk epidemic" and relates it to the growing belief that we can and should control all the risks to our safety, to our health, and to our existence [577]. Others have pointed out that we live in a "risk society" [578–579].

This kind of attitude has never existed before and we can attribute it to the combination of discoveries in science and the ability of computers to meet enormous statistical challenges and calculate all kinds of relationship among variables. Unlike our forebears who carried a reasonably fatalistic attitude toward our inevitable demise, a prevalent social attitude—backed up by many legal proceedings—is that people can identify and eliminate risk factors through proper "risk management" and can thereby prevent disease and of course, death [577; 580]. What unfortunately accompanies this notion is the linkage of risk factors with causal hypotheses. And if knowing someone is at risk leads to a supposed cause for a problem that medical professionals are assigned to treat, then failure to control supposedly high-risk situations leads to malpractice claims and rising unrealistic expectations of health care, social services like child welfare, and mental health care. As Brian describes it:

> We operate in a very risk-aversive society, where mistakes, oversights, and misstatements are often blown out of proportion. This has us all on pins and needles, and in organizations we may overreact to even small missteps. It is impressive sometimes to see what some of the things are that make us crazy. They are problems to be sure, but they are not catastrophes. When we overreact, staff are left scratching their heads and feeling terribly unsafe. As a result, they may become more secretive about what might be going wrong, and problems can escalate to the point that things become dangerous.

Risk and Risk Avoidance in the Mental Health System

Nowhere is the problem of risk assessment, risk management, and risk avoidance more evident than in the delivery of mental health services. To assess risk, it is necessary to classify risk, and in mental health this means classifying people into various forms of mental disturbance. This would not be so problematic if, as in pneumonia or heart disease, we were able to take a blood test or a radiology study of some sort and scientifically diagnose a problem. But psychiatry is not a science based on hard, quantifiable data but on the subjective determination of more-or-less skilled and experienced clinicians. As pointed out by the author of the Study Guide to *DSM-IV*, "*the diagnoses in DSM-IV are like ready-made suits that come in a variety of standard styles and sizes. They fit many patients well, others adequately, and some barely at all. The clinician's task, like the clothier's, is to fit individuals with specific characteristics into standard, predefined categories...The art of diagnosis depends on the clinician's ability to find and fix the patient into the appropriate diagnostic category even if he or she has atypical signs and symptoms*" (pp. 175–176) [581].

A significant problem with this approach is that the diagnostic label defines reality, even when the person does not actually fit the label very well at all. Although mental illness has and still does exist, each new version of the *Diagnostic and Statistical Manual* has expanded the number of categories that are considered to be mental disorders until virtually everyone could be seen as having some symptoms typical of some disorder that may or may not be causing some form of debilitation. Since mental health professionals are presumed to be expert at providing the remedy for the mental versions of medical disorders, then mental health professionals become responsible for preventing the problems related to or caused by the individuals bearing these diagnoses. And if problems still occur, even though these diagnosed individuals are under the care of medical experts, then the medical experts can be held responsible for the failures in "treatment." Given that every kind of behavior can fit into this nosology, individual choice is largely superseded by a definition of medical disorder.

This becomes a particularly pressing issue when people in certain kinds of diagnostic categories do harm to themselves or harm to others. Relatively few mental health professionals will quibble over the responsibility they carry when treating someone who is acutely psychotic, manic, or psychotically depressed. But what about the "liminal" disorders, the people who carry diagnoses of personality disorders, particularly borderline personality disorder [582]? Sometimes recognized as "sick," other times as "bad," these patients are notoriously at high risk for harmful and destructive behavior and yet they are generally considered to be neither legally insane nor incompetent. Nonetheless, a significant amount of time, resources, and energy in all mental health practices is spent on trying to figure out how to assess and manage the risks these individuals pose. The ever-present danger is that they will act destructively in some way—a horrific circumstance for everyone involved—and that the mental health professional and his or her system will be held liable for the patient's conduct.

Several investigators reviewing the issue of risk management have noted that the behavior generally focused upon as risky is selective and narrow. Never is there a thorough investigation of the risks to the patient of risk management or of the risk to the clinician of not resorting to the *DSM-IV* diagnostic system [581]. In reality, an overemphasis on risk management is likely to lead to "treatment" environments within which real treatment is impossible because the possibility for the individual actually taking risks and thereby engaging in the process of change is so minimized that stagnation occurs. And it is impossible, unless there is some source of private funding, to even enter the systems of care without having a diagnosis. And relatively little attention is paid to the risk of using psychotropic medications despite a large body of evidence supporting the established dangers of many of these medications [583].

In many settings, the confusion is profound and frequently results in restrictive, controlling mental health settings that at times may minimize the risk of some forms of danger but also minimize the possibility that anything will change. As we discussed in Chapter 4, the underlying mental model that holds up the mental health system is a fundamental part of the problem. As long as troubled and troubling people are either "sick" or "bad" (or both), the definitions of what constitutes sickness and the legal wrangling surrounding these definitions will inevitably continue.

A model that views most psychological dysfunction as a sign of "injury" can lead to very different premises upon which to make sounder judgments [1]. Regardless of how divergent their point of view, injured people—as long as their basic cognitive functions are intact—are seen as having agency and as individuals who are responsible for their own choices. Risky risk avoidance happens when social service and mental health organizations become so risk avoidant that they inhibit therapeutic change and instead insist on trying to "control behavior." The only way we can control someone else's behavior is to completely restrict that person's freedom, and when we do that we also eliminate that person's capacity to make the choice to change. The issues of power, control, and risk become steadily and significantly more critical when an organization is in crisis.

Chronic Crisis, Centralized Control, and Terror Management

When a crisis occurs, centralization of control is significantly increased with leaders tightening reins, concentrating power at the top, and minimizing participatory decision making [533]. Even where there are strong beliefs in the "democratic way of life," there is always a tendency in institutions, and in the larger containing society, to regress to simple, hierarchical models of authority as a way of preserving a sense of security and stability. This is not just a phenomenon of leadership; in times of great uncertainty, everyone in the institution colludes to collectively bring into being authoritarian organizations as a time-honored method for providing at least the illusion of greater certainty and therefore a diminution of anxiety [362].

From an evolutionary standpoint, this makes a great deal of sense. As we mentioned in Chapter 4, terror management theory has experimentally shown that reminding people of their own mortality enhances and strengthens their existing worldview, religious beliefs, group identifications, and their tendency to cling to a charismatic leader [292]. When danger is real and present, effective leaders take charge and give commands that are obeyed by obedient followers, thus harnessing and directing the combined power of many individuals in service of group survival. Fear-provoking circumstances within an organization are contagious. Within a group, emotional contagion occurs almost instantly, and predictable group responses are likely to emerge automatically [383].

Threatened groups tend to increase intragroup attachment bonds with each other and are more likely to be drawn to leaders who appear confident, take control, and are willing to tell other people what to do. Interpersonal conflict decreases within the group, while the threatening person or group becomes the dehumanized enemy. Everyone pulls together toward the common goal of group survival, producing what can be experienced as a wonderful state of oneness and unity with a group, leading to a willingness to sacrifice one's own well-being for the sake of the group. This is a survival strategy ensuring that in a state of crisis decisions can be made quickly and efficiently, thus better ensuring survival of the group, even while individuals may be sacrificed.

Under crisis conditions, the strong exercise of authority by leaders coupled with obedience to authority by followers may be life-saving. In a group confronted by new, unique, and dangerous conditions, if someone in a position of authority—or someone with the confidence to assume authority—gives orders that may help us to survive, we are likely to automatically and obediently respond. But when a state of crisis is prolonged, repetitive, or chronic there is a price to be paid. The tendency to develop increasingly authoritarian structures over time is particularly troublesome for organizations.

Chronic Crisis and Authoritarian Behavior

Chronic crisis results in organizational climates that promote authoritarian behavior, and this behavior serves to reinforce existing hierarchies and create new ones. Under stress, leaders are likely to feel less comfortable in delegating responsibility to others and in trusting their subordinates with tough assignments when there is a great deal at stake. Instead, they are likely to make more decisions for people and become central to more approvals; this in turn builds a more expensive and expansive hierarchy and bureaucracy [109]. Communication exchanges change and become more formalized and top down. Command hierarchies becomes less flexible, power becomes more centralized, people below stop communicating openly and as a result, important information is lost from the system. *"It is the increased salience of formal structure that transforms open communication among equals into stylized communications between unequals. Communication dominated by hierarchy activates a different mindset regarding what is and is not communicated and different dynamics regarding who initiates on whom. In situations where there is a clear hierarchy, it is likely that attempts to create interaction among equals is more complex, less well learned, and dropped more quickly in favor of hierarchical communication when stress increases"* (p. 138) [518].

The centralization of authority means that those at the top of the hierarchy will be far more influential than those at the bottom, and yet better solutions to the existing problems may actually lie in the hands of those with less authority. *"There is a tendency to centralize control during a crisis period, to manage with tighter reins and more power concentrated at the top. The need for fast decisions may preclude participative processes. But this is risky. Centralization may transfer control to inappropriate people; if top managers had the ability to take corrective action, there might have been no crisis in the first place"* (p. 243) [533]. As Brian sees it:

> *What I am seeing a lot here is that decisions are often being made one level above where they should be made. Each level seems to be abdicating responsibility to the manager above them. I have to believe we are cueing people to do this because it is so prevalent. So decisions are being made by people with less direct knowledge than those actually facing the problem.*

In this way, *"the same process that produces the error in the first place, also shapes the context so that the error will fan out with unpredictable consequences"* (p. 140) [518]. Lipman-Blumen has studied the dynamics of leadership and has recognized that *"Crises can create circumstances that prompt some leaders, even in democratic societies, to move beyond merely strong leadership to unwarranted authoritarianism. In tumultuous times, toxic leaders' predilection for authoritarianism fits neatly with their anxious followers' heightened insecurity.... Set adrift in threatening and unfamiliar seas, most of us willingly surrender our freedom to any authoritarian captain"* (pp. 99–100) [584]. Many observers have noted this sequence of shared behavior occurring at a national level after the events of September 11, 2001[548–551; 585].

In mental health and social service delivery, crisis situations typically are instances in which a client's life, health, safety, or well-being is seriously endangered. In these circumstances, both uncertainty and risk are high, and the penalties (consequences) for errors in decision making are severe—factors that greatly increase practitioner stress [586]. In situations of chronic crisis and high costs for errors, leadership positions are likely to keep or attract people with strong authoritarian tendencies in their personality makeup, while more democratic leaders will find such situations unsatisfying and even toxic. As this occurs in human service delivery systems, there may be a progressive isolation of leaders, who tend to become more autocratic over time, a dumbing-down of staff, less participation of staff in decision-making processes, and a loss of critical judgment throughout the organization. Without anyone intending it to happen, or even recognizing that it is happening, the organizational culture becomes toxic.

Everyone knows that something is happening that is all wrong, but no one feels able to halt the descent that is occurring. As time goes on and the situation feels increasingly out of control, organizational leaders are likely to respond by becoming even more controlling, instituting ever more punitive measures in an attempt to forestall what appears to be a slacking off of staff and an increase in disciplinary problems, all signaling impending chaos. Helplessness begins to permeate the system; staff become helpless in the face of their clients, clients feel helpless to help themselves or each other, and administrators helplessly perceive that their best efforts are ineffective. As we will see, in our ever more complex world, this tried-and-true evolutionary adaptation to crisis can easily backfire because of the untoward effects of centralization of authority and authoritarian states of mind.

The Inherent Problem of Authoritarianism

Compared with others, authoritarians have not spent much time examining evidence, thinking critically, reaching independent conclusions, and seeing whether their conclusions mesh with the other things they believe. Instead, they have largely accepted what they were told by the authorities in their lives. (p. 93)[587]

Bob Altemeyer, The Authoritarian Specter

The nature of people who were recognized as highly authoritarian was studied in the late 1940s after Hitler's totalitarian regime had caused such enormous global suffering. Most recently, Dr. Robert Altemeyer has been studying authoritarian behavior for the last 25 years, and his work illuminates the central cognitive problems in authoritarian behavior that pose significant challenges when people high in these traits become employed in the mental health and social service systems, particularly in positions of power [587].

In his research, Altemeyer has noted three fundamental and interrelated characteristics of people who are high in authoritarian traits: *authoritarian submission*, which is a high degree of submission to the authorities who are perceived to be established and legitimate in the society in which one lives; *authoritarian aggression*, which is a general aggressiveness, directed against various persons, that is perceived to be sanctioned by established authorities; and *conventionalism*, which is determined by a high degree of adherence to the social conventions that are perceived to be endorsed by society and its established authorities. These traits hold great significance and danger for human service environments when people high in authoritarianism achieve significant levels of power over other people, namely clients or staff.

People who are high in authoritarian submission generally accept the statements and actions of established authorities and believe that those authorities should be trusted and deserve both obedience and respect, by virtue of their positions. They place narrow limits on other people's rights to criticize authority figures and tend to assume that critics of those authority figures are always wrong. Criticism of established authority is viewed as divisive and even destructive and motivated by little except a desire to cause trouble. For such people, when authority figures break the law, they have an inherent right to do so, even if the rest of us cannot.

Those who are high in authoritarian aggression are predisposed to control other people through the use of punishment, and they advocate for physical punishment in childhood and beyond. They deplore any form of leniency toward people who diverge from established authority and advocate capital punishment. Unconventional people and anyone considered to be socially deviant are believed to pose a threat to the social order and therefore aggression toward them is justified, particularly when condoned by authority figures.

Conventionalism indicates a strong acceptance of and commitment to the traditional social norms of one's society. Anything that is based on long-standing tradition and custom and that maintains the beliefs, teachings, and services in their traditional form is preferred. Such people reject the idea that people should derive their own moral beliefs to meet the needs of today because moral standards have already been established by authority figures of the past and should be obeyed without question. This requires endorsing traditional family structure within which women are subservient to men and "keep their place" and that the only proper marriages are between men and women. Other ways of doing things are simply wrong and potentially dangerous.

Authoritarianism in Human Services

For all the problems connected to authoritarian behavior, it is the impact on mental functioning and the behavior associated with authoritarianism that has the most bearing on the functioning of the mental health system. In investigating the cognitive behavior of authoritarianism, Altemeyer found that authoritarians do not spend much time examining evidence, thinking critically, reaching independent conclusions, or seeing whether their conclusions mesh with other things they believe. They largely accept what authority figures have told them is true and have difficulty identifying falsehoods on their own. They copy other people's opinions without critically evaluating them if those opinions come from someone with established authority. As a result, they end up believing a number of contradictory things without even being able to see the contradiction. They do not mentally reverse situations and put themselves in "the other person's shoes." They examine ideas less than other people and tend to surround themselves with people who agree with them and do not contradict them. They show a "hefty double standard" when testing whether something is true: if evidence supports what they believe, they accept it unquestioningly as truth; if evidence fails to support what they believe, they tend to throw out the evidence. Since thinking independently is not easy for them, they are vulnerable to mistaken judgments and can be astonishingly gullible when an insincere communicator bears the trappings of authority [587].

This inability to think critically, synthetically, and diversely is an enormous handicap in trying to assist those with complex physical, psychological, social, and moral difficulties secondary to exposure to repetitive stress, trauma, and violence. If authoritarian leaders assume key administrative positions within human service organizations, the result is likely to be highly detrimental to true trauma-informed change because they will be unwilling to shift away from what are now "fundamentalist" explanations of emotional problems embodied in the *Diagnostic and Statistical Manual* and 30 years of behaviorism and biological reductionism. There are strong links between authoritarianism and fundamentalist belief systems, meaning any literal-minded philosophy with pretense of being the sole source of objective truth forever, in all places, at all times, religious and otherwise. Fundamentalism always requires people to reject information that is or may be inconsistent with established dogma, and this is an extremely dangerous position to take when it comes to dealing with the complexity associated with trying to help complex and diverse human beings to heal in a changing world [588].

Leaders who are high in authoritarian traits are likely to insist on a centralized and traditional hierarchy, discourage true staff participation, be unable to facilitate team treatment, punish dissent, and surround themselves with people who will agree with their view of the world. Authoritarian leadership then encourages the same leadership style throughout the organization. As a result, the organizational norms for all staff are likely to endorse punitive behavior, empathic failure, and traditional methods for managing difficult situations. It is hard to imagine a situation more detrimental to long-lasting, positive change in the lives of trauma survivors. As for the staff, when authoritarian behavior comes to dominate a situation, the result can also be devastating. Unchecked authoritarians can become bullies at any organizational level, but when they are given power, they can become "petty tyrants."

Dangers of Authoritarianism Under Stress

The twentieth century bears witness to the potential horrors of authoritarian systems, particularly when they become totalitarian as well. But we don't have to look at the large global scene to understand the inherent dangers of combining authoritarian systems with stress. In his recent book *Outliers,* author Malcolm Gladwell has described the way that the aviation industry is trying to prevent airplane crashes by addressing the dangers inherent in authoritarian cultures [589]. Gladwell describes work done by Dutch psychologist Hofstede in the 1960s and 70s looking at cross-cultural differences along a number of dimensions. The one of most interest here was what he called the "power distance index," which is concerned with attitudes toward hierarchy, specifically with how much a particular culture values and respects authority. Different cultures rank differently on this index as do different jobs. Captains of planes, like captains of ships, have ultimate authority in the air. It has been shown that co-captains can be quite hesitant to challenge the authority of the captain, despite the fact that this is precisely why there are two pilots in a plane: so that the safety of the passengers does not depend on one person. In examining crashes, this tendency to respect authority too much, to not dissent or assert another opinion, has cost too many lives to be ignored. In commercial airlines, captains and first officers split the flying duties equally, and yet historically, crashes have been far more likely to happen when the captain is in the "flying seat." The conclusion is that planes are safer when the least experienced pilot is flying because it means the second pilot isn't afraid to speak up. As a result of these findings, major airlines now give training in what is called "Crew Resource Management," designed to teach junior crew members how to communicate clearly and assertively with superior officers and to standardize that training cross-culturally. Human services would be well-served by adopting a similar training program.

Bullying in the Workplace

Workplace bullying has been defined as "repeated and persistent negative acts towards one or more individual(s) which involve a perceived power imbalance and create a hostile work environment [590] or *"the repeated, malicious, health-endangering mistreatment of one employee (the Target) by one or more employees. The mistreatment is psychological violence, a mix of verbal and strategic assaults to prevent the Target from performing work well. It is illegitimate conduct in that it prevents work getting done. Thus, an employer's legitimate business interests are not met"* (p. 3) [591]. Another authority on the subject, Einarson points out that it is *"the systematic persecution of a colleague, a subordinate or a superior, which if continued, may cause severe social, psychological and psychosomatic problems for the victim* (p. 17) [592].

Bullying behaviors may include social isolation or the silent treatment, rumors, attacking the victim's private life or attitudes, excessive criticism or monitoring of work, withholding information or depriving another person—particularly a subordinate—of responsibility, and verbal aggression. They may include changing work tasks or making them difficult to perform, personal attacks on the person's private life by ridicule, insults, gossip, verbally humiliating workers in public, and threats of violence [592]. The main difference between "normal" conflict and bullying is not necessarily what and how it is done, but rather the frequency and longevity of what is done and the power differential that exists between people.

Increased fear and authoritarian behavior combined with a breakdown in communication is likely to lead to an increase in workplace bullying and gives license to those employees who are already prone to engage in bullying behavior to continue and escalate their negative behavior toward others. Bullying has been shown to be associated with higher turnover, increased absenteeism, and decreased commitment and productivity. It has been reported to result in lower levels of job satisfaction, psychosomatic symptoms, and physical illness as well [590]. Research has shown that workplace bullying is commonplace in many different organizations and professions, including health care and mental health care settings. Brian has seen his share of bullying behaviors:

> Let me describe the typical pattern of bullying I have seen. Some of our more aggressive staff can also be our most effective at managing the behavior of very difficult and aggressive children. While we may claim to deplore heavy-handed techniques, it is possible to turn a blind eye when faced with a really challenging kid. If a worker is particularly effective with this child, managers and coworkers may be relieved and not ask a whole lot of questions about how this particular worker is able to limit destructive or troubling behavior. It is not a leap at times to assume that the staff members who are most assertive with the children are also assertive with their coworkers. They get either direct or indirect messages from their managers or teammates that they are very reliable, maybe to the point of being indispensable. Staff members with this somewhat inflated sense of self-worth may begin to take some short cuts because they feel entitled. They get the toughest assignments, so if they duck out a little early, raise their voice, use some coercive techniques, cut corners, they feel they have earned the right to do so. The message to coworkers, at times, either directly or indirectly is that the other staff had better not question what they do or they might get hung out in a crisis situation or maybe even be targeted by the kids, at the suggestion of this bullying staff. Coworkers may complain anyway, but in the long run managers may value this bully of a worker more than the worker who is complaining, because when it is all said and done, it is the bully who runs a smoother shift. Managers may in fact be critical of the worker who complains and suggest that the bully needs to be more assertive to compensate for the passivity of his or her teammates. It becomes pretty clear over time that the manager may be saying one thing but doing another, talking about one value, but acting on another. It does not take new workers long to figure out what is really going on and what we really value.

In one large survey, 8.6% of respondents experienced ongoing bullying and nonsexual harassment at work during the 6 months prior to the survey [592]. There are no comparable figures available for U.S. health care settings, but in a survey of 217,000 National Health Service staff in the United Kingdom, 10% of those surveyed had been bullied and harassed by colleagues in the 12 months to March 2005. This figure rose to 37% when abuse from patients or their relatives was included. Additionally, 1% had been physically assaulted by fellow employees, 42% of these workers across the United Kingdom said they would not report incidences of bullying in the workplace; 39% of managers in the United Kingdom say they have been bullied in the past 3 years; and 70% of managers believe misuse of power or position is the number one form of bullying [593]. We suspect the results would be worse if we surveyed the U.S. health and mental health care environment. Many different forms of bullying behavior have been supported, encouraged, and condoned for decades in every domain of our society. As a result, our social norms have radically altered in the direction of actually admiring and even advocating for increasing levels of bullying, authoritarian, and violent behaviours.

Organizational factors are clearly important in the emergence, maintenance, prevention, and response to bullying behavior. Thirty years ago Brodsky studied over a thousand cases of work harassment in the United States and concluded that for harassment to occur there must be elements in the organizational culture that permit or reward such behavior [594]. Bullying will only occur if the offender believes he or she has the overt or more usually covert support from superiors for his or her behavior. Organizational tolerance for, or lack of sanctions against, bullying serves to give implicit permission for the bullying to continue. Aggressive or predatory behavior that starts on a one-to-one level can end up splitting an organization into opposing camps. Conditions that serve as enabling structures and processes that make it possible for bullying to occur include power imbalances between the victim and perpetrator, low perceived costs of bullying from the point of view of the perpetrator, and dissatisfaction and frustration in the workplace. One of our Sanctuary Institute faculty describes an example of a bullying manager:

For many years we tolerated the worst behavior from one of our senior leaders. This manager consistently abused power, maintained high levels of secrecy in his work operations, triangulated colleagues and subordinates, and alienated funders and vendors with his bullying and arrogance. Leaders in the organization, including the CEO and the COO, felt quite trapped. Because of the high levels of secrecy employed, we had a poor handle on the area of the operation this manager directed. If his behavior was confronted he would act out and his reactions would spill all over the place and do significant damage to other people as well as the functioning of the organization, but failing to address the behavior suggested the behavior was condoned. At a point in the organization's development when we were trying to get staff to communicate more openly and confront problems using the Sanctuary Model, we were not able to model this behavior at the executive level. Staff members take their cues from leadership and we had leaders who were badly behaved and were unable to challenge each other on these shortcomings. The stress of this arrangement was troubling and mirrored a domestic violence situation. There would be a terrible transgression, followed by a gentle reminder that this behavior was inappropriate. Like a batterer, the problem manager would inevitably have a brief expression of guilt or remorse and a pledge to do better in the future. That pledge would be honored until the next time something displeased or threatened this manager and then the cycle would be repeated. What is fascinating about this is that it occurred when we were well into implementing Sanctuary. We knew full well what the right thing was, but it was too hard to do it. When under stress you can convince yourself that something is the lesser of two evils or the situation is really not that bad. It is this kind of denial in the face of authoritarian destructive behavior that leads to terrible things happening in families, organizations, and whole societies.

One of the obstacles in dealing with bullying in the workplace is that the organization frequently treats the victim, not the perpetrator, as the problem, tending to accept the prejudices of the offenders and blaming the victim for his or her own misfortune [592]. One investigator has pointed out four key organizational factors that are prominent in eliciting bullying behavior at work: *(1)* deficiencies in work design; *(2)* deficiencies in leadership behavior; *(3)* a socially vulnerable position of the victim; and *(4)* low moral standards in the organization [595].

Toxic Leaders and Petty Tyrants

Unhealthy environments lend themselves to the emergence of what have been described as "toxic leaders" [584]. Toxic leaders are subtly or overtly abusive, violating the basic standards of human respect, courtesy, and the rights of the people who report to them. They tend to be power-hungry and appear to feed off of the use and abuse of the power they have. They play to people's basest fears, stifle criticism, and teach followers never to question their judgment or actions. They lie to meet their own ends and tend to subvert processes of the system that are intended to generate a more honest and open environment. They compete with rather than nurture other leaders, including potential successors, and tend to use divide-and-conquer strategies to set people against each other. Brian recalls a conversation with a colleague:

I remember some years ago talking to someone from a facility that had some major incidents and ended up with a cottage that was totally out of control. The unit was obviously run by someone with major problems, and he was permitted to behave in really terrible ways in an effort to maintain control. Things like making children strip to their underwear, depriving kids of sleep, and other forms of coercion were commonplace. Several of the more aggressive residents became the "lieutenants" of the lead staff person. He gave them special favors and position in the pecking order. These kids then kept the other children and sometimes the staff in check through a more overt campaign of fear and intimidation. The cottage code became "what's done here stays here." People bought in because it was the safest way for them to proceed. The program became increasingly corrupt and because everyone was sworn or pounded into secrecy, agency leadership didn't realize what is going on. Nothing was reported and to the casual observer, things appeared to be in check. Unfortunately when things are in check, we often don't pay much attention. In this case the sad ending came when two children were arrested for sexually assaulting a third child and a staff person was arrested as well for allegedly holding the child down while his peers assaulted him. How on earth can these things happen in a treatment program? They happen when values deteriorate and the organization becomes too stressed and too preoccupied to even see the drift. The temptation to look for authoritarian solutions is very seductive.

In order to distract attention from their own misbehavior, toxic leaders will not hesitate to identify scapegoats and then direct followers' aggression against the designated scapegoat rather than themselves. They frequently promote incompetence, corruption, and cronyism and exploit systems for personal gain [584]. We both have seen our share of toxic leaders in organizations. In for-profit companies, toxic leaders may eventually be extruded because of their detrimental effect on worker morale and ultimately on the bottom line. Unfortunately, in the public and nonprofit sector, toxic leaders can hide for a very long time because their impact is often less directly tied to inefficiencies or negative behavior on the part of workers. Instead, the worker becomes the problem. Additionally, the lack of ability to consistently judge outcomes based on worker or consumer satisfaction tends to create situations where it is less clear exactly what managers are accountable for. And command-and-control agendas within organizations support behavior that often leads to toxic behavior on the part of leaders.

Under what is arguably the worst conditions, an organizational leader, predisposed to authoritarian behavior and acquiring power, may evolve into a "petty tyrant" [596]. A petty tyrant is someone who arbitrarily and in a small-minded way, exercises absolute power oppressively or brutally. Petty tyrants believe certain things about their employees, a set of beliefs that have been termed Theory X—that the average person dislikes work, lacks ambition, avoids responsibility, prefers direction, and is resistant to change [597]. They do this in definable ways. They use their authority in ways that are unfair and that reinforce their own position or provide personal gain. They play favorites. They belittle subordinates and humiliate them in front of others. They lack consideration and tend to be aloof, cold, and unapproachable. They force their own point of view on others and demand that things be done their way. They discourage participation of others and discourage initiative. They are likely to be critical and punitive toward subordinates for no apparent reason.

Barriers to Empowerment in the Workplace

In order to counter the tendency for increased bureaucracy, the abuse of power, and the inability to deal with complex problems that accompanies an increase in authoritarianism, we need to create more participatory environments.

Workers at every level must be empowered to make better decisions. But if we are to get better at more democratic forms of participatory governance, we will have to attend to a number of significant challenges that arise in any participative group, including managing time, handling the frequent and intense expression of emotion, and coping with the reality of certain inequalities [598]. Another interesting challenge is the potential loss of individual autonomy as peers in a more democratic workplace become responsible for monitoring each other, which can too often feel like colleagues are "looking over each other's shoulders" resulting in conflict-laden issues of social control [599].

Organizational size can be a substantial barrier to a more participative, democratic workplace. Limitations on human cognitive capacity make it difficult for human beings to manage a great number of relationships simultaneously so that even with a group of 10 the number of relationships that one must keep track of begins to become staggering (see Chapter 8).

The formula that represents the number of face-to-face contacts possible is $n(n - 1)/2$ where n indicates the number of people in a social group. So with a group of five people, the number of linkages is 10, but for a group of 10 people, the number jumps to 45. As a result, social science research has demonstrated that *"the intense, face-to-face interaction required by real, direct democratic participation cannot be maintained in something larger than what we call a small group"* (p. 174) [600]. Larger groups, therefore, must contain smaller subunits and develop systems of representative decision making, thus immediately confronting the distinction between direct democracy and representative democracy—an inevitable consequence of growth. Earlier we mentioned the "iron law of oligarchy," proposed by Michels in the early twentieth century. Michels proposed that all large organizations, beyond the 3000–5000 member range, inevitably move toward control by a few. He believed that regardless of the commitment to democracy and participation, large organizations incline toward the increased concentration of power [550]. It certainly makes sense that this concentration of control would happen, given the current extraordinary pressures on all organizations—most acutely felt in large organizations—to change rapidly, compete in an ever-condensing global structure, and survive in an exceedingly stressful world climate. If, as terror management theory suggests, a primary role of culture, including organizational culture, is to manage existential terror, then situations that arouse threat are likely to increase the centralization of control and diminish the likelihood of democratic participation, which is always complex, messy, and conflict laden.

Time itself can pose barriers to democratic workplaces—time to engage in the processes necessary to encourage and support participatory processes and the longevity of the organization. Currently, sustaining democratic processes requires charismatic leaders who inspire the change necessary for individuals and groups to move beyond hierarchical, top-down control structures to flattened hierarchies and democratic participation. Inadequate succession plans often leave organizations barren of inspiration and absent a clear mission once the founder or charismatic leader is gone.

Bureaucracies are often put into place to create order as an organization ages and grows, but all too often bureaucracies that were originally intended as deeply democratic, egalitarian structures become depersonalized and dehumanized with, yet again, the concentration of power that tends to diminish or destroy participatory processes [600]. This can be witnessed in many social service and mental health programs and institutions where the initial organizational vision was revolutionary, but which over time, and as a result of neglect and increasing levels of stress, have become stagnant bureaucracies that dehumanize workers and clients alike. As various leaders and orators have reminded us over the years, the price of liberty is eternal vigilance.

Democracy is, at least in our present state of evolutionary development, fragile wherever it appears. As Professor Cheney observed, *"a question persists about what if anything a specific organization can do over time to resist the temptation to formalize, centralize, standardize and otherwise reduce the spontaneous and dynamic aspects of life within it....In any event, collective and careful reflection on the goals and practices of non-traditional, democratic organizations must be a regular part of an organization's decision-making process"* (p. 177) [600]. Brian describes his experience:

> We have more than once felt that we have disengaged from our staff during a difficult time and convinced ourselves that this was in service of democratic processes. But leaving folks to their own devices is not the same thing as democracy. Democracy is about participation, participation of everyone, not just the line staff or the clients. It is no more desirable for the leadership to check out than it is for anyone to check out. In fact, it is far less desirable and far more destructive. Leaders certainly do not always have the answers, but they play a crucial integrative role in the organization. Leaders have the power and authority to get the right people to the table and ensure the right conversations are happening. When leaders check out, people might be able to continue to function in their various work groups, but they will struggle to reach across department or functional lines to improve things.

Managers often freely embrace the rhetoric of democracy, empowerment, and participation but are reluctant to actually share power, grant autonomy, disclose information, or include employees in substantive decision making. And workers have not always been eager to participate in decision making when they will be held accountable for the changes that occur as a result. The result, as organization theorist Chris Argyris has written is that *"despite all the best efforts that have gone into fostering empowerment, it remains very much like the emperor's new clothes: we praise it loudly in public and ask ourselves privately why we can't see it. There has been no transformation in the workforce, and there has been no sweeping metamorphosis"* (pp. 98–99) [601].

Bogus Empowerment

Workplace participation can mean many things, and unfortunately, democratic participation in the workplace is all too frequently a cover for the same old authoritarian leadership structures. Very few organizations actually allow employees at all levels of the organization to have a shaping influence on policy; as a result, employees who are promised participatory structures can become easily disillusioned. Quality circles and similar programs are often used to pacify employees and defuse potential resistance to employment practices that may actually be harsh or even abusive.

This kind of behavior is not limited to the for-profit sector. Organizational scholar George Cheney describes his involvement with a large and highly visible peace movement dedicated to ending the nuclear arms race during the 1980s that conducted its meetings as virtual monologues. The director barked out orders, dictated entirely the flow and specific nature of work, unilaterally assigned all roles and tasks, and pressured paid staff and volunteers to work unreasonably long hours—all of which Cheney interpreted as a kind of organizational violence. But when confronted, the director refused to recognize the painful contradictions between the organization's mission and its internal practices. All he could say was that the ends of the organization entirely justified the means [600].

The term used for worker empowerment that does not really empower anyone at all is "bogus empowerment" defined as *"the use of therapeutic fictions to make people feel better about themselves, eliminate conflict, and satisfy their desire to belong, so that they will freely choose to work toward the goals of the organization (control of individualism) and be productive (instrumentalism). Leaders who offer bogus empowerment are unauthentic, insincere, and disrespectful of others. They believe that they can change others without changing themselves"* (pp. 64–65) [602]. The sociologist C. Wright Mills offered one of the clearest articulations of bogus empowerment early in the twentieth century: *"The moral problem of social control in America today is less the explicit domination of men than their manipulation into self-coordinated and altogether cheerful subordinates"* (p.69) [602].

So what does true empowerment look like? When you empower others you do at least one of the following: you help them recognize the power that they already have, you recover power that they once had and lost, or you give them power they never had before. In his study of grassroots organizations, Richard Cuoto says there are two main kinds of empowerment. The first kind he calls *psychopolitical* empowerment. This increases people's self-esteem and results in a change in the distribution of resources and/or the actions of others. In other words, empowerment entails the confidence, desire, and most important the ability of people to bring about real change. This is probably what most people think of when they think of empowerment. Cuoto calls the second form of empowerment *psychosymbolic* empowerment. This raises people's self-esteem or ability to cope with what is basically an unchanged set of circumstances. More often than not, leaders promise or appear to promise *psychopolitical* empowerment but actually deliver *psychosymbolic* empowerment (p. 60) [602]

Psychosymbolic empowerment can become just another form of manipulation in service of authoritarian values—just a little more subtle than the use of actual force. Americans can easily be drawn into notions of empowerment because we are known to treasure democracy and its accompanying values of liberty and equality. If Americans "walked the talk" about democracy, we would have the most democratic workplaces in the world, *but we don't.* Democratic participation is difficult and requires sophisticated social skills. Empowerment doesn't just mean people assuming power over or with other people or organizations; it also means the assumption of more responsibility. Democratic processes are messy and often very disordered, at least for a while. As Tom Wren points out, ever since American independence, there has been a conflict between the values of equality and authority [603].

> *Thomas Jefferson, in declaring for liberty in 1776, grounded his call on the premise that "all men are created equal." While this appears axiomatic in our political and social system, our commitment to equality is rife with leadership implications, for it makes problematic the maintenance of good order in society. Establishing and maintaining a delicate balance between equality and order have occupied intellects since at least the time of Plato, and remain a challenge which has been central to the American experience. In today's corporate world, the challenge of empowering workers while maintaining organizational coherence poses precisely the same value conflict experienced by the Founders as they sought to pilot the ship of state among the shoals of quality and good order* (p. 1) [603]

In a society where people value individualism and freedom, the challenge of leadership in organizations is the challenge of *"leading a flock of cats, not sheep"* (p. 61). In the world of for-profit business, the issue of participation and order are frequently in conflict. Getting the job done and making money trumps everything else in our market economy. The market is *"a mean and ruthless boss"* (p. 62) [602]. When making profit is more important than the means and people used to get it done, then leadership is effective if and only if it gets profitable results. In this kind of cultural framework, there is little if any room for things that have intrinsic value but do not necessarily serve the interests of profit. *"As a result, the greatest of all impediments to empowerment in business and increasingly in all areas of life is economic efficiency. It acts on rules that refuse to take into account anything but the short-term bottom line* (p. 62) [602].

Although financial profitability is not the main motivator in many components of the social service delivery system, the rationing of services over the last 25 years, and continuing and even worsening today, has compelled organizations to employ many of the same tactics and strategies as the for-profit, market-driven economy. But lacking the corrective of competition and the tangible assessment instrument of profitability, or even consumer satisfaction, social service organizations have no real measure for whether what they are doing is effective. Criteria for service delivery may be things like adequacy of paperwork, or recidivism, or number of home visits made. But does paperwork have anything at all to do with whether their client improved? Does it mean that service delivery was a failure if someone returns to a short-term hospital unit? Or does it mean it was a success? Does the number of visits made have anything to do with whether children are being adequate protected? Maybe, maybe not. But when dealing with chronic complex problems and prevention it is astonishingly difficult to assess effectiveness. How do you prove a negative? If prevention of any sort of problem or worsening of problem has been prevented, no one will ever know that it has. To some degree, these are inherent problems of doing the work that we do.

In the mental health system, the desire for empowerment has arisen out of the multiple historical abuses of the mentally ill. The consumer-driven movement seeks to empower clients to determine what is effective treatment for them and what is not. Unfortunately, however, it is impossible to have a democratic system when only one component of the system has a voice. It is time to move beyond just client empowerment and include staff empowerment. To do that we will need leaders in our social service system who have learned the skills of democratic leadership.

Conclusion

Authoritarian behavior is dangerous in situations that demand complex problem solving, but authoritarian pseudosolutions are likely to increase under the influence of chronic stress, as is the sense of helplessness and disempowerment that accompanies it. Without deep systemic change, what we end up with are systems that are punitive and organizations that are unjust, both of which are subjects we will focus on in the next chapter.

Chapter 10

Punishment, Revenge, and Organizational Injustice

SUMMARY: *As leaders become more authoritarian and their efforts to correct problems are ineffective, organizational stress increases further, and the organization is likely to become more punitive in an effort to control workers and clients. Organizational practices that are perceived as unjust evoke a desire for vengeance. As in the case of the chronically stressed individual, shame, guilt, anger, and a desire for justice can combine with unfortunate consequences. When this is happening, the organization may become both socially irresponsible and ethically compromised. We explore what happens when good people do bad things, including when otherwise decent people stand around and watch unjust behavior and do nothing.*

The Problem of Revenge

Revenge can be defined as *"the infliction of harm in righteous response to perceived harm or injustice"* (p. 803) [604] or as *"the attempt, at some cost or risk to oneself, to impose suffering upon those who have made one suffer, because they have made one suffer"* (p. 862) [605]. Revenge can be differentiated from normal defensive aggression in two ways: it occurs after the damage has been done, and hence is not a defense against threat; and it is of much greater intensity, and is often cruel, lustful, and insatiable [606]. The quest for revenge can be seen as *(1)* a motivation for aggression; *(2)* as a source of psychological distress; and *(3)* as a key factor in the philosophical discussion of punishment and justice [604].

The search for vengeance poses enormous problems for humanity. An injured individual is rarely in the position of applying a balanced solution to a wrong that has been perpetrated against him or her. The problem of vengeance is a social problem that must be resolved in the complex interaction between the victim, the perpetrator, and the social group. Acts of "wild vengeance," therefore, can be seen not only as the failure of the violent individual but also the failure of the social group. Revenge is justice gone awry and takes over when society's institutions fail. If, as a society, we are to eliminate violent perpetration, then we must socially evolve systems of justice that effectively contain and manage the human desire for revenge. A sense of justice is so basic to humanity that the origins can be found in early childhood.

Development, Trauma, and Revenge

The beginnings of a sense of justice occur early enough in human development that we can consider it part of our basic biological programming. At about 18 months of age, children first exhibit prosocial altruistic behaviors—reaching out, wanting to help, and offering comfort. During the second or third year of life, children become very concerned about issues of fairness, although their initial concern is with being treated fairly. Children begin to protest against unfair treatment as early as 1 year of age. Around age 4, they become capable of learning how to treat others fairly [607]. As researcher Paul Bloom observes, *"A growing body of evidence suggests that humans do have a rudimentary moral sense from the very start of life. With the help of well-designed experiments, you can see glimmers of moral thought, moral judgment and moral feeling even in the first year of life. Some sense of good and evil seems to be bred in the bone"* (p. 46)[608].

Studies have looked at how children make decisions about retaliation after an intentional or accidental injury to their property. The average age of the children was almost 9 years for boys, and a little over 9 years for girls. Even at that age, children were capable of making very subtle discriminations between intentional acts and accidental acts that shaped their responses to a perpetrator's actions. They also made subtle discriminations between types of retaliation, the age of the perpetrator, and the relationship of the victim to the perpetrator [609]. In this way, gradually and in interaction with significant others in their social environment, normal children learn how to modulate and manage their normal desires for retaliatory vengeance and channel these desires into socially acceptable behavior. Children certainly compete with each other, but they also learn how to cooperate with each other as a fundamental social strategy, even when adults aren't around to tell them what to do.

Even so, studies of normal populations tell us that the urge to retaliate for perceived injustice lingers throughout adulthood. Any kind of unfair treatment or abuse—physical, sexual and emotional—is likely to provoke retaliatory behavior unless a sufficient number of mitigating factors impact on the desire and action of seeking revenge. Whether in interpersonal relationships or the workplace, human beings retaliate for perceived injustice if they continue to be treated poorly, if there is no apology for misconduct, and if they feel morally justified in their outrage.

As we discussed in Chapter 3, the psychobiology of trauma offers a useful way of understanding why people act out violently toward themselves and others, once we understand that the roots of violence lie in exposure to child-hood adversity. It is not difficult to understand how things could go very wrong, how people who are badly treated by others, especially when that bad treatment originates in childhood, could become excessively violent. The normal devel-opmental process of learning about fair and unfair treatment, or acting on or inhibiting retaliatory desires does not occur. Instead, these children are exposed to injustice, often from the time they are born.

When Good People Do Bad Things

Evil consists in intentionally behaving in ways that harm, abuse, demean, dehumanize, or destroy innocent others—or using one's authority and systemic power to encourage or permit others to do so on your behalf (p. 5) [548]

Philip Zimbardo, The Lucifer Effect

Given that a sense of justice appears to be embedded in the human psyche and evokes such powerful feelings of outrage and vengeance on the part of indi-viduals and groups when mobilized, how is it that injustice is so often being perpetrated? And why isn't there more of a reaction to injustice when it occurs? To understand more about this, we need to look at what happens to people under the influence of a group. Since World War II and the Holocaust, research-ers have been trying to understand how otherwise good people could become so irresponsible as to commit unjust and wrongful acts or allow others to do so. Every day, on the political stage, in corporations, in social service settings, in hospitals, in clinics around the country, bystanders are watching their friends and colleagues break the rules, hurt people, act irresponsibly, and sometimes break the law. In social circumstances, we frequently do not approve of other people's conduct and yet we do nothing, say nothing. Why not? What is the psychology of those who deliberately do wrong and what is the psychology of people who are onlookers?

There are, of course, psychopaths in every walk of life, more than many of us care to admit [559]. People high in psychopathic traits are distinctly different from other people in that they do not register feelings in the same way and are particularly deficient in the involuntary experience of mirroring other people's feelings and thus lack empathy. Evidence is beginning to accumulate that they have brain abnormalities that may help explain their conduct [557]. But psy-chopaths comprise only a small fraction of the population, and they cannot account for all the irresponsible and cruel behavior that happens every day. To acquire an understanding of that, we need to reach beyond the individual and focus attention upon the social world and the impact that social circumstances can have on us.

In most circumstances that arouse concerns about justice and responsibility, attention is exclusively focused on the victim and the perpetrator. But there is a missing component to virtually every situation: the bystander. Who is a bystander? Bystanders are the audience. They are all those present at the scene of an incident (physically or psychologically present), who provide or deny support for a behavior. The victim and perpetrator form a linked figure, and the bystanders form the ground against which the injustice is either carried out or prevented. It is useful to note that among acts of perpetration that have been studied, it is the behavior of the bystanders which determines how far the perpetrator will go in carrying out the act of violence [610–612].

Obedience to Authority

In his seminal experiments immediately after World War II, psychologist Stanley Milgram wanted to understand how so many otherwise reasonable people could have willingly participated in the Holocaust. What he found was startling and disturbing: the powerful influence of the group was found to be an important determinate of whether otherwise healthy people could be persuaded to become sadistic and abusive [613].

Milgram set up an experimental situation in which a subject (the "teacher") on orders from an authority figure, flips a switch, apparently sending a 450-volt shock to an innocent victim (the "learner"). Subjects were told they were participating in a study of the effects of punishment on learning. Every day the teacher arrived at the laboratory with another person who would be the one receiving the shocks, (the learner), someone who was actually an accomplice in the experiment. They were instructed to administer the shocks whenever the learner—the actual accomplice—gave a wrong answer to a series of questions. The shocks began at low levels of 15 volts and progressed with every incorrect answer to 450 volts.

As the experiment proceeded, the teacher could hear cries coming from the learner, and the teacher actually believed that he or she was inflicting serious injury to the learner. Many became visibly upset and wanted to stop, but when the authority figure told them to keep going, most of them did so, despite the tortured outcries from the victim. In fact, 65% of experimental subjects conformed to the demands of authority to the point at which they supposedly inflicted severe pain or possible death on another human being. Milgram concluded that this was the "I was only following orders" defense of the Nazi leaders. Milgram repeated the experiments many times, in different countries, and the results were consistent: two-thirds of people were willing, under orders of an authority figure, to shock to the limit [614]. When assured by apparently legitimate authority that there was a good cause for the experiment, subjects overrode their own sensory impressions, empathic responses, and ethical concerns and automatically obeyed authority without questioning the grounds on which this authority was based or the goals of established authority.

In his conclusion, Milgram warned, "*A substantial proportion of people do what they are told to do, irrespective of the content of the act and without limitations of conscience, so long as they perceive that the command comes from a legitimate authority*" (p. 189) [613].

More recent experiments concerning decisions to dump toxic waste or manufacture defective automobiles has demonstrated that people perceive themselves as less responsible for such acts when the transgressors are conforming to company policy or obeying the orders of a superior than when they are acting alone [615]. It is also true that researchers have found that small groups of people sometimes collectively rebel against what they perceive as unjust authority [616].

The Lucifer Effect

Philip Zimbardo rose to fame in the early 1970s, when, influenced by Milgram's work, he conducted the Stanford Prison Experiment, one of the seminal studies into human nature and brutality. Student volunteers at Stanford University were subjected to what was supposed to be 2 weeks of false imprisonment to see how students, some of whom played the role of "prisoners" and others as "prison guards," would react to the situation and to each other. The study had to be curtailed after only 6 days because of the remarkable and entirely disturbing impact the study situation had on these otherwise healthy, normal, male college students. In less than a week, pacifist students were behaving sadistically toward their peers when they played the role of guards, and normal kids were breaking down emotionally while playing the role of prisoners.

During the 6-day simulation, the experimenters found that the guards began—and quickly escalated—harassing and degrading the prisoners "*even after most prisoners had ceased resisting and prisoner deterioration had become visibly obvious to them*" (p. 92), and they appeared to experience this sense of power as "*exhilarating*" (p. 94) [617]. Zimbardo concluded that the effect of power over others can become so intoxicating that *(1)* power becomes an end in itself, *(2)* the power-holder develops an exalted sense of self-worth, *(3)* power is used increasingly for personal rather than organizational purposes, and *(4)* the power-holder devalues the worth of others [618].

In reviewing his own experiments and those of other social psychologists, as well as immersing himself in the study of the Abu Ghraib scandal and other wartime phenomena, Zimbardo concluded that it is dehumanization that is at the core of much human cruelty, consistent with our discussion in Chapter 8. "*Dehumanization occurs whenever some human beings consider other human beings to be excluded from the moral order of being a human person. The objects of this psychological process lose their human status in the eyes of their dehumanizers. By identifying certain individuals or groups as being outside the sphere of humanity, dehumanizing agents suspend the morality that might typically govern reasoned actions toward their fellows"* (p. 307) [548].

How often in behavioral health and other social service settings are diagnoses and the descriptors associated with those diagnoses actually used as a way of dehumanizing the very people we are supposed to be helping? Dehumanizing human beings is a slippery slope and inevitably leads to destructive outcomes. Brian has seen this occur:

> *Sometimes we do dehumanize the kids as if we are better than them in some way. I have seen staff walk in 10 minutes late for work and then ream a kid out for getting down late to breakfast. I have seen staff eating in the living room and tell a kid who comes in with a snack "you cannot eat in here" while they are putting a fork in their mouth. When you ask about this, there is a rationalization. They respond by saying something like "I will not make a mess" or something goofy like that. At the bottom of this is an attitude—"I have power over them and so the rules do not apply to me in the same way." This can become a rationalization for just about any hypocrisy.*

Sanctioned Perpetration

Lessons from soldiers in wartime teach us that traumatization occurs when we participate in the infliction of harm, particularly when there is no cause or sense of a higher purpose to help us rationalize the act. Even when we can momentarily persuade ourselves that we are unaffected, we find haunting images and memories become a part of our psychological baggage, persisting until we resolve them. Researchers studied the My Lai Massacre that occurred in 1968 during the Vietnam War. The massacre was investigated and charges were brought in 1969 and 1970, while trials and disciplinary actions lasted into 1971. This massacre was considered to be a "crime of obedience," committed by average soldiers representing a cross-section of American men. This incident came to be an example of a "sanctioned massacre," an act of indiscriminate, ruthless, and often systematic mass violence, carried out by military or paramilitary personnel while engaged in officially sanctioned campaigns, the victims of which were defenseless and unresisting civilians, including old men, women, and children.

Three social processes tend to create these kinds of conditions: authorization, routinization, and dehumanization. Through authorization the situation is defined so that the individual is absolved of the responsibility of making personal moral choices. Through routinization, the situation is organized so that there is no opportunity to raise moral questions. Through the process of dehumanization, the target of the proposed aggression is structured so that it is neither necessary nor possible for the individual to view the target as a true human being [619]. These three processes—authorization, routinization, and dehumanization—can be seen in some mental health treatment environments, hospitals, nursing homes—anywhere where these familiar consequences of bureaucratic treatment are in play. Brian recalls that:

> A few months ago a staff person at another agency was arrested for putting a kid in care in a choke hold. The provocation—and I am not making this up— was that the kid was being disrespectful while the staff person was teaching an anger management class. Anyway the staff person was arrested and the story hit the papers. The newspaper website had a blog and folks responded to the story. Most of the entries on the blog railed about what a bunch of animals the kids in that facility are and how they deserve a beating. Even when the kid was the victim, he was wrong. He was less than human and of course the staff person would need to choke him. Hmmm…how slippery is that slope?

The Dynamics of Violence and the Bystander

Bystanders share elements of both victimization and perpetration in the dynamics of violence. Healthy attachment generates empathic connections among people: we cannot observe abuse and violence without being affected. The very circuitry of our brain means that our social relationships, our representations of our ourselves, and the pain we experience are interrelated, connected pathways [556]. We identify at one end or the other and through this identification, we are inducted into the traumatic event. The phenomenon of "secondary traumatization" refers to the toxic effects of a violent act upon the community of bystanders [620–621]. Not to act to prevent harm undermines our sense of efficacy, reinforces powerlessness, and often results in profound feelings of guilt and shame.

How do we cope with our considerable exposure to violence as witnesses? Many of the same psychological processes for victims of trauma come into play with secondary trauma. The human mind can handle only so much before primitive defensive strategies are activated. As we are finding with cigarette smoke, passive exposure to noxious agents can be debilitating. Attribution theory teaches us that our psychological state influences our perception of responsibility and agency in acts of violence. Many, for example, upon learning of an instance of rape, find themselves driven by personal distaste and powerlessness to discounting the crime in an effort to feel less uncomfortable. We find ourselves wondering "if she brought it on herself."

Researchers have explored other people's willingness to listen to and support a victim's need to disclose information about his or her experience [514]. It is quite clear that the bearers of disturbing information and negative emotions are suppressed in various ways. Listeners switch the topic away from trauma. They attempt to press their own, less upsetting perspective of the trauma upon the victim. Listeners tend to exaggerate the victim's personal responsibility in the traumatic situation. If these strategies do not work to get the victim to stop talking, then the listener will avoid contact with the victim altogether. The reasons for this behavior are fairly clear. The suffering of victims can threaten the listener's assumptions about a "just world" in which people get what they deserve and this can arouse great anxiety in us. The feelings of a trauma victim can be so relentless in their intensity and negativity that even the most empathic person becomes overwhelmed. Victims are usually quite aware of the reluctance of people to listen and will often cease talking in order to protect their social connections.

Devaluation is another example of this trick of distorted perception. When a murder happens involving a highly valued member of society, there is strong reaction; when a homeless person is killed, little notice is paid. Countries in which anti-Semitism was strongest were those in which Nazis executed the largest number of Jews.

Denial is another delusional mechanism that may arise as a bystander attempts to cope with violence. In all of its forms—minimization, rationalization, projection—denial assists the uncomfortable bystander to manage the painful observation by bending and twisting reality into a more digestible form. That "bad things happen to bad people" is a rationalization we are conditioned to believe through a childhood of messages telling us that we deserve what we get.

But a key finding with respect to research on the bystander effect is this: we cannot detach ourselves from another's suffering and hurt without paying a high price. We are inevitably interconnected and failing to help another suffering being means we have failed ourselves, that our own humanity is slowly, pervasively, and insidiously ebbing away.

So, if dehumanization, devaluation, denial, authorization, minimalization, routinization, sanctioning of violence, rationalization, and projection are all defenses used by ordinary people to inflict horrific cruelty on other people, what is the potential in the mental health and social service system for abuse? The potential is extraordinarily high. Our system of compulsory psychiatric labeling—for all its good intentions—has the unintentional effect of setting people apart so that they *become* their diagnoses and are thereby dehumanized. This is particularly true for the least professionally trained workers who are likely to have no theoretical basis for understanding the complex and disturbing behavior they witness and with which they must contend. This systematic dehumanization process is itself devaluing. Then within institutional settings, obedience to authority, the minimalization of personal responsibility, the routinization of attitudes and behaviors toward needy clients all serve to support the continuing devaluation of human worth.

Aggression is one of the immediate reactions of dehumanized human beings, but since their behavior cannot be understood within a human context, once they have been dehumanized, violence against them can be sanctioned and rationalized as "treatment" or deserved punishment. In the criminal justice and juvenile justice settings, the dehumanization and devaluation process is taken even further by the bad and incorrigible labels they acquire, by the desire to punish and exact retribution, and is supplemented by the way in which they themselves devalue themselves and others. These powerful tendencies within individual human beings and within our own human service system to dehumanize others have been demonstrated repeatedly throughout history in the abusive and condescending treatment of the mentally ill and the socially disenfranchised. In any institutional settings we are both actors and bystanders. As Brian reminds us:

> We have tended to devalue or dehumanize parents of children in residential care as well. We see them as incompetent. We resent when they question our interventions and we suggest they are intrusive when they want information on how their child is doing. In reality, any parent with any sense of responsibility would be frantic about his or her child being in an RTC.

Bystanders Beware

As bystanders become increasingly passive in the face of abusive behavior, action becomes increasingly difficult. Just as there is a deteriorating spiral of perpetration in which each act of violence becomes increasingly easy to accomplish, so too is there a deteriorating cycle of passivity. As the perpetrators actively assume control over a system without any resistance on the part of bystanders, their power increases to the point that resistance on the part of bystanders becomes extremely difficult if not useless except to the extent that such behavior serves as an example for others. It has been repeatedly demonstrated that the more people there are who could respond to a situation, the less likely it is that anyone will. What follows is the emergence of a group norm of passive non-action.

Even willing helpers can be derailed by social propaganda, by coercion, and by the influence of others who want to deny the perpetrator behavior and who offer an alternative outlook with such explanations as "He deserves what he gets," "She's just trying to get attention," "People can always find a job if they look hard enough," "People just want to blame their parents," "Welfare recipients are just lazy and don't want to work," "There's more crime because we've gotten too soft on criminals." Note the ways in which all of these sayings reduce the humanity of the person or group that is targeted. And note the way the word "just" is always used to minimize a far more complex explanation.

If people who are willing to help can get past the propaganda and see the flaws in thinking, they still have to feel that they have some responsibility for solving the problem and that they are able to choose something to do to help and put their plan into action. The fundamental question is whether witnesses to the mistreatment of other people have an obligation to act. What is our moral responsibility to each other? Are we, in fact, "our brother's keeper?" Until quite recently in human history, the family group or the tribe was the only group to which we felt the kind of loyalty that demands protective action. If bullies are allowed to bully, if liars get away with lying, if free-riders get away with loafing, then it is because all of us who knew about the behavior said nothing and did nothing. This is what happened in Abu Ghraib, in the Holocaust, in the Catholic Church—that those who knew and believed the conduct to be wrong gave consent by their silence.

Why Organizational Injustice Matters

The sense of injustice is the sympathetic reaction of outrage, horror, shock, resentment, and anger, those affections of the viscera and abnormal secretions of the adrenals that prepare the human animal to resist attack. Nature has thus equipped all men to regard injustice to another as personal aggression. [622]

E. Cahn *(1949) The Sense of Injustice (as cited in DeGooey, 2000, p. 61)*

Injustice arouses powerful feelings in most human beings, and the more relevant that injustice is to our own lives and experience, the more outraged we are likely to become. In real-life work environments, people do not usually keep their feelings about being unjustly treated to themselves. They talk to their peers, seek social support, and in the process, individual views of justice are combined to create collective views about the "organizational justice climate." Talk about what is fair and not fair in the workplace is a primary way that people have of making sense out of their reality and perceptions. Feelings about organizational justice are contagious, communicated from one individual to each other and maintained across groups [623]. Just hearing about someone else's experience may color the subsequent viewpoints of the listener. People tend especially to rely on other people in situations that are ambiguous, and evaluations of what is fair and not fair in an organizational context are often ambiguous and open to interpretation.

Types of Organizational Justice

Researchers have demonstrated that three kinds of justice need to be addressed in workplace situations and are all aspects of overall fairness that tend to interact with each other. *Distributive justice* deals with how resources are allocated and what some get and others do not. Employees regularly do a sort of internal calculus balancing what we put into the job and what we expect to get out of it. We feel justly treated when inputs and outputs are balanced. We feel unjustly treated if we work harder than we are rewarded for, and this can lead to worker sabotage and to employee theft, as people try to "even the score" on their own terms. We are likely to feel guilty when we are rewarded more than we feel we have earned and may overwork in order to establish a more acceptable equilibrium. When what we receive is equitable, we are rewarded based on our individual contribution and this tends to reward high performance. When it is equal, we all are treated alike, and this tends to build esprit de corps among teammates [624–625].

Procedural justice refers to the means by which allocation of rewards and punishments occurs. This form of justice establishes principles that govern decision-making processes. A just process is one that is applied consistently to everyone, is free of bias, accurate, representative of all relevant stakeholders, correctable, and consistent with ethical norms. When employees believe that a process is fair, they tend to trust their leaders more and are more committed to the organization. Procedural injustice creates distrust and resentment [624–625]. If procedures are believed to be fair, even if the outcome is unfavorable, the employee is more likely to remain loyal and behave in the interest of the organization. In a study of over 1000 employees a major determinant of whether employees sued for wrongful termination was their perception of how fairly the termination process was carried out. Only 1% of ex-employees who felt that they were treated with a high degree of procedural fairness filed a wrongful termination lawsuit versus 17% of those who believed they were treated with a low degree of process fairness [626–627].

Interactional justice refers to how one person treats another: if he or she appropriately shares information (informational justice) and treats the other with respect and dignity (interpersonal justice). Because these three forms of justice interact and influence each other, one component can be low but if employees perceive that the other two forms are present, the negative effect can be offset [624–625]. Brian has encountered dilemmas over about organizational justice frequently in his managerial role:

> *In a stressed organization it seems to me that justice is elusive. Even if a manager wants to behave justly, it is likely, given the conditions, that he or she will not always be consistent, timely, neat, and clean across the board. A simple misstep is easily interpreted by someone as unjust. Additionally, most staff will never know the whole story. Sometimes a process may be viewed by the staff involved as unfair because they believe their situation is unique. Their impressions of what happened may be shared with others in the organization, but the manager may not be able to talk about the situation because of privacy issues. As a result, the whole story never gets out. Without open communication, which is often impossible when it comes to personnel issues, justice is in the eye of the beholder.*

Organizational structure is defined as the recurrent set of relationships between organization members, and the kinds of organizational structure that exist can be broadly divided into two categories: "mechanistic" and "organic." Mechanistic structures tend to look like traditional bureaucracies: power is centralized, communication follows rigid hierarchical channels, managerial styles and job descriptions are uniform, formal rules and regulations direct decision making. Organic organizations are more flexible, loose, and decentralized while authority lines are less fixed and more flexible with a decentralization of power and communication channels. Rules are created in a more flexible and less formal manner, all designed to help employees achieve the organizational goals [628].

In mechanistic organizations, procedural justice is extremely important. Formal procedures are part of the normal organizational landscape in such organizations and when fairness of these procedures is violated, it disturbs trust in the entire organizational structure. In less formal, more organic kinds of organizations, it is interactional justice that is a more influential determinant of trust, particularly trust in supervisors. Because of their reliance on less formal, face-to-face communication, interpersonal interactions count for even more than in mechanistic organizations. Additionally, when interactional justice is low, individuals in organic organizations report lower levels of trust than do their mechanistic counterparts [628].

When Organizations are Perceived as Unjust

Managers often must contend with what has been termed a "justice paradox"— that what might in fact be a useful screening mechanism from the point of view of the organization may appear to be very unfair to the employee. For example, testing cognitive ability and personality does relate to how well the person will fit into the organization, but such devices are often perceived as unfair to the employee. However, job interviews have been demonstrated to be fairly useless in predicting who is a good fit and who is not, and yet applicants often perceive the interview as a sign of fairness and its absence as injustice in hiring practices [625].

Reward systems need to accomplish two goals that may sometimes feel mutually exclusive. They need to motivate individual performance, and they need to maintain group cohesion. It is important to reward high performance, but it is also important that people experience the workplace as providing rewards that are equal when individual performance depends on group performance. The key to resolving this perpetual difficulty is making sure that the procedures used to make these kinds of decisions are fair. Employees who report less pay satisfaction are less satisfied at work. But when they feel that the methods for deciding on pay are decided fairly, they experience high organizational commitment and positive reactions to their supervisors. Everyone hates pay cuts but when interactional fairness is perceived, employees are much more likely to accept the bad news and less likely to engage in behaviors like stealing or resigning. When workers understand why things have happened, are treated with respect and consideration, they tend not to vent their anger on the organization [625].

Managers may spend as much as 20% of their time settling—or trying to settle—conflicts between employees, and when both parties are intransigent a manager may simply have to impose a settlement upon them. As long as any component of justice is present—distributive, procedural, or interactional— the arbitration is likely to improve the situation. Managers can make hard choices, but they must do so in a just fashion. *"If you can't give people the outcome they want, at least give them a fair process"* (p. 43) [625].

Layoffs are so devastating to people—the ones that lose their jobs and the ones left behind to pick up the extra work—that there is inevitably a sense of distributive injustice. As it turns out, downsizing as a cost-cutting measure is highly risky to an organization, and the costs of workforce reduction often outweigh the benefits. But when a layoff is handled with procedural and interactional justice, victims are less likely to be derogative about their former employers and less likely to cause lawsuits. Among those who felt unjustly treated, 66% contemplated litigation but among those who felt justly treated, the number dropped to 16%. Sincerely apologizing to people for what's happening to them does not admit guilt; it shows compassion and may help the organization survive a crisis with its reputation intact [625]. When downsizing occurs, those left behind may be profoundly affected by a form of survivor guilt. If attention is paid to providing them with accurate information and other forms of interactional justice in regard to those who are gone, employees who remain respond less negatively.

Performance appraisal is another place where organizational justice plays a significant role in determining whether employees feel they are fairly treated. Performance appraisal is tricky business and provides abundant fodder for feelings of injustice. It is important to approach performance evaluations with a deep understanding of their subjectivity. In a meta-analysis of 27 field studies evaluating employee participation in performance appraisals, researchers found that significant problems arose when employees did not feel they had a voice and when they saw the process as unfair. Three core elements create a sense of injustice if they are not available: people feel unjustly treated if they do not have adequate notice that they will be appraised and given the criteria by which they will be evaluated (*adequate notice*); if the feedback review is not limited to performance, but includes personal attacks and inadequate time for the worker to provide his or her own interpretation of events (*just hearing*); and if the standards for making these decisions are judged to be erratic or unfair (*judgment based on evidence*) [625].

Justice, Trust, and Emotions

Maintaining a just environment has been shown to profoundly affect organizational function in a number of key ways. Justice builds trust and commitment. All three components (distributive, procedural, and interactional) predict trust, and trust predicts organizational commitment. Workplace justice has been shown to predict the effectiveness with which workers discharge their job duties. There are indications that the emotional response to injustice is aroused first, followed by cognitions and interpretations of the events that precipitated the emotions, and retaliatory behaviors may follow closely on the heels of this complex response. As Cahn noted in 1949, the response to injustice is a powerful one that closely resembles the fight-flight response, and given all we have discussed in this book, individual and group judgment can be, and often is, profoundly affected by stress.

The relationship between injustice, stress, and aggression is an intimate one. In a study of Department of Veterans Administration programs, 67% of employees responding in 2000 and 63% in 2002 identified "being treated in a rude and/or disrespectful manner" as the most frequently experienced form of workplace aggression. In this study, stress was associated with aggression and injustice with stress. Stress creates a state of readiness to instigate aggression, bad feelings have been found to be associated with reduced helping behavior, people with high levels of stress are known to be more likely to have emotional outbursts during the workday and more likely to express anger to others. And research has shown a relationship between work-related stressors and interpersonal aggression, hostility, sabotage, and complaints, including claims for stress-related illness and injuries [395].

Organizational Injustice and Health

Some research indicates that the organizational justice climate can affect individual physical health. Research has indicated that employees who reported high justice at work had a 45% lower risk of cardiovascular death than their counterparts who had experienced low or intermediate organizational justice [629]. Other research has shown that low perceived workplace justice is related to other factors that influence susceptibility to illness, including elevated unfavorable serum lipids, high diastolic blood pressure, insomnia, and other health problems, possibly secondary to the impact of chronic anger, uncertainty, loss of control, and psychophysiological stress that often accompany experiences of injustice [630–632].

Evidence also is accumulating that employee mental health is related to characteristics of the work group's justice climate. Low levels of organizational justice are associated with significant increases in psychological distress as well as anxiety and depression, all of which are associated with lower work performance [633–634]. *"This research supports the premise that a socially constructed, collective view of justice has implications for understanding the psychological well-being of employees… Managers should be aware of perceptions that develop and are shared in a work group. Water cooler and break room talk can coalesce to have important effects on individual members of the group, specifically in relation to justice judgments"* (pp. 746, 748) [633].

Impact of Organizational Injustice on a Group

As a result of the impact of chronic stress, an entire group of people confronted with a presumed condition of injustice doled out to even one individual member of the group can become rapidly mobilized and polarized to experience feelings, thoughts, and behavior that are not measured or even entirely rational. In reviewing the literature on emotional contagion as it applies to the perception of organizational injustice, DeGooey summarizes three key aspects of this research: *(1)* people tend to be motivated to affiliate with others when faced with a distressing or threatening event; *(2)* they do so in order to receive social validation for their emotional reactions to and interpretations of the event; *(3)* affiliation may alleviate feelings of emotional distress (and potentially, soften people's interpretations of the sources of distress), but it can also exacerbate these feelings and interpretations due to polarization, social facilitation, and/or emotionally contagious effects [623].

Moral retaliation occurs when people make fairness judgments and are motivated to react to mistreatment without being directly and personally victimized or disadvantaged [635]. Once the emotional reaction to perceived injustice occurs, people start making interpretations and assigning blame. Interpretations of any organizational event are highly influenced by people's social environment—what other people have seen, heard, experienced. Individuals may at first perceive that they have had a bit of hard luck, and then other people convince them that they have been unjustly treated. Blame attribution may also be influenced by an individual's previous experience with injustice and his or her level of self-esteem. Rumination about the perceived injustice sets in, and then thoughts and sometimes actions follow. These actions may be ones that produce collective protest, and the organization may act to right a wrong even if by only providing information. This sense of moral outrage on the part of people who did not themselves experience the events but perceived them may negatively impact an organization's standing in the community, employment applications, and legal proceedings against the organization. As investigators have discovered, *"these studies show that perceptions of unfairness and one's subsequent reactions do no depend solely upon personal experiences—they can be initiated vicariously"* (p. 382) [635].

Organizational Retaliation

If acts of injustice that are perceived to be significant are not addressed, there is an increased likelihood of vengeful behavior, sometimes to the point of sabotage. Organizational retaliation has been defined as *"reactions by disapproving individuals to organizational misdeeds"* (p. 384) [635]. The goals of retaliation can be multifaceted. One objective may be to restore a balance between involved parties. Another might be to educate the offender—to "teach them a lesson." Another may be to restore social order between parties—to "even the score." People may be motivated to address threats to the well-being and safety of the organization that arise from whatever injustice is perceived. Or people may be concerned with protecting or restoring social norms and organizational cultural values [635].

Retaliatory behavior can take many forms. It can be directed at one person, directly or indirectly, or at the entire organization. The behavior can be active, as in boycotting, or passive, as in withdrawal. It may take the form of verbal aggression, such as spreading rumors or gossip. Or direct action may be taken. Employee perceptions of injustice have been associated with a variety of vengeful acts, including organizational petty theft, spreading rumors and damaging equipment, doing sloppy work, and engaging in excessive absenteeism [636]. Brian notes that:

> This is a real challenge in managing an organization because perception is as good as reality. If someone feels mistreated, slighted, or disrespected, it is not really relevant whether you meant to make the person feel that way or not. In a healthy organization it may be possible to discuss these feelings, explain yourself and move on. But unfortunately, in most cases, people hang on to the bad feelings and it does not get talked about directly. It just stews.

Organizational sabotage is defined as behavior intended to damage, disrupt, or subvert the organization's operations for the personal purposes of the saboteur by creating unfavorable publicity, embarrassment, delays in production, damage to property, the destruction of working relationships, or the harming of employees or customers. It is most likely to occur when the injustice is experienced in several domains, when there is a sense of cumulative injustice, and when the saboteur believes that he or she has been unjustly treated interpersonally. But in the end, the main motive of the sabotaging behavior is retaliation [637]. As we mentioned earlier, there are psychopathic people in workplaces at every level—as managers and as staff—and people with antisocial tendencies are more likely to commit antisocial acts, particularly when they feel that they have been unfairly treated.

Punishment in the Workplace

As institutional stress increases, workload intensifies, employee frustration and helplessness rise, and interpersonal conflict escalates, it is likely that workers will express their anger, frustration, and resentment in a variety of ways that have a negative effect on work performance. When changes are rapid, there is likely to be a clear statement of new principles. But when change is gradual and slow—as has been the case in the health, mental health, and social service sectors—there may be no real clarity of intention and managers adjust to the changes by interpreting the changes individually and idiosyncratically. Frequently, bureaucracy is substituted for participatory agreement on necessary changes, and the more an organization grows in size and complexity, the more likely this is to happen [638]. When this occurs, leaders become more desperate to achieve rapid and positive responses to a changing environment and are therefore likely to institute increasingly punitive measures to exact control. Research has demonstrated that the lower performance gets, the more punitive leaders become and that very possibly just when leaders need to be instituting positive reinforcing behaviors to promote positive change, they instead become increasingly punitive [639]. As one investigator summed it up, *"decreased worker performance led to increased punitive and autocratic leader behavior"* (p. 135) [639].

Is Punishment Effective?

Punishment has been defined as the presentation of an aversive event or the removal of a positive event following a response which decreases the frequency of that response [640]. But is punishment effective? In studies that look at the impact of punishment, there appear to be key variables that determine the effectiveness of punishment. The first is timing. An aversive stimulus can be introduced at different times—while the negative behavior is occurring, immediately after the behavior, or some length of time after the behavior. According to the research, the sooner the aversive event is delivered the more likely it is to be effective [641].

This is one significant contributor to why punishment usually fails to be very effective in most organizational contexts and certainly in those related to social services: rarely do the problematic behavior and the consequences of that behavior occur close together in time. Because of other factors that are likely to be in play such as in-group loyalty, distrust of supervisors, distrust of the system, and bureaucratic inefficiency, there are likely to be protracted time periods between infractions and response. By the time the employee actually experiences the punishment, so much time has elapsed that he or she is likely to perceive the response as unfair and even abusive instead of an appropriate and even helpful corrective response.

Another fairly well-demonstrated proposition is that moderate levels of punishment are more effective than low- or high-intensity levels [641]. But how do we define low, medium, and high intensity? This is likely to be individually variable and if the match between person and punishment is not correct, it is likely to lead to adverse outcomes rather than a desired change in behavior.

Another variable is the relationship to the punishing agent, and this reflects research taken directly from work with children. Warm and affectionate parents achieve greater effectiveness with punishment than cold and unaffectionate parents, but it is unclear whether this is a result of the punishment or the withdrawal of affection. The implication for organizations is that punishment is likely to be most effective when administered by warm and friendly supervisors [641].

The effects of punishment also depend on the schedule of punishment. In laboratory experiments, punishment is most effective if administered on a continuous schedule after each negative behavior. In at least one study, absenteeism decreased when employees received punishment every time they were absent compared to those who received punishment for the same behavior intermittently. To be effective in administering punishments, managers must be consistent over time, punishing the same behavior each time it occurs; consistent across employees; and every manager must be consistent with every other manager. But this demand for consistency may interfere with the individual reasons for problematic behavior, and if a manager always must be viewed by others as both fair and equitable, an individual approach must be entirely eliminated [641]. These demands for consistency are virtually impossible across a large, complex, frequently understaffed and poorly funded organization, when a manager may have to hold on to fractious or incompetent staff simply because there is no one else to hire and the manager cannot afford to have the position vacant. A former medical director told us:

> At times I have been forced to hire and keep on board psychiatrists who I thought were barely competent, socially impaired, with poor language skills, and who were unsupervisable simply because there were so few people to pick from. Punishment, reward, it didn't matter – these were people who should have been working by themselves, on machines, not trying to help people. But like ours, many of the areas of the country have suffered from shortages in psychiatric care for years. At the same time, the system is dependent on psychiatric evaluations and even routine psychiatric care. So unless I wanted to work 24 hours a day, 7 days a week, 365 days a year, I had to hire—and keep—somebody who would sign the forms and make the phone calls the insurance companies required. It was an absurd situation, but there was little I could do except to go around after the person, cleaning up as many messes as I could.

The effects of punishment, at least on children, are improved when children are offered clear, unambiguous reasons explaining why the punishment occurred and what the future consequences will be if the behavior recurs. This kind of reasoning may make late-timed punishment and low-intensity punishments more effective than they would otherwise be. Effectiveness of punishments is also greatly enhanced when there are clear alternative responses that are available to people [641]. Unfortunately, because of delays in timing, inadequate or absent management training, and avoidance of conflict, employees are often not given any clear reasons, nor is there consistency from time to time, from person to person in human service delivery environments. At the interface between government regulations and programs, relationships have become increasingly punitive and often the punishment appears to be arbitrary, capricious, and counterproductive. Unambiguous reasons are often never given and vary from program to program.

Punishing Unconscious Reenactment

There is another key recognition that must be taken into account, particularly when we focus on punishment within the context of a care giving organization. The rate of exposure to adverse childhood experiences (ACEs) is likely to be extremely high within these settings, in the clients and in the staff. As mentioned in Chapter 2 in the discussion of the ACE's Study, if that study can be generalized to a broader population, only a third of adults, at best, have an ACE score of zero. This being the case, we can assume that many workers in the human services will have been victimized at some point in their own lives and are likely to get triggered by the reenactments of the children or adults who enter their treatment environments. They are vulnerable to becoming drawn into reenactment scenarios with the clients and with each other that may lead to the breakdown of discipline and a wide variety of behavioral problems.

Knowing this changes the responsibility of the supervisory system and the organization as a whole. How can we expect to see change in our clients if we remain as resistant to change as they frequently are? How can treatment be successful if we continue to unwittingly reenact our own early childhood scarring experiences through our negative behavior and punitive responses toward them? People who have been unfairly treated and punished as children are likely to respond to punishment in the present as further evidence of a fundamental injustice that they have been exposed to since childhood, while at the same time setting themselves up to be punished over and over again. For them, untimely, harsh, non-relational punitive systems are likely to be further damaging.

Managers' perceptions of fair punishment practices have been shown to be associated with their belief that the subordinate knew that the behavior was wrong and expected to be punished [640]. But managers hold a variety of beliefs about their employees and may attribute far more conscious awareness about the wrongness of the behavior than is warranted. This is particularly true when supervisors have more professional training than the people they supervise. It is difficult to imaginatively go back in time and remember what we once did *not* know. Supervisors may mistake ignorance for a conscious and deliberate decision to engage in wrongful behavior. Cultural, class, and religious beliefs and practices may also vary greatly and therefore organizational norms and expectations must be exceedingly clear and consequences for varying from those norms must likewise be clear and consistent.

Additionally, employees who through their misbehavior are reenacting some earlier and largely unconscious conflict are unlikely to be able to describe the role this played in their behavior because such automatic behavior is just that: automatic. But even so they may still respond quite negatively to what is internally experienced as an unfair response that they do not really understand. They may be unable to take full responsibility for their actions simply because they do not truly have control over their own behavior. For them, the early experiences of injustice may have been fundamentally traumatizing, and further experiences with perceived injustice may compound existing problems and lead to even more aggression. This is particularly likely to happen when managers' punishment decisions are based not on constructive, forward-looking dialogue with the problematic employee but instead is motivated by a desire to "make an example" of him or her. When this is happening, it is likely that the same staff members are then reenacting these punishing scenarios with the clients who may have very similar backgrounds. Brian has noticed this scenario unfold:

> I have worked with some staff who seem hell-bent on getting a punitive response. They will push a simple issue to the point of absurdity. Like parking their car in a no-parking area time after time, talking on their cell phone when they are supposed to be taking care of children, again and again. They seem to be begging for a punitive response. And even if the response is measured, it is seen as punitive. This is very tough to handle. What I think happens is that managers anticipate that a confrontation will evoke bad feelings, so they ignore the behavior repeatedly, which gives permission for the behavior to occur. When they finally have had it, they intervene, but their tone is not what it could be and it is seen as an overreaction, especially when the behavior was ignored for weeks or months. The staff member is angry then and may pull others into their reenactments in a rescuer role. If someone feels wounded, he or she may try to engage others in their experience of being mistreated or into his or her quest for justice and pretty soon an individual problem terms into a collective disturbance.

Punishment to Change Behavior or as Revenge?

The ideas that most people have about punishment originate in their early experiences of childhood and the definitions that parents give to children. There is a frequent confounding of notions of punishment—sometimes applying to the idea of achieving justice and retribution which is a "past orientation," and at other times being applied instrumentally as a way of changing or modifying behavior which is a "future orientation" [641]. In the laboratory these two fundamental ideas about punishment may be easy to separate. In the practical application of punishment in the complex situation that defines an organization, these two concepts may easily appear simultaneously and interactively.

Since "getting even" is likely to produce unethical behavior in the workplace, while aiming at changing behavior may have no untoward ethical implications, when they are intertwined the result is likely to produce negative consequences. These are particularly problematic scenarios for organizations that treat troubled children or adults because the ways in which organizations respond to employees may mirror the damage originally done to the clients; by doing so, they may set up parallel processes that create toxic environments within which healing cannot take place. Here Brian reflects on his own experience at Andrus:

> It is quite clear we cannot travel along the same pathway we have always traveled and expect to blaze a new trail for the children and families we serve. For years we ignored the punishing physical and emotional pain our kids had already experienced so our response to problematic behavior in residential care was to induce some kind of pain. The idea was that problematic behavior needs to be punished and punishment will discourage future events. We believe this because this is what has been engrained in those of us who remember being punished by our parents. If punishment or pain does not correct the problem or modify the behavior, it is probably because the punishment was inadequate and the pain was insufficient to really make an impression. In this way of thinking the pain and punishment need to be ratcheted up. This is how things can begin to spiral out of control and how we easily become engaged in reenactment after reenactment.

Managers may have other reasons for punishing an individual besides trying to actually bring about a change in the behavior within that person. They may be very concerned about the other employees in the environment and use punishment as an example-setting experience to reinforce behavioral standards, making an example of the violator, and thus maintaining that the organization is a place where people "get what they deserve." Effective disciplinary action can, in fact, result in important learning for everyone in the organization, but managers do not always think about whether the employees are learning what they want them to learn, no more than the employees consider whether the children or adults in their care are learning what they want them to be learning.

If employees see punishment administered unfairly, inappropriately severe, non-contingently, without cause, in an untimely way, with a disregard for privacy or constructive suggestions for improvement, they are likely to see the manager involved, and the system as a whole, as unfair and untrustworthy [640]. Such an environment promotes secret keeping, cliques, mutual protectiveness, and retaliatory actions. As a result, conduct can go wildly wrong before management even is aware of the problem.

Punishment and Performance

Studies over many years have demonstrated that the behaviors that leaders reward generally correlated positively with performance in employees. In fact, the relationship between what gets rewarded and how people perform is much stronger than the relationship between punitive behavior and performance [639]. In one series of studies, punitive behavior had no correlation with performance for professional and technical groups, and in administrative and service groups, punishment was *inversely* correlated with performance, meaning the more people were punished, the worse their performance [639]. In many other studies, punitive behavior on the part of supervisors was associated with lower productivity, higher turnover, and aggressive feelings on the part of employees [642].

Disciplinary actions taken to correct workplace problems are frequently put into effect long after the events have actually taken place, do not necessarily take into account individual differences that could account for the failures in discipline, are vulnerable to the exercise of favoritism by managers, and are often viewed as unfair and capriciously applied by workers. As the psychological distance grows between an employee and management, arbitrary punishments are likely to emerge to cope with workplace problems. Many of these interventions designed to punish the employee actually compound the problem by seeming to punish innocent people—if an employee is suspended, demoted, or fired, the result is more work for everyone else. Brian describes what he sees in the environment that he manages:

> It is not uncommon in our setting for some of the more credentialed staff to see some of the milieu staff as overly aggressive or heavy handed with children, and in fact some may be more directive and confrontational. At the same time it is not uncommon to construct a plan for children who are struggling that consists of having them staffed by these very same people, with very limited support. Although it may not be spoken aloud, staff who may be assertive and confrontational, at times are more successful in keeping a child's problematic behavior under wraps. More often than not the more credentialed staff attributes the success of these workers to their ability to strike fear in the hearts of these children. In fact, it is more complicated. What I see is that they are not afraid to engage with children, even when their behavior is very disruptive. I believe it is the engagement, not intimidation, that is the hook. So here are these staff who are seen as heavy handed and confrontational and they are given the assignment hour after hour and day after day of containing this very dysregulated child. On some level the staff person knows that his or her value to the team and to the organization is to contain this child, and at times the staff person is given little help and support in this activity. So days pass, maybe weeks go by, and this staff person continues to be charged with the care and containment of our most

difficult client. The child may be doing better, but at a great price to the individual worker. The stress and strain may be enormous.

After this prolonged assignment, the worker finally does something counter-aggressive. Yells at the child, grabs him by the shirt, or calls him a name. Clinical staff may end up saying, "I knew he was too aggressive, he does not appreciate the nuance of working with a traumatized child." In fact, the worker's failure was staged from the beginning. He was placed in that role because he was rough and tumble, he was given very little support, and then when he takes a wrong step because of hours or days of unrelenting pressure he makes a bad choice, we jump all over him. Prophecy fulfilled. It is becoming clearer and clearer to us that we are missing the boat by focusing on change in the clients that we serve. Obviously this is the ultimate goal, but it is becoming more and more apparent to us that the systems in which care is delivered and the individuals who deliver care need to change. While we may not need to change as much, we do need to change first. The children that we serve come to us with some very established patterns of behavior, learned through years of mistreatment and misunderstanding. We also come to this work with our own patterns and baggage. The children's behavior induces a set of responses in us and our choice of response either reinforces the child's old patterns or perhaps begins to create some new pathway for the child.

It has been demonstrated that in the workplace, punishment of infractions only works under certain conditions. As one early investigator put it, *"Experience indicates that even severe punishment achieves nothing to redirect behavior into more desirable channels, at least in the large majority of cases... the troubles experienced in our [workplace] seem more consistent with the hypothesis that, in adults, punishment generally produces many undesirable—and few, if any, desirable—results"* (p. 65) [638]. In fact, unless the person punished—child or adult—believes that the punishment is just, he or she is likely to be driven by a desire for vengeance, a basic retaliatory response of an injured human being. As a manager, Brian draws an important distinction:

I think we need to understand a distinction between power and influence here. Displays of power are really quite useless in our settings. At the end of the day a manager has the power to exit someone from the organization and that is really all the power the manager has. You can make someone miserable, but why would you want to make an employee who is in your shop miserable? That is certainly not going to help the kids. Managers should focus on "influencing" workers. Influence is more about training, coaching, mentoring, communicating, and clarifying. If someone does not respond to being influenced, then maybe it is best to employ power to just move them on. If you need to continuously remind people you have power, you probably should not have it and you are likely to abuse it, just to prove you have it.

Ethical Paradigms, Ethical Dilemmas

In any human service delivery organization there are different kinds of ethical dilemmas because there are a variety of concerns that have to be taken into account. Four ethical paradigms have been described. First, there is an *ethic of justice*, which focuses on fairness and equity and is informed by the whole body of rules, regulations, and laws that have accumulated over time. Then there is an *ethic that critiques the ethic of justice*, raising questions about class, race, gender, and other areas of difference and asking: Who decides what is just and unjust? Who benefits from those rules? Who has the power and who is silenced? The *ethic of caring* requires individuals to consider the consequences of their decisions and actions on the welfare of others: Who will be hurt? What are the long-term effects? And then there are the *ethical codes* that are a foundation of every profession, which may vary somewhat from profession to profession and which may pose special dilemmas when a professional must interact in a decision-making capacity with nonprofessionals. Confidentiality is one example of this; another is the injunction that all physicians have, as does everyone in the helping professions, to "do no harm" [643].

As discussed in Chapter 1, there are profound conflicts inherent in the ideological framework of present-day health care and the provision of social services. The effects of these conflicts are often not direct, but instead comprise a background "noise" that can eat away at the fiber of a professional's existence, creating such unrelenting moral distress that they may be compelled to use a wide variety of protective conscious and unconscious defenses that interfere with their capacity to deliver high-quality service. Or they may leave the professions they are in entirely. Over time, the departure of those most concerned about moral distress may leave a system morally bankrupt.

In a larger social context within which caring for others has gone from being a sacred obligation to a commodity that is delivered for the lowest possible dollar in service of the greatest amount of profit, moral distress is virtually inevitable. As a result, the larger culture has set up a pressure-cooker environment that serves no one well. Demands to carry increasing caseloads with an attendant increase in paperwork combined with significant decreases in staffing and resources have made many health care and social service settings almost unbearable. Under such conditions, it is increasingly difficult for caregivers to find the time or psychic energy to provide the level of compassion that victims of violence require if they are to take the first steps in recovery. Placed in untenable moral dilemmas, caregivers often feel powerless to effect change and as a result professionals may succumb to both physical fatigue and compassion fatigue.

One key issue that creates significant tension in many treatment environments and that creates significant ethical dilemmas as well as safety concerns is the role of punishment as a form of, or at least acceptable part of, treatment.

There are strong currents within the larger culture that wax and wane around rehabilitation versus retribution and that then emerge in our criminal justice system, correctional institutions, juvenile justice facilities, mental health organizations, and school settings. The arguments are as old as humanity, reflected in the Biblical injunction to "spare the rod, spoil the child." Nonetheless, an enormous body of scientific research makes clear the dangers of punitive responses, particularly corporal punishment showing that there is little research evidence that physical punishment improves children's behavior in the long term, there is substantial research evidence that physical punishment makes it more, not less, likely that children will be defiant and aggressive in the future, clear research evidence that physical punishment puts children at risk for negative outcomes, including increased mental health problems, and consistent evidence that children who are physically punished are at greater risk of serious injury and physical abuse [305; 644–645].

Environments—and the people in them—tend to become more punitive under stress as tensions rise, emotions flare, and people become increasingly fearful and threatened. Under conditions of chronic stress, punitive measures become institutionalized and may be then called "treatment" with entire systems of rationalizations built up to demonstrate why punitive and coercive measures are absolutely necessary. The problem, of course, is that punishment is inevitably linked to justice and if a person–child or adult-does not feel that the punishment is just, it tends to escalate his or her anger and the desire for retaliation, leading to a seemingly endless cycle of escalating bad behavior and escalating punitive responses.

This applies to the people who work in human service delivery environments as well. The typical response to some kind of infraction is punishment, although often the administration of punishment is actually distant in time from the actual infraction. The fear of punishment often drives other problematic behaviors like denial of responsibility, fear of taking any risks, lying, and covering up. And whenever people feel unfairly treated, they are likely to become vengeful.

Moral Development and the Ethical Organization

Recently, some ethics researchers are taking the issue of reward and punishment in the workplace a step further, and it is work that has immediate implications for treatment as well. Using Kohlberg's stages of moral development, they propose that the heavy reliance on rewards and punishments fosters low levels of moral reasoning and in the long-term contributes to unethical behavior. In exploring why some employees behave unethically, although there are admittedly some "bad apples" as individuals, management researchers conclude that corporations elicit, inculcate, or even encourage unethical behavior by employees [646].

According to these ethics researchers, organizations, like individuals, have stages of moral development. Kohlberg divided the progression of moral reasoning into six stages. Stages 1 and 2 he called "pre-conventional" usually achieved in elementary school; Stage 1 is represented by obedience and punishment, and Stage 2 is represented by individualism, instrumentalism, and exchange best summed up in the ideas behind "you scratch my back and I will scratch yours" and "do onto others as they do onto you." Stages 3 and 4 he called "conventional" and he believed were typical of most people in society. In Stage 3 what is right is understood as whatever is represented by the expectations of one's society or peers. This is represented in "being a good boy or girl," and individual vengeance is no longer acceptable. In Stage 4 respect for laws and authority is paramount. Justice revolves around criminal justice and demands that the wrongdoer be punished and must "pay his debt to society." For Stage 5 and Stage 6 he used the term "post-conventional" and claimed that relatively few members of society reach this level of moral development. Stage 5 is represented by the social contract meaning that moral action in specific situations is defined by universal, abstract moral principles based on human rights and responsibilities. In this stage the idea that justice demands punishment is viewed as nonsense because retributive punishment is neither rational nor sane for the society. Individual freedom should be limited by society only when it infringes on someone else's freedom. In Stage 6 people behave based on a set of universal principles grounded in the equality and worth of all human beings and are guided by principled conscience [647].

Organizations that are operating at Kohlberg's lowest levels of moral reasoning have specific design mechanisms that shift employees' focus from ethical behavior toward stakeholders, to acting in ways that generate rewards or avoid punishments. Performance appraisal systems usually assess behaviors that contribute to profitability or achievement of the organization's strategy and goals and may lower employees' moral reasoning by focusing their attention on behaviors that result in rewards and avoid punishment, regardless of whether it is ethical behavior. In the case of human service systems, particularly managed behavioral health systems, the managed care companies are usually perceived as the punishing agent and as a result, organizations are likely to do things that they do not feel are effective, fair, or even adequate simply to avoid punishment. Premature discharges, changed diagnoses, and changes in medication—all of which may be dictated by the insurance company—may not be clinically indicated, but unless compliance occurs, they may lead to heavy penalties—for the organization and for the clients. The disengagement between the people who deliver services and the people who fund services, along with ever-increasing productivity demands, promotes unethical behavior that is then denied.

Reward and punishment systems may create workplaces that are low in trust, in which people feel controlled and are not encouraged to learn, progress, or consider ethical positions. Size matters as well; large organizations in which an employee only has a small part of a task may discourage moral reasoning because they have little role in decision making and because they are simply a small cog in a very large wheel. Access to information may be denied some people and when this is the case their reasoning cannot be complete because they lack sufficient information to make complex judgments. Codes of ethics may focus on nothing but adhering to rules and regulations, which encourage Stage 4 moral reasoning [646].

Leaders may model a low level of moral reasoning. Research has supported that a group's moral reasoning decreased when the group leader operated at a low level of moral reasoning [646]. It is clear that employees make more effort to understand and follow top management's ethical values and guidelines if the organization rewards people who follow desired ethical practices and punishes or sanctions those who fail to behave ethically [648]. Unfortunately, according to young managers who were interviewed, very few companies embodied values consistent with those they hoped to live by [649]. Gaps may actually exist between a manager's level of moral reasoning and the organization's level of moral reasoning, and this may put the manager in conflict with the organization's system of rewards and punishment [650]. According to some investigators, research suggests that reward and punishments systems may sometimes reward unethical behavior and punish ethical behavior.

Communities socialize employees and make them aware of their relationship with and responsibilities to each other and the larger society, not just as self-interested individuals. Heavy reliance on a system of rewards and punishments assumes that employees will only work on this basis and that they cannot be counted on to "do the right thing" for its own sake. In more corrupt institutions, the system of rewards and punishments implies that employees can be counted on—with sufficient incentives—to do the *wrong* thing. Organizations that are designed with many layers of bureaucracy, with rigid control systems, complex sets of ever-expanding rules and regulations, and limited access to information and compliance systems all signal employees that they cannot be counted on and are not responsible for moral reasoning. This is particularly relevant to care giving organizations, where outcomes are very unclear, as when the desired outcomes focus not on permanent change in the clients but instead on controlling the clients. When everything becomes focused on control, then it gives license to engage in behavior that may otherwise be quite damaging. Brian recalls his own experience with a set of twisted ethical norms:

When I was a young childcare worker I worked in an institution in which the way you first "earned your stripes" was when you did your first restraint. After the first time you held a kid to the ground, your colleagues would give you a look like "welcome to the club, now you're one of us" and that was how you really got to be a reputable staff member. And all of this was framed as "treatment" of the kids and was completely condoned and supported by the organization. It was the proper way to do things.

When organizations react to wrongdoing or perceived wrongdoing with a tightening of controls, increased suspicion, and supervision, as well as more rules and regulations, they simply reinforce these notions without ever considering what the employees are really learning [646]. Brian has noted a very specific tendency to try to include every "exception to the rule" to the point of absurdity:

Many organizational policies are directed at the least common denominator. When you read through most human resources handbooks, the rules, regulations, and policies are pretty common knowledge or just good manners. Several years ago we terminated an employee for urinating in a movie theater parking lot in front of the kids. He filed for unemployment and the hearing officer asked us if we had ever told the worker not to do that. We managed to resist the temptation to add "there will be no public urination in front of children" to our codes of conduct.

Some commentators are urging that organizations must be designed and operated as ethical communities. According to them, it is clear that organizations:

… are typically designed for the few individuals who might behave unethically and take advantage of the organization rather than for the majority of employees who can be trusted to conduct themselves responsibly and ethically… When we view a corporation as a community—or more specifically, as an ethical community—we begin to focus on how the organization shapes and develops the character of employees working within it. (pp. 362–363) [646]

In the private mental health and social service sector, where profit has to be made, and in the nonprofit sector where the bottom line is also increasingly the standard by which performance is judged, service employees may find themselves in serious ethical conflicts quite frequently. Demands to cut services, cut the number of sessions, see a fixed number of people within an unreasonable amount of time, and to get people in and out of service despite enormous obstacles may all put enormous pressure on professionals who are accustomed to having the client as the central focus, not the amount of income the organization is making.

Conclusion

The search for justice is a fundamental human aspiration in our personal lives and in our workplaces, but similarly so is a desire to seek vengeance, to "even the score." Stressed people and stressed environments are more likely to become punitive. Professional standards of ethical behavior are ancient norms for the healing community. People who enter the professions have other motivations for doing human service work besides profitability. When the only way they can make a living and support themselves and their families is to participate in unethical behavior, they experience a profound sense of loss that is rarely acknowledged. Signs of unresolved grief and organizational decline are in evidence all around us. That is the subject of the next chapter.

Chapter 11

Unresolved Grief, Reenactment, and Decline

SUMMARY: *Exposure to trauma always means loss—even if it is the loss of invulnerability that protects us from feeling helpless. People in organizations and organizations as a whole suffer many kinds of loss. Staff, leaders, and programs depart. Neighboring systems close. Standards of care deteriorate and quality assurance standards are lowered in an attempt to deny or hide this deterioration. Over time, leaders and staff lose sight of the essential purpose of their work together and derive less and less satisfaction and meaning from the work. People begin to question whether they are actually successful at what they do or just permanently failing. When this is occurring, staff feel increasingly angry, demoralized, helpless, and hopeless about the people they are working to serve: they become "burned out." Unresolved loss increases the tendency of human beings to repeat the past and reenact tragedy and loss.*

Loss of Attachment in the Workplace

In the norms of the world of work, all losses become disenfranchised, because emotions and feelings are discounted, discouraged, and disallowed... Even mourning as it relates to death is severely constrained by narrowly defined policies that govern acceptable behaviors. (p. 92)

A. J. Stein & H. R. Winokuer, *Monday Mourning:*
Managing Employee Grief

Wherever there is attachment behavior, there is the potential for loss of attachment. We are complexly interdependent on each other for our entire lives and any disruption in normal attachment relationships, particularly those being established in early childhood, is likely to cause developmental problems [210]. Dr. John Bowlby's description of grief responses that proceed through protest, despair, detachment, and finally personality reorganization holds true for many different kinds of losses because any significant loss is likely to arouse childhood fears of loss of attachment regardless of our age or life experience.

327

Although there are no clear "stages of grief" that people inevitably work their way through, nor is there likely to be anything like "closure" after a significant loss, there do appear to be tasks of grief work. The first task is to accept the reality of the loss. After a sudden or traumatic loss people are likely to be "in shock," an acute state of denial that buffers people from the reality of the loss and gives them the time to adjust to this reality. Different people need different amounts of time to make this adjustment. In many situations, denial may serve the needs of survival in the moment and therefore accepting the reality of loss may be delayed.

Grieving is, by definition, painful, both physically and emotionally, and may be accompanied by a number of other distressing emotions, including anger, shame, and guilt. The mourner must adjust to life without whomever or whatever is missing and lost and then must emotionally relocate whatever or whoever is gone and move on with his or her life. Grief occurs within a sociocultural context which varies greatly from culture to culture and will be affected by a number of factors, including the extent of the loss and the damage to the community as a whole. There is no set timetable for grief; everyone grieves in a different way, and every new loss opens the door again onto every other loss that has ever occurred. Organizations that do not grieve for their losses can remain stuck in the past, unable to adequately adapt to the present and create a better future.

Many people spend at least as much time in the workplace, with workplace colleagues, as they do with their families. The result is that workplace relationships assume a vital part of each worker's support network and any loss of that support is likely to result in reactions typical of anyone who has a real or threatened loss of an attachment bond [651]. In the protest phase, employees may hold on to what was lost through a wide variety of real and symbolic behaviors [652]. They may try to hold on to old work equipment, resist a move to a new office location, go out to lunch only with former colleagues, file grievances or other actions to stop change, and engage in other forms of written and vocal protest [651]. One of our faculty consultants shared this story with us:

> The CEO had worked long and hard to achieve a long-held dream of a new school. Finally the new facility was ready. It was gorgeous—all new structures, new equipment, and lots more space. She was perplexed then after the move, when the staff seemed to do little except complain about missing the old, broken-down, decrepit building they had left. No one had thought about bringing a symbolic part of that well-worn and highly remembered building with them to the new facility.

For as long as they possibly can employees may deny that the change that is anticipated is really going to occur. When the prospective changes are brought up, they typically change the subject, continue to use old forms, old procedures, and old labels. Employees may attempt to bargain with their supervisors, trying to hold on to previous attachments: "Can I keep my desk?" "Can I stay in my office?" "Can we use the old software?" "Can I go to lunch at the same time?"

When new people are added to the organization as part of organizational change, veteran employees may keep their distance from them. These behaviors must be understood as reluctance to let go of what has been so much a part of who we are regardless of whether that is other coworkers, a sense of safety and trust, predictable routines, or familiar surroundings. *"To let go is to let a part of ourselves die. This is painful and we want to delay it, push it away, and pretend it isn't happening. We hope for a last-minute rescue, a change of heart by the Board of Directors, or a miraculous new contract"* (p. 38) [652]. Individual reactions to loss will be influenced by experiences of previous loss.

Despair and disorganization may be seen in decreased work effort, many complaints, and active expression of distress, including feelings of anger, hurt, fear, guilt, and shame. When any kind of attachment bonds are broken, people experience an aching emptiness. The physical and emotional pain of grief that occurs along with anger is a part of the process. *"For people who have made their work and the workplace their social environment the most important part of their lives, the loss or threat of loss of what has been can result in devastating pain"* (p. 46) [652]. Because fractured attachments are experienced at a gut level as a threat to survival, the result may be fear rising to the level of panic and even terror. Employees may express fears about security and their future. Trying to contain fear and anxiety may lead to an increase in both physical and emotional symptoms. One of the programs in our Sanctuary Network shared this experience with us:

> Daniel had been the executive director for years and was loved and admired. We were shocked when we learned he only had a few months to live and when he died within weeks of this announcement. I am not sure any of us ever had a chance to really grieve for his loss. There was so much to do just to keep the organization together that we had no time. We went to the memorial service, of course, but I know I for one was focused on how I was going to do the job I wasn't really ready to do yet. I think we can still see evidence of unresolved loss throughout our organization.

Rage, resentment, bitterness, sabotage, and violence can represent the anger phase of loss and grief. Anger may be displaced onto someone else: other managers, coworkers, family, or the family pet. Anger may be directly expressed through hostile attitudes, words or behaviors, or through grumbling, excessive questioning, complaining, angry facial expressions, arguing, fighting, insubordination, destruction of property, theft, and in the worst cases, physical violence. Other people may express their distress through passive-aggressive behavior: lateness, absenteeism, work slowdown, less teamwork, poor communication, increased errors, decreased cooperation, lack of follow-through, and diminished self-direction. *"Take a title, desk, parking space, job security, workplace friend, or feeling of trust away from an employee and anger is a natural reaction"* (p. 45) [652]. We express anger whenever we are denied something we want or we perceive obstacles to our goal. Frustration converts to anger very quickly and is a natural, normal release of an inner emotional state. Depression may characterize the whole environment. People may withdraw from normal routines and relationship patterns, and give off nonverbal signals that say "just leave me alone."

Both managers and line staff may feel guilt, the former over the role they may be playing in the decisions that are resulting in change, and the latter over surviving the changes when some of their colleagues have not. Deep feelings of shame may dominate the employee who is demoted or otherwise loses status in the organization. When the mourning process is neither complicated nor delayed, employees can then begin to envision an end to the transition and begin to develop a new identity and a new set of skills. They may not be entirely happy with the changes, but they are beginning to accommodate to the changes. They are likely to reconcile themselves cognitively before they completely work through the loss emotionally. Brian shares his own feelings about leading through loss:

> *Change can be very hard. People I liked a lot both professionally and personally have left. I have felt very bad about those changes at times. But in my position of leadership, my "love" can't be unconditional. If a person isn't meeting the needs of the organization—and that is to serve the welfare of the children— then that person has to go, regardless of my personal feelings about him or her. So when someone leaves, or is forced out, I end up feeling a mixture of confusing feelings: relief that the problems the person was causing are over, sadness because someone I care about has left the organization, and guilt because I had to make a tough decision or could not help the person get on track. It's always hard for me, too, because as things are changing, those steady and predictable relationships that I felt I could rely on change as well, and you can't be sure where it is all going until it goes.*

Complicated Mourning

The concept of "complicated grief" applies to people and situations where bereavement exceeds the expected norm and creates additional problems. The subject has been extensively covered by Theresa Rando and she highlights seven high-risk factors that predispose individuals to complicated mourning.

These include sudden, unexpected death, especially when traumatic, violent, mutilating, or random; death from an overly lengthy illness; loss of a child; the mourner's perception of the death as preventable; a premorbid relationship with the deceased that was markedly angry or ambivalent, or dependent; prior or concurrent mourner liabilities such as other losses, stresses, or mental health problems; and the mourner's lack of social support. All of these factors result in greater numbers of people experiencing complicated mourning [653].

Childcare organizations and the employees that work in them are at risk for complicated bereavement when a death of a child occurs while the child is in the care of the organization. Children who enter residential treatment facilities are likely to arrive there after multiple experiences with disrupted attachment and as a result suffer from complex physical, emotional, cognitive, and social problems. These children have much to grieve for and few internal resources available to them. They have a history of unsafe behavior, which is the usual precipitant which leads them to be admitted to intensive treatment environments. They have profound difficulties managing distressful feelings and a history of unresolved loss. With little ability to envision a better future for themselves, these children may be a threat to themselves or to others.

The fundamental job of the treatment environment is to keep these children safe. And sometimes the staff fail. On rare occasions, children succeed in seriously harming themselves, others, or even dying from being forcibly restrained or from suicide. In virtually all of these cases, government officials, regulatory agencies, and the providers themselves will perceive these injuries or deaths as unexpected, horrific, and preventable. The staff members involved are likely to experience significant guilt and are not likely to receive much social support throughout the course of the legal and sometimes criminal investigations that follow.

Ambiguous Loss

Ambiguity means being driven in at least two ways at once, or experiencing conflicting feelings that cannot be synthesized. Pauline Boss has extensively explored the concept of "ambiguous loss": *"My basic theoretical premise is that ambiguous loss is the most stressful kind of loss. It defies resolution and creates long-term confusion about who is in or out of a particular couple or family. With death there is official certification of loss, and mourning rituals allow one to say goodbye. With ambiguous loss, none of these markers exist. The persisting ambiguity blocks cognition, coping and meaning-making and freezes the grief process"* (p. xvii) [654].

Boss defines two main groups of ambiguous loss: *(1)* when loved ones are physically absent but are kept psychologically present, especially when the loss is not verified by evidence of death, such as when someone is missing in action or the person's body has never been found, but it also applies to cases of adoption, divorce, or work relocation; and *(2)* when people are physically present but psychologically absent, as when their affliction is denied and they are expected to act as they were, as in the case of dementia, chronic mental illness, addiction, head injuries, and obsessive preoccupations. According to Dr. Boss, her premise is that ambiguity coupled with loss creates a barrier to working through loss and leads to symptoms such as depression and relational conflict that erode human relationships.

Although Dr. Boss is referring to situations where actual physical death is involved, the notion of ambiguity has applications to the workplace as well. Workplace loss often manifests with signs of ambiguous loss. In the corporate world, people sometimes just "disappear"; one day they are there as usual, and the next they are gone and all of their personal things missing from their desks/cubicles. These disappearances may be good for the overall financial stability of the organization, but for people who are connected to others in the dense web of connection that is often created in workplace settings, particularly those where relationships are at a premium, the hole left by the person who is no longer there may be filled, at least for a time, with the person's psychological presence. This may present challenges to managers who believe the person is well and truly gone, while colleagues are acting as if he or she is still present, still exerting influence on the environment.

Disenfranchised Grief

Disenfranchised grief has been defined as grief that is deemed as inappropriate, that cannot be publicly acknowledged, openly mourned, and socially supported and which is thereby refused the conditions for normal resolution through the work of grieving. When someone has been involved in what is considered an illicit affair and the lover dies, or in many cases, when a homosexual partner dies, the person may experience disenfranchised grief [655]. The term has been extended to apply to the workplace in general, serving to indicate that any loss becomes disenfranchised if we are not allowed to express grief in the one place where most of our waking hours during the week are spent. This is particularly important since at any point in time, 16% of the workforce experiences a personal loss within a given year. Brian notes a particularly difficult situation for staff:

> *I think the best example for the disenfranchisement of grief in the workplace is when someone is fired. I think we consider it ok to grieve the loss of coworkers for other reasons, but when someone is fired I think there is a sense you need to keep your grief to yourself. If you really miss that guy who hit a kid or falsified his time sheet, what kind of person does that make you? And if you openly express grief after your manager has fired a guy, what will the manager do*

to you? I always say that everyone in an organization is loved by someone. Even in the most obvious cases of termination, someone feels bad about what happened.

Grieving in the workplace can lead to decreased individual productivity, and anything that inhibits the grieving process and thus causes the mourning period to be lengthened, more severe, or entirely postponed, is likely to negatively impact the organization. Nonetheless, little attention has been paid to this issue in the social service workplace [656].

In the mental health system, particularly in residential treatment settings for children, we often hear about a staff member who has been accused by a child of some form of abuse. In the worst cases, the accusations are demonstrated to be true and the staff member is fired. But not all accusations are true, and all accusations must be investigated. During the period of investigation, the staff member is removed from the setting and no one at that point knows for sure what is going to happen. The loss of that individual is often experienced painfully and acutely by colleagues and by other children, but the circumstances cannot really be discussed when the case is under investigation. Unfortunately, investigations can drag on and on for weeks, sometimes months. Even if the staff member is found guiltless, the effects of the trauma and loss—and the inability to set in motion any healing actions at the time—may be long lasting. It's a very tough call. Children must be protected. In this book we certainly have not pulled our punches about just how dysfunctional a treatment environment can be. On the other hand, in our experience there is little attention paid to the overall well-being of everyone in the program and how they are being affected by the critical incident.

But even apart from such difficult circumstances, grieving in the workplace, even for losses associated with death, has been actively discouraged. Typically, the amount of grieving in the workplace that is "allowed" is determined by the perceived closeness of the relationship. On the average, organizations give employees about 3 days off to grieve for the death of a loved one and after that time they are expected to get back to work and resume normal activity. And the amount of allowable grief may be determined by the person's role in the organization. Leaders are expected to go on working as if nothing had happened in their private lives. People who deal with life and death issues all the time are expected to keep tight control in their workplace and this of course includes physicians, nurses, and social workers [656]. Perinatal deaths or the deaths of the elderly are often easily dismissed. Grieving over the loss of someone who is still alive but is no longer the same person, such as in dementia or brain injury, may be minimized. Losses that are a result of abortion, sudden infant death syndrome, suicide, homicide, AIDS, or "preventable" accidents may be stigmatized. The problem, of course, is that grief often refuses to comply with the organizational timetable. Grieving is not linear and does not decrease steadily over time. The more that normal grief is inhibited and the longer the grieving process is postponed, the more likely it is to become problematic and even pathological. When this happens and performance is affected, corrective measures are often directed at the symptom rather than the cause, and the individual may become increasingly alienated from the organization [656].

Unresolved grief can result in an idealization of what has been lost that interferes with adaptation to a new reality. Individual employees and entire organizations may distort memories of the past just as individuals can. Organizations may selectively omit disagreeable facts, may exaggerate or embellish positive deeds, may deny the truth, and engage in what has been termed "organizational nostalgia" for a golden past that is highly selective and idealized and when compared to the present state of affairs, surpassingly better. It is a world that is irretrievably lost, with all of the sense of inexpressible grief associated with such loss, and the present is always comparably poorer, less sustaining, less fruitful, less promising. In this way the organizational past—whether accurately remembered or not—can continue to exert a powerful influence on the present. The failure to grieve for the loss of a leader may make it difficult or impossible for a new leader to be accepted by the group. In fact, one author has noted that *"Nostalgia is not a way of coming to terms with the past (as mourning or grief are) but an attempt to come to terms with the present"* (p. 132) [657]. The former medical director of a psychiatric inpatient program had to confront nostalgia, up close and personal:

> I didn't realize how much I was in the grip of nostalgic feelings and years of unresolved loss until a new medical director joined us who was young and just out of her training. One day, after listening once again to all of us reminisce about the way things used to be in out treatment program, she interrupted us and said, "You know I care about all of you, and I admire the work you have done, but really…. I just can't stand one more discussion about 'the good old days'! I have to make the most of what is here now."

Traumatic Loss, Chronic Loss, and Organizational Change

> Losing the comfort of a safe and reliable work environment creates an ongoing sense of the loss of trust. Loss is the factor that determines our grief. Loss— whether from a death or a death-like change in our life circumstances—hurts. (p. 27) [652]
>
> <div align="right">J. S. Jeffreys (2005), <i>Coping With Workplace Grief:
Dealing With Loss, Trauma, and Change</i></div>

The losses associated with organizational change are significant and impact the lives of the individuals within the organization as well as the organization as a whole. Organizational change can be a result of downsizing, mergers, restructuring, reorganization, and transitions secondary to traumatic events. Some employees describe the constancy of organizational change as "permanent white water" [652]. Brian has experienced that at Andrus:

> *This place really was a family when I first got here. It was very intimate. We had a 56-bed residential program and the children were higher functioning than the children we see today. We used to have staff parties or a luncheon and people watched 55 kids. Now, with 150 kids you need 100 staff to watch them. The whole climate has changed. The people who are "old timers" remember it when everyone knew everyone, but those days are gone forever. It's not a product of choice and people don't always understand that. The industry changes and we have to respond to those changes or close our doors. What we once were is no longer. We are different. As I see it now, everyone reacts differently to loss. Recently one of our key organizational leaders has been acting out a lot, being arbitrarily divisive and obstructing everything I try to do. She is questioning things that she would not have questioned before and being just difficult about things she doesn't need to be difficult about. Interestingly, she is not even someone who is affected by the things she is questioning. This all started after her reporting relationship changed. As I think about it, this is the way she is managing the losses she has experienced, including her reporting relationship; that has never really been addressed. Systems are funny. Every time you add something you lose something. We added a diagnostic center and a day treatment program and after all the planning, we—the administrators—were excited about the new programming. But the primary programs felt like there was someone else leeching off them, depriving them of their resources, and the new programs felt like second-class citizens. You are always contending with that: the new people feel like stepchildren and the old people think the new kid is taking up their space.*

What are the losses that employees experience? Losses include changes in organizational structure that means adjusting to new managers or supervisors, changes in employment status and job description, changes in physical locations, salaries, benefits, job security, dependable colleagues, and resources. As one author has pointed out, *"Whatever we left behind after we went through the transition represents loss. Even if the new situation is a desired change—promotion, new office—we still lose the way it used to be, and the reaction to this loss is grief"* (p. 15) [652]. This is the way good managers at one level can become the dreaded "micromanagers" at another level. Brian can personally relate to this:

> *I think I have been trying to hold on to some things myself. As C.O.O. I am no longer able to manager day-to-day operations. I enjoyed doing this in my*

previous roles and to some extent I have continued to do this ...to hold on to certain operations for too long. As a result, I have not allowed the people who report directly to me the space to manage their own affairs. It is only recently that I am coming to grips with this and becoming a leader rather than a manager. I do miss many aspects of my former job, but that is not my job anymore.

Organizational restructuring may mean that people with whom other people have bonded are suddenly gone. One's status in the organization may suddenly be changed. Familiar procedures, surroundings, and trusted reporting relationships may be lost. Employees may lose the ability to do the work they were trained to do and must spend more time doing paperwork than they are developing relationships with clients. The result of all this may be the loss of safety, security, control, and some basic assumptions about what they can expect from the organization, which jeopardizes the sense of basic trust [652].

Downsizing has been called *"a pervasive form of organizational suicide"* (p. 31) [658]. According to previous research, 80% of the organizations studied that were involved in downsizing suffered morale problems. Under such circumstances, people feel insecure and their organizational commitment is decreased. They fear taking any risks and thus innovation is dampened. They must work harder for the same pay or, worse, accept pay cuts. Anger and grief over the loss of colleagues may lead to a false sense of hope that the lost coworker will eventually come back or will be rehired. The emotional toll is high on everyone [415]. As one executive reported, *"while layoffs may provide a short-term boost to profits, over the long run downsizing begins a cycle in which companies falter because of loss of talent and a decay of morale that constrain economic performance for years afterwards"* (p. 32) [658].

It is clear that the ways in which grief, loss, and termination are handled have a significant impact on employee attitudes. There is evidence that when employees are given permission to grieve for the"end of what was," the readjustment to new conditions is likely to be less problematic [659]. But unfortunately, in the human service sector, time to grieve for losses in the workplace has become a rarity that has enormous consequences: *"Our society in general, and the business world specifically, has typically not granted enough permission for people to grieve. As a result, many grieving employees are given little time to be off balance, sad, angry, scared, unmotivated, and unproductive. When there is a lack of time to mourn what was, employees are less free to bond to the new situation"* (p. 16) [652].

Deaths by suicide or homicide are acutely traumatic, particularly to a mental health or social service setting where the fear of recriminations for a failure to anticipate or prevent the deaths may be a major component of the event as it is experienced by the members of the organization. Sudden firings or other departures of key personnel may be experienced as organizationally traumatic, as may the sudden death of a leader or otherwise influential employee. A former program director at a residential facility where a child was killed shares her experience:

> *It's over 15 years ago and I still have never really recovered from the death of that child on my watch. When I got the call that he had been killed, it was like time stood still and the world dropped out underneath me. I had to identify the body, call the family, go through multiple investigations, support the staff, calm down the executives above me, and represent the institution in the media. It was a nightmare and I still worry about something like that happening every day. I orchestrated ceremonies, rituals, and a memorial for the child, but nobody ever really helped me work through my grief and that still makes me really angry when I think about it.*

When individuals become a member of an organization, the individual surrenders some of his or her own individuality in service of the organization. As a result, losses to the organization are likely to be experienced individually as well as collectively [660]. For the same reason, failures of the organization to live up to whatever internalized ideal the individual has for the way that organization should function, are likely to be experienced individually and collectively as a betrayal of trust, a loss of certainty and security, a disheartening collapse of meaning and purpose. Brian talks about his own experience with the loss of the ideal collective image of our ability to maintain safety:

> *Several years ago a child who was in our care was discharged to another agency. Several weeks after he left us, he was killed by another resident in that agency. Our staff felt terrible. We held several meetings to talk about it and many staff expressed anger that we had let the kid and family down because we did not have a high school program. If we really cared about our kids, they seemed to be saying, we would not discharge them to some other program. We would have our own. In reality everyone will move on eventually—we cannot protect children forever, much as we might like to. But this was a terrible tragedy and very upsetting, particularly upsetting to our sense of control that we can and must protect kids from harm.*

As workers in this field have determined, "*the relationship between employee and organization are: deep-seated; largely unconscious; intimately connected to the development of identity; and have emotional content*" (p. 429) [660]. Because of this connectedness between individual and collective identity, and because all change involves loss, organizational change and grieving tend to go hand in hand [660].

Traumatic Reenactment: Never Having to Say Goodbye

Our individual identities emerge out of a group context; we have a social brain and we begin mirroring other people when we are only hours old. This mirroring, in healthy people, never stops. When people expect something of us, we give it to them. We have stable and relatively predictable relationships with other people as a result, until our expectations change. Changed expectations ring the death knell for many relationships because the other person has difficulty adapting to changed expectations and simply continues playing the role he or she already knows, those well-rehearsed lines. Changing these roles, once we are in them, is difficult usually because the present role has been and still is reinforcing patterns of relationships and roles that we have been replicating since we were children. How many times have you had a friend or colleague who got through a terrible divorce only to meet and marry someone who was virtually the same person, and yet the friend couldn't see that? This is the power of reenactment: that other people see the roles we play long before we see them ourselves. If we fail to see them and fail to ask, "Why is this person doing this— what happened?" we are likely to retraumatize the person because the social response that he or she needs—the ritual reenactment that changes the story— is not forthcoming. Brian tells a poignant story about reenactment:

> Many years ago long before Sanctuary and before we knew anything about trauma, we had a young girl in our care who challenged us at every level. She was aggressive and very dysregulated. She would run away and take rides from strangers after she left the property. She scared us to death, because she was going to get herself killed. When she would return from an elopement, she was placed on house or room restriction for days and watched closely by a variety of staff. Inevitably she would run again, either when the staff was not looking or once the close restrictions were lifted. Each time she ran, the restrictions got longer, tighter, and harsher. For some time we staffed her in a room with only a small window, which resembled a prison cell.
>
> This little girl was terribly injured, but we never took that into account. We never gave much thought to her past, a past that included physical and sexual abuse and neglect. Although we did not inflict the same kind of abuse on this child, we did mistreat her. In our effort to contain her, in our effort to manage our own feelings of fear and anger, we treated her not as a little girl who was scared and hurt, but like a kind of monster who needed to be contained and controlled. While this did not characterize her entire stay with us, it was certainly not our finest hour and we ultimately failed to make substantial changes in the way this little girl viewed the world around her.

Without an understanding of our basic group nature and our deeply programmed need to express our distress to our social group, it is impossible to understand why traumatized children and adults keep repeating their traumatic and traumatizing relationships with other people, even when they could make other choices. Our persistence in continuing to utilize ineffective strategies reflects the incredible resistance that a highly individualistic culture has to recognizing group effects, both conscious and unconscious. Here are some comments from a childcare worker that reflect the inherent difficulty in addressing this issue:

> It has been so difficult to change the behavioral management system that has been in place here for a long time, even though from what I can see, it doesn't really change these kids' behavior. The staff want to respond to everything with some punitive consequence and from my point of view, it just seems to reinforce the kind of treatment the kids have received their entire lives. But when I even try to bring this up, that it isn't working and that it may be hurting the kids, the pressure to go along with the rest of the staff is enormous. It's intimidating for me. They make me feel that any change in a different direction will make them less safe and it will be my fault.

Enactment in Our Evolutionary History

As we discussed in Chapter 3, traumatic reenactment is the reenactment of a traumatic past that has not been laid to rest, that remains unintegrated as a complete biographical narrative. Reenacting strategies that harm the chances of survival rather than enhance the chances appear to be backward, pointless, and crazy if we narrow our point of view to include only the individual. From what we know about reenactment, particularly it's universality and perseverance across the centuries, we can conclude that perhaps our neurobiology and our deep psychology have prepared us with some methods to heal from traumatic experience. However, these are not *individual* methods but *group* methods, historically necessary for the survival of a very traumatized species. If we realize that enactment is essentially a communicative act, then we can begin to understand that traumatic reenactment may itself be an important survival strategy in our evolutionary history, even if it fails us now [661].

The great American poet W. H. Auden has pointed out the importance of enactment in human functioning, *"Human beings are by nature actors, who cannot become something until first they have pretended to be it. They are therefore to be divided, not into the hypocritical and the sincere, but into the sane, who know they are acting, and mad who do not. We constitute ourselves through our actions"* (as quoted in Driver, 1991) [662]. We *were* actors long before we were talkers in our evolutionary history, and enactment remains a nonverbal form of communication with others of our kind. As we have discussed, the tendency to repeat, to reenact, the past is an intrinsic part of all life. If we have survived yesterday, then it makes sense to use the same survival strategies today. We all repeat the past all the time—as individuals, as groups, and as institutions. If we have survived, if we have even prospered, then repetition is logical and survival enhancing.

Collective Reenactments

If traumatic reenactment is a clear and possible outcome to a traumatic experience of the individual, is it possible that traumatic reenactment can also occur at the level of the group? And if reenactment behavior does affect entire groups of people, is it possible that a group's "character" can also become maladaptive as a result of repetitive stress? An organization that cannot change, that cannot work through losses and move on, will, like an individual, develop patterns of reenactment, repeating past strategies over and over without recognizing that these strategies may no longer be effective. This can easily lead to organizational patterns that become overtly abusive. Corporate abuse comes in many forms, including discrimination, demotion without cause, withholding of resources, financial manipulation, overwork, harassment, systematic humiliation, and arbitrary dismissal [663].

Our assumption in this book is that something emerges out of the collection of individuals that comprise any sustained group that becomes a collective living being, with feelings and with memories. Because we are still at such a primitive state of fully understanding this emergent being, much of what happens occurs completely outside of the conscious awareness of the individual members. At its worst, this is what happens when a mob reacts violently. But these effects are likely to be happening all the time in group settings. When a person behaves in such a group context, he or she may be representing aspects of the group's unconscious mind without recognizing it. If so, the individual is seen as a living vessel through which unconscious group life can be expressed and understood.

The group as a whole is conceptualized as having a life different from, but related to, the dynamics of the individuals within the group. Groups are living systems and the individuals in the group are subsystems of which the group is comprised. The group-as-a-whole concept implies that individual behavior in groups is largely a result of group "forces" that channels the individual action. From this perspective, when a person speaks, he or she does so not only for herself but also voices the unconscious sentiment of the group. This position implies that if a group as a whole can be a repository of hopes and fears, then it can also become a repository of secrets, of what is fragmented, denied, cast off, and suppressed [664]. Such a dynamic system paves the way for individual reenactment behavior; so too does it pave the way for group reenactment. Here is a story from one of our faculty consultants:

> *The staff of an inpatient unit were under considerable stress due to staff reductions and leadership changes after years of a controlling, and sometimes abusive leader. A woman was admitted with suicidal ideation and a number of serious*

medical problems. She had managed to get away from her abusive partner but in doing so had lost her job and had no place to live. The staff perceived the patient as needy and dependent and took an immediate dislike to her. There was little discussion about the nature of her problems. Shift to shift, day to day, the word was that she was too needy and should be discharged. Little time was spent talking to her and the belief system about her took on a life of its own. The patient then began having escalating symptoms of psychosis and only then did she get attention from the staff. Her medical problems, which were previously attributed to attention-seeking behavior, worsened and more medical attention was obtained for her. Meanwhile, the staff kept talking about how she really did not deserve to be in the hospital and should be discharged. Only when the psychiatrist was able to get the woman's entire story and share it with the staff were they able to see this patient as deserving of care. He was able to frame her neediness as posttraumatic and pointed out to the staff how much the woman needed to be empowered to take care of her own medical problems that formerly had been under the charge of her abusive husband. Once the patient began being heard, her psychotic symptoms resolved without antipsychotic medications and all of her symptoms improved enough to support discharge.

This patient was a victim of domestic violence. By the time she entered treatment she was feeling literally and emotionally beaten down after years of abuse. She expressed neediness probably because she was, indeed, needy but she also conveyed to the staff her expectations that she would be punished, just as she had been in her marriage, while secretly hoping for rescue. The staff members then walked right into her personal drama, bringing into it their own sense of being victimized by the larger system and therefore angry at her for asking anything more of them. As a result, they began persecuting her by denying her needs and rejecting her reasonable requests, thus reenacting her marital situation. All of this went on completely outside of the realm of any conscious or deliberate planning or even conversation. Fortunately, her psychiatrist was enough outside of the group unconscious at that moment that he could evaluate the situation, recognize the disturbance that was unfolding, and help the staff into conscious awareness of this patient's very real plight—both physical and emotional. Once the roles shifted for the staff, they automatically also shifted for the patient, who finally got the help she needed.

But recognition of these recurring patterns is often missed so that with every repetition there is further deterioration in functioning. Knowledge about this failing is available, but it tends to be felt before it is cognitively appreciated. Without the capacity to put words to feelings, a great deal of deterioration may occur before the repetitive and destructive patterns are recognized. Healthier and potentially healing individuals enter the organization but are rapidly extruded as they fail to adjust to the reenactment role that is being demanded of them. Less autonomous individuals may also enter the organization and are drawn into the reenactment pattern. In this way, one autocratic and abusive leader leaves or is thrown out only to be succeeded by another, while those who have been involved in the hiring process remain bewildered by this outcome [665]. Here is an example shared by a board member of a family shelter:

> After the founder of the organization died, we couldn't seem to find someone adequate to run the place. We would interview people, they would look good on paper, but when it really came down to it, every successive manager seemed to make things worse. They would come in, try to "lay down the law" to the staff, and when it didn't work, each one would leave, and it would start all over again. I don't think any of them ever asked us to review the past history of the organization or took a particularly sympathetic approach to the staff.

Reenactment patterns are most likely to occur when events in the past have resulted in behavior that arouses shame or guilt in the organization's representatives. Shame and guilt for past misdeeds are especially difficult for individuals and organizations to work through. The way an organization talks to itself is via communication between various "voices" of the organization. If these voices are silenced or ignored, communication breaks down and is more likely to be acted out through impulse-ridden and destructive behavior [665]. The clinical director of a pediatric inpatient unit described it in this way:

> I have been trying so hard to get the staff to stop putting the kids into holds. It's clear to me that they do it many times when the kids should be dealt with in an entirely different way, but instead they escalate the problem. Every time I push them, it comes back to the same discussion about the kid who seriously injured a staff member a number of years ago and they aren't taking any chances of that happening again.

For human beings, grieving is a social experience. It would appear that on an evolutionary basis we are set for reenactment behavior and that this behavior has important signal importance to our social support network. The nonverbal brain of the traumatized person signals through gesture, facial expression, tone of voice, and behavior that something is amiss, that there is some rift in the social fabric that connects the individual to the social group, a rift that must be healed because individual survival depends on the group and group survival depends on individuals. The behavior of the individual triggers a ritual response in the group in order to help the person tell the story, reexperience the emotion, transform the meaning of the event, and reintegrate into the whole, while simultaneously the group can learn from the experience of the individual. The amount of social support that is offered is often enormous, with an entire tribe participating in escorting the injured party back into the fold through any means necessary to do so [360].

But in the workplace, although employees may indeed be constantly reliving the losses they have experienced, there is likely to be little time or attention given to the need to provide individual employees the sustained social support they require. Nor is it likely that a stressed organization will pay attention to the losses it sustains and allow any natural ritualized forms of working through organizational loss to unfold. The mental health system has sustained enormous losses over the past decade as leaders and staff have left, programs have been dissolved, communication networks destroyed, and meaning systems abandoned. Yet there has been little discussion of the unrelenting signs of unresolved grief that now plagues the system. Instead what remain visible are abundant signs of organizations in decline. Brian describes the way loss can interfere with a healthy merger with an organization that had lost a great deal but had even more to lose if the merger was unsuccessful:

It was this unresolved grief I think that was at the core of the reenactment that we found ourselves in over and over again. It would go something like this. "We used to do this level of staff development and supervision back when, and it made for a much better place to work and much better treatment." To which I would respond, "Well, things have changed and we can no longer sustain this amount of time for training, case conferencing, and supervision." To which staff would respond, "The work is so stressful and we need this kind of activity to refuel and bolster ourselves against the stress of the work." To which I would respond, "Well, we could do that, but then in relatively short order we would not have much to talk about since we would be out of business." Their response: "All you care about are billables; you do not care about quality." To which I would say, usually in a more sophisticated way, "Grow up."

We operated on two different planes for a long time. I did not feel we had time to feel bad or mourn; we had to get moving. Each of us had our own pain, and we managed it by simply getting angry and frustrated with each other. What I failed to realize then was that there was no way to move forward until folks could properly mourn the past and somehow make peace with what they had lost. Although I know I acknowledged the loss and pain at times, I think it was generally experienced as lip service. "I know this has been hard. I know you wish things were like they used to be. Can we move on now?" I am quite sure the majority of staff felt I could care less. In spite of all I knew about trauma, I could not see the reenactment triangle that had been created and created mostly by Andrus. In the early days we presented ourselves as the rescuers. We were going to save this organization. I believe the interpretation of this message is we were going to rescue them from something that had already happened. The change in funding that had wreaked havoc on their system was done and there was no way anyone was going to save them from that. You can't ever rescue people from something that happened 10 years ago.

So not only did we not rescue them, but we did not even acknowledge their pain. The more we tried to move things to another place, the more resentful people became and the more victimized they felt. It did not take long for the rescuer to become the perpetrator, and we would rail about how stuck everything was. Over time, I began to feel like I could not get anywhere and no one appreciated how hard I was trying. I felt hopeless, helpless, and abused. Misery loves company and we all had plenty of company. When I look back, I shake my head because we missed so many opportunities. I was so eager to get moving that I never really listened. What if I had taken a few weeks to ask people, "What are you most proud of?" "What makes this a great place to work?" "What do you miss most about the way things used to be?" "Who do you miss most and what do you miss about them?" "What was it like working here back when?"

I never had these conversations because I saw such conversation as regressive. "Can we stop dwelling on the good old days?" was my general reaction. "We have things to do." This was exacerbated by the fact that their "good old days" were not my good old days. I wonder how things would have been different if we had taken the time up front to really hear the story, supported them in mourning their losses, and sincerely empathized with them.

Costs of Not Addressing Normal and Complicated Loss

There is a high price to be paid individually and collectively when the process of grief is inhibited or arrested. The grief does not go away but instead turns into feelings and attitudes that can severely disrupt productive work. An overall feeling of distrust and resentment toward the organization may lead to hostile acts, counteraggression, destructiveness, stealing, poor work product, and chronic anger. Shame and an inclination to "play it safe" can lead to stagnation, an unwillingness to take any creative risks, avoidance, and isolation. Chronic fear lowers creativity and increases stress-related physical and emotional problems. As one authority states it, "*Unresolved anger can lead to chronic bitterness, self-hatred, grudges, and an ongoing sense of helplessness. It some cases, it can also lead to physical aches and pains, symptoms of stress, depression, and other emotional disorders*" (p. 45) [652]. Under these circumstances, similar to their repetitively and chronically stressed clients, employees may overreact to even minor provocations.

On the other hand, "*Anger that is constructively managed can fuel productive change and bring about motivation to develop new skills and to complete important tasks*" (p. 45) [652]. Feelings that are not allowed appropriate expression through grieving are unavailable for productive purpose and productive work is likely to plummet with morale sinking and errors compounding.

In this discussion of organizational change and loss it is important to remember that as we discussed in Chapter 4, we expect our institutions to help contain anxiety. When instead, they generate more angst, the terrible distress that human beings are so vulnerable to—feelings of disintegration, annihilation, chaos, and death—are unleashed. We organize our social institutions to accomplish specific tasks and functions, but we also utilize our institutions to collectively protect us against being overwhelmed with these anxieties that underlie human existence. A faculty consultant shared this experience with us:

The CEO and the COO had previously worked closely together, although always in subordinate positions, and had developed a close personal and professional relationship. When the CEO moved up, he became more distanced from his talented COO geographically and practically. Neither of them expressed the experience of personal loss over these changes, nor was any attempt made to process organizationally what it meant to have the CEO so distanced from the daily operations that he had so lovingly and carefully managed before. When a client murdered another client shortly after leaving the institution and not long after these major management changes had occurred, the CEO conveyed a mixture of feelings to the COO but mostly expressed anger, frustration, and disappointment that the COO hadn't done a better job in keeping the institution safe. The COO was already feeling severely wounded by the reality of the situation she had to deal with, but compounding this was a sense of betrayal and overwhelming loss at not being able to turn to her friend for support. Over the next several years, the performance of the COO declined, she was demoted, and ultimately, she left the field entirely.

Vicarious Trauma, Secondary Traumatic Stress, Compassion Fatigue, and Burnout

As we have discussed earlier, human beings are sociobiologically connected to each other. Witnessing another person's suffering is so traumatic that torturers frequently force their victim to observe the torture of another in order to elicit information. It has long been recognized that emergency workers, physicians, nurses, police officers, firemen, journalists, clergy, social service workers, colleagues, family members, and other witnesses and bystanders to disasters and other trauma can experience secondary symptoms themselves. Currently the terms that are used most frequently to describe these symptoms are secondary traumatic stress, compassion fatigue, and vicarious traumatization. Although there are some differences, these terms are often used interchangeably. Secondary traumatic stress is defined as the natural, consequent behavior and emotions that result from knowledge about a traumatizing event experienced by another and the stress resulting from helping or wanting to help a traumatized or suffering person. The symptoms are almost identical to those of posttraumatic stress disorder (PTSD) [363]. Compassion fatigue is described as the natural, predictable, treatable, and preventable unwanted consequence of working with suffering people [666].

Vicarious traumatization is a term that describes the cumulative transformative effect on the helper of working with survivors of traumatic life events. The symptoms can appear much like those of PTSD but also encompass changes in frame of reference, identity, sense of safety, ability to trust, self-esteem, intimacy, and a sense of control. The presence of vicarious traumatization has been noted in many groups of helping professionals who have close contact with people who have experienced traumatic events. Caregivers are at even higher risk if they have a history of trauma in their own backgrounds and if they extend themselves beyond the boundaries of good self-care or professional conduct [667].

There is a relationship between terms used to describe this reaction to dealing with people exposed to trauma and the more traditional terms of "burnout" and "countertransference." The more familiar term, "burnout," refers to a collection of symptoms associated with emotional exhaustion and generally attributed to increased workload and institutional stress, described by a process that includes gradual exposure to job strain, erosion of idealism, and a lack of achievement [668]. Burnout may then be the result of repetitive or chronic exposure to vicarious traumatization that is unrecognized and unsupported by the organizational setting. In contrast, "countertransference" is a far broader term, referring to all reactions to a client and the material he or she brings. Countertransference reactions are specific to the particular client and are tied to interactions with that client. In this case, vicarious traumatization can be seen as a specific form of countertransference experience, differentiated from other countertransference reactions in that vicarious traumatization can continue to affect our lives and our work long after interactions with the other person have ceased [621].

People working in a wide variety of social service organizations are vulnerable to vicarious trauma and, ultimately, to burnout. A considerable body of research is accumulating to demonstrate just how much of a problem this is for our settings and individual well-being. But it may not be the immediate contact with trauma survivors that is so chronically damaging as much as it is the contextual factors, the chronic and unrelenting pressures to produce more and more with less and less—the toxic stress—that make effective work so difficult.

Burnout

The most commonly accepted version of burnout is comprised of three components: (1) *emotional exhaustion*, a lack of energy and a feeling that one's emotional resources are used up; (2) *depersonalization* (also known as cynicism), marked by the treatment of clients as objects rather than people, detachment and callousness toward clients, cynicism toward clients, coworkers, and the organization; and *(3) diminished personal accomplishment*, the tendency to evaluate oneself negatively [669].

The burnout concept began being actively discussed and evaluated in the late 1970s and 1980s but initially was viewed as a problem of particular individuals. Now, it is becoming increasingly clear that burnout is not a problem of individuals but of the environments within which people work. Burnout occurs in "normal" people who have no previous history of psychopathology. Recent research has also differentiated burnout, which is related to work content, from depression, which is multifaceted. It is also clear that burnout negatively impacts effectiveness and work performance [670].

Burnout has a negative effect on worker performance, including absenteeism, job turnover, low productivity, overall effectiveness, decreased job satisfaction, and reduced commitment to the job [671]. Some research has indicated that burnout may also have a negative effect on people's home life as well. And burnout has been associated with heart attacks, chronic fatigue, insomnia, dizziness, nausea, allergies, breathing difficulties, skin problems, muscle aches, menstrual difficulties, swollen glands, sore throat, recurrent flu, infections, colds, headaches, digestive problems, and back pain. The Japanese even have a word, *karoshi*, for sudden death that results from overwork [670].

It is of interest to note that although there are numerous references to the effect burnout has on mental health professionals in published articles over the last 5 years, most of these come from England, Wales, Australia, Japan, Canada, Ireland. China, Sweden, Norway, Greece, the Netherlands, and very few from the United States, despite the enormity of the changes that have impacted mental health care here and the crisis in mental health care that has frequently been cited. Burnout is most likely to occur when there is work overload [670], when employees do not feel they have any control [670], when there is insufficient reward for their work, when there is a breakdown in the sense of workplace community, when there is an absence of fairness [185], and when there are conflicting values—all symptoms of the present human service delivery system.

Organizational Decline

Organizations attempt to anticipate and adapt to environmental changes, but the larger, more rapid, and harder to predict the changes are, the more difficult it is for the organization to adapt. This failure to adapt then leads to organizational decline and, possibly, dissolution. *"Decline begins when an organization fails to anticipate or recognize and effectively respond to any deterioration in*

organizational performance that threatens long-term survival" (p. 94) [672].
Brian describes the toll that constant adaptation to change takes:

> *It is very difficult to think about change and innovation when you are just trying to keep your head above water. It is not uncommon for our staff to respond with skepticism whenever we suggest the idea of change. Even when the current way of doing business is clearly inefficient and ineffective, it seems impossible to fathom where we will find the time to plan to do something different. We have likened the change process to trying to change the fan belt on your car while the car is moving. We cannot just change things; we usually have to maintain a current flawed process while we invest the time and effort in planning a new way to operate. I have scratched my head for years wondering why staff people do not take the initiative to solve problems or improve processes when it is clear they know what needs to be done and they know how to do what needs to be done. It can be exhausting, and at times, easier to just live with what we have always done. Innovation takes time to think, plan, and experiment, all of which are in short supply in our terribly stressed systems.*

One of the most pronounced effects of decline is to increase stress, and under stressful conditions, managers frequently do the opposite of what they need to do to reverse decline by relying on proven programs, seeking less counsel from subordinates, concentrating on ways to improve efficiency, and shunning innovative solutions. Their responses are dictated by what they believe caused the problems, but their causal explanations are likely to be overly simplistic. Just when people need to be pulling together, interpersonal and intraorganizational conflict increases and becomes difficult to resolve and as a consequence goal setting, communication, and leader–subordinate relationships decline [673].

As we discussed in Chapter 7, studies have shown that institutions, like individuals, have memory. Once interaction patterns have been disrupted, these patterns can be transmitted through an organization so that one "generation" unconsciously passes on to the next norms that alter the system and every member of the system. But without a conscious memory of events also being passed on, organizational members in the present cannot make adequate judgments about whether the strategy, policy, or norm is still appropriate and useful in the present [674]. This process can be an extraordinary resistance to healthy organizational change [665]. Organizational decline is said to be caused by a dysfunction in organizational learning and organizational learning is seriously impaired by failures of organizational memory. Regression may occur so that previous levels of achievement, knowledge, training, and service delivery are no longer remembered and appear to play little if any role in the organizational culture. A colleague shared his memories of just such an experience:

> *I had worked for years in inpatient settings in the early 1990s and had decided to move from outpatient work back into inpatient work because private practice*

had become so lonely and I wanted to work with a team again. I was appalled and disheartened by the changes that had occurred in the inpatient program where I had previously worked, despite the fact that some of the same people I knew as social workers and members of the nursing staff were still working there. I first noticed that the physical condition of the program had radically altered. The place was dark and dingy. The carpets were stained and the furniture was battered and dirty. Regardless of what the cleaning staff did, the place never really looked clean. Many of the patients were dressed in hospital gowns, rather than street clothes. Likewise, some of the other psychiatrists insisted on wearing white coats and all that was missing was a stethoscope around their neck to convey the medical nature of the program. The unit, previously unlocked, was now carefully locked and off-duty policemen were often called in to manage "security" problems, sometimes wearing their weapons and accompanied by police dogs—and not the friendly ones. The staff had come to view a patient restraint as a form of treatment and congratulated themselves when a restraint went well; and they had frequent opportunities to exercise their skills.

I was also disturbed by the nature of the patient information in the charts. Apparently, because of the excessive regulation instituted by the combined forces of managed care and increased risk management, the charts had become "dumbed down" to such an extent that they were largely worthless in providing any useful clinical information about the client. That is not to say that the charts were empty of paper. In fact, if anything the charts had expanded in size but not in meaningfulness. There was a great deal of detailed reporting about exactly what the patient said, detailed charting of their bathroom and dietary habits, particularly when they were on some kind of special monitoring. What was lacking was any assessment or synthesis of what the information meant. There was no case formulation, no evidence of a thought process, no true clinical assessment.

The staff appeared unable to think, and instead just wanted me to tell them what to do, give them a set of directions, point them in the direction of a manual they could use. I picked up one chart in which a nurse had noted that there was a client—a "frequent flyer"—meaning a patient who had been in and out of the hospital many times. The nurse had written a note that the patient was threatening to kill himself by jumping into traffic. Nowhere had she drawn upon her own knowledge of the patient and his past history to note that he was a known heroin addict who had previously not followed through on treatment recommendations and was probably drug seeking, using suicidal ideation as his ticket into inpatient treatment and the hope that he could find someone to give him narcotics.

On another chart, there were careful recordings about what a woman said about her compulsion to self-mutilate. In the social service history there was brief mention that this woman had been repeatedly sexually abused as a child. But nowhere was any connection made between the sexual abuse and the *self-mutilation, nor was there any formulation that the two problems could be related. For me, these examples and many other experiences helped me to recognize how previous standards of care had deteriorated dramatically, although none of these negative changes were reflected in existing standards of quality assurance. The unit had just passed national and state inspections with flying colors. I came to believe that this "dumbing down" of the whole process of treatment were signs of unresolved grief in a system that had numbed itself to the anger, sadness, shame, and despair associated with downsizing, loss of resources, and loss of status.*

Working in this place, I felt like I had gone into a time warp and was back in the early 1950s before the ideas of milieu treatment had permeated the system. It is a terrible thing to see the extent of regression that has occurred in our field and no one seems to be willing to talk about it. They don't even seem to notice. But this unit still passes all the inspections. What in the world are these regulatory agencies calling quality care at this point?"

Many dysfunctional behaviors characterize organizational decline. Increases in conflict, secrecy, scapegoating, self-protective behaviors, loss of leader credibility, rigidity, turnover, decreases in morale, diminished innovation, lowered participation, nonprioritized cuts, and reduced long-term planning are common problems associated with periods of decline [675]. All of these behaviors can be seen as inhibitors of organizational learning and adaptation—both necessary if the decline is to be reversed [676]. And put together, these lead to burnout of individual employees.

In discussing organizations as living systems, "theorists are preoccupied with when organizations are 'born,' what species they are (their forms), and when they have changed enough to be termed dead" (p. 52) [677]. Organizational death can be more difficult to define than biological death. It may come when an organization ceases to operate, when it loses its corporate identity, when it loses the capacity to govern itself, or it experiences any combination of these situations. An organization may die when it successfully merges with another organization, so that organizational death may not be equated with failure [677]. Brian comments:

I think some agencies are dead, but no one has told them. It is like those movies when someone is a spirit—a person who has died but has not passed on for some reason, but just continues to roam around. Many agencies continue to exist, but they no longer matter or do effective work.

Successful or Permanent Failure: Is This the Future We Want?

A German professor of political and administrative science, Dr. Wolfgang Seibel, upon looking at what was happening in the nonprofit social service sector in his own country, explored the idea of "successful failure" when an organization or social sector continues to be funded, albeit inadequately, despite its apparent failure to solve the fundamental problem it has been created to solve:

> One prerequisite of continuous resource mobilization despite low performance is that the principals at both levels (board and public) are interested in failure rather than in achievement of the organization they are in charge of....Second, another prerequisite of continuous resource mobilization despite low perfor-mance is that the principals at both levels prefer not being confronted with dilemmas that the organization has to cope with. Consider the organization's job being something terrible, disgusting, or just puzzling. Again, the mere remoteness from public attention may facilitate forgetting about those jobs. (pp. 99–100) [678]

Many of the organizations and systems we work in seem to be "permanently failing" yet continue to operate for years on end [679]. And many of these can be considered "successful failures," meaning that the true, albeit unconscious social objective is to keep a troubling issue out of the public eye while creating the illusion that something is being done [678]. It is this kind of "successful" or "permanent" failure that best defines large components of the existing mental health and social service system. The mentally ill, the poor, the homeless all bring up distasteful reminders of what is wrong and socially unjust in our pres-ent social, political, and economic system and arouse anxiety about life's uncer-tainties. The people that work to help the sick, poor, and underprivileged then must fail to actually accomplish much, while still being held to the account-ability and efficiency standards of modern society.

It is this unseen and denied but real "successful" failure that most confounds people who dedicate their lives to the health, mental health, and social service professions. When young professionals first enter the helping professions, they are motivated by a desire to serve, a willingness to sacrifice financial gain for the satisfactions they assume to be found in helping other people get well, seeing people change, and bettering the lives of suffering humanity. What they fre-quently find instead are bureaucratic systems designed to "control the behavior" of children and adults and keep them from causing any difficulty for the society, rather than systems designed to facilitate healing and empowerment.

In this book we have tried to read what is going on in our society, below the level of conscious awareness. Put it all together and it becomes disturbingly clear that the job we have been delegated to do as human service delivery work-ers is to successfully fail and to prove to the rest of the culture that nothing really has to change: that capitalism as an economic system is not the problem; that it is perfectly acceptable to have less that 1% of a society controlling 99% of its wealth; that vast overpopulation of the planet is not killing us; that violence, insensitivity, constant conflict, secrecy, authoritarian control, injustice, and grief are the inevitable outcomes of the one and only world that is possible; and that during the times of radical decline ahead, survival will be just as it was in our primal past—brutal and violent.

Professor Seibel notes that the probability of successful failure increases for a number of reasons. He surmises that the probability of successful failure increases if organizations find themselves in a peripheral position outside the dominant spheres of the public and private sector. This certainly describes the mental health and social service sectors of this country. The mental health system has yet to achieve parity within health care, although legislation moving in that direction was finally enacted in October 2008, and perhaps health care reform will improve the situation. But it will come as no surprise if little is done to improve the financial position of these services as belts are tightened under the influence of economic downturns. As the economic system ratchets down, the rich continue to get richer but human services and education pay the price and funding is repeatedly and consistently reduced.

Seibel raises the question about whether those providing resources to the organization are really interested in failure rather than in achievement. In our social service system there has been little accountability for performance if that means actually seeing change in the human beings we are serving, not just adjustments to the budget. There is now considerable talk in the human services about "evidence-based practice," but until quite recently there have been no performance standards that insist that the clients in human services have made significant change.

Seibel believes that successful failure is more likely if those providing resources to the organization prefer not to be confronted with dilemmas the organization has to cope with. As we assert repeatedly in this volume, mental health services and other social services have been progressively underfunded, destabilized, and regressing for the past thirty years. In that time little has been done about the social disparities that create the kind of allostatic load that produces physical, psychological, and social illness and injury. It is currently politically incorrect to focus on poverty, racism, and child maltreatment as the etiology of mental illness; it is not possible to address the complexity of problems confronting our system because of funding limitations, because a diagnosis that would reflect that complexity is not currently available, and perhaps most importantly because we seem to lack the imagination for anything better than what we already have.

Seibel goes on to propose that the probability of successful failure is increased if there are plausible ideologies available that protect the organization against the "inappropriate" application of efficiency and accountability standards, thus mitigating the cognitive dissonance caused by the gap between poor performance and the standards of organizational efficiency and accountability.

If psychological and social problems are due to disturbed genetics or neuro-transmitter function, then we do not have to act now to change social condi-tions but instead need to wait until the scientists and psychopharmacologists have found what will inevitably be expensive and profitable "cures."

We believe that this is exactly what has happened to the human social service sector. If, as a society, we really wanted to solve the social problems that generate the childhood and adult adversity and trauma that have been the substance of this book, we would make sure that the institutional segment delegated to resolve those problems would be able to do so. As Seibel wrote, *"Why delegate [particularly pressing problems] to an institutional segment whose resource dependency, governing structure, and ideology imply weak rather than strong performance? ... we may assume the public at large to be interested in weak rather than strong organizational structures when coping rather than problem-solving is requested"* (p. 103) [678].

Scary to think of that, isn't it? Successful failures. Is that all we are? These very deep individual, organizational, and systemic conflicts about what generates mental illness and social dysfunction and how to deal with them are chronic, underlying, and largely hidden sources of chronic stress within every compo-nent of the human service system. How often do we ask ourselves whether what we are doing is really working? What do we really mean by "working"? Do the standards and regulations demanded of each component of our systems truly reflect success that is expressed in the functioning of the clients? What does it mean if most of the mental and social illness that we encounter was at some point in time, entirely preventable? Is it possible for any of us to be effective without engaging and speaking up at a social and political level?

Conclusion: Chronic Disaster

We have been describing a public health nightmare. As it stands now, we are not doing much about the source of the problem to see if we could keep people from becoming ill. We know enough when it comes to other public health problems to do things like washing our hands to prevent the spread of disease. But when it comes to exposure to trauma and adversity, it's as if there are people standing at the edge of a high cliff, throwing children over the cliff and into the dangerous rapids below, and all of us in health care, mental health, and social services are running around dragging those kids out of the water one by one. And, in some way or another, we are blaming them for ending up in the water in the first place. When are we going to start working upstream? When do we initiate a "Manhattan Project" for bearing and raising healthy children in the context of healthy families?

Disasters usually occur quickly—a tornado, a tsunami, an earthquake, a plane crash, a terrorist attack. The worst is over then and recovery efforts can begin. We desperately need a healthy human service delivery system capable of responding to what amounts to a public health disaster—a slow-moving disaster that just keeps rolling out, passed on generation to generation. It needs to be a system that can respond to injured children, adolescents, adults, and families and that is able to engage in primary, secondary, and tertiary prevention efforts.

But we are in the midst of what Kai Erikson has defined as a "chronic disaster," one that "...*gathers force slowly and insidiously, creeping around one's defenses rather than smashing through them. People are unable to mobilize their normal defenses against the threat, sometimes because they have elected consciously or unconsciously to ignore it, sometimes because they have been misinformed about it, and sometimes because they cannot do anything to avoid it in any case*" (p. 21) [355]. In individuals this manifests as "*a numbness of spirit, a susceptibility to anxiety and rage and depression, a sense of helplessness, an inability to concentrate, a loss of various motor skills, a heightened apprehension about the physical and social environment, a preoccupation with death, a retreat into dependency, and a general loss of ego functions*" (p. 21) [355].

As this slow-moving disaster rolls out over expanses of time, "*the mortar bonding human communities together is made up at least in part of trust and respect and decency and, in moments of crisis, of charity and concern. It is profoundly disturbing to people when these expectations are not met, no matter how well protected they thought they were by the outer crust of cynicism our century seems to have developed in us all....The real problem in the long run is that the inhumanity people experience comes to be seen as a natural feature of human life rather than as the bad manners of a particular corporation. They think their eyes are being opened to a larger and profoundly unsettling truth: that human institutions cannot be relied upon*" (p. 239) [355].

Our institutions are failing us. They are failing our clients and making too many of us sick in body, sick in mind, and sick in spirit. If you have reached this point in the book, we know it has been unrelentingly depressing. But you cannot deal with a slow-moving disaster until you recognize there is one. And that has been our intent: to recognize the magnitude of the problem. In the next volume, *Restoring Sanctuary,* we will share with you some ideas we have about changing things for the better. In the final chapter, we will briefly introduce some of the concepts of the Sanctuary Model.

Chapter 12

Restoring Sanctuary: Organizations as Living, Complex Adaptive Social Systems

SUMMARY: *This concluding chapter represents both an ending and a beginning: the conclusion of this volume and an introduction to what will be more fully covered in a forthcoming volume. We briefly introduce the central concepts of the Sanctuary Model, a change in the operating system for the organization we liken to a parallel process of recovery for human service delivery systems. After briefing describing the Sanctuary Commitments, we discuss how the Sanctuary Model is being implemented via the Sanctuary Institute, the Sanctuary Network, and Sanctuary Certification.*

There Is So Much at Stake

If you have come all this way, read these chapters, and it has given you an opportunity to think about, and perhaps develop a better and more empathic perspective on the human service delivery system, on mental health work, on the places you have worked in or where you work now, we will have accomplished our goal. Maybe you are feeling some relief that somebody has put pen to paper and actually said all these things. But you may be feeling a variety of more distressing feelings—anxiety, disgust, sadness, shame, depression, fear, anger. We know because those are the feelings—all of them—that motivated the writing of this book. Maybe you are now questioning yourself as a leader or the people who lead you, your coworkers, and even yourself.

We have not written this book with the purpose of leaving our readers dejected. We started with a vision of a different mental model, a different way of understanding how to work together in this ever-changing world. We suggested that we need a new Organizational Operating System—a Living System approach—to completely change the way we view our clients, each other, and the mission we must accomplish in and for our world.

We have walked you through the successful failures that represent so many of the organizational climates of human service environments today. We did this so that we could share a trauma-informed, human-informed language and understanding of what must change. What we didn't say yet is this: human service delivery systems are societies' most important and underutilized social laboratories. Within our psychiatric hospitals, shelters, residential treatment centers, juvenile justice programs, and prisons reside—at least for a short time—the human beings who have suffered the most serious injuries to another being that it is possible to sustain. On the one hand they are badly injured and often do terrible and unfair things to themselves, their children, and other people. But they are also survivors. They have descended into hell and they have something to tell us about the journey. We need to listen. We need to help them heal because in that healing lies the potential healing for our world. It is urgent that our species learn to overcome and transform many of the adaptations that guaranteed our survival in our primeval past but that now guarantee our anni-hilation in the present unless we make radical change. Sandy recounts a recent experience:

> *I was doing a presentation for a local court system—lawyers, judges, advocates, and court officials. After everyone left at the end of the day, a woman walked back into the room, sat down with me, and asked me if she looked familiar. I told her that she did, but I did not know why. She proceeded to tell me that she had been on our original Sanctuary unit for 10 days 17 years ago and that "those 10 days changed my life." She was working and was doing well except for some medical problems. She also told me that a group of the people who were on our unit at the same time back then had continued to meet at least once a year to keep up with each other. She commented on the importance of the ACEs Study and how pleased she was that our work was now being applied to children. She said, "We all have medical problems similar to what you described in that study. If only we had been able to get help when we were kids."*

We are going to leave you with the good news that there is currently the beginnings of a different organizational operating system, one that connects with and honors the past but posits the possibility that a new transformed social service system could help lead all of us out of the mire, the apparent evo-lutionary dead end threshold that beckons us and from which there is no return. We call this operating system The Sanctuary Model. It represents a trauma-informed, theory-based, evidence-supported, whole-system, long-term, still-evolving methodology to help transform mechanistic organizations and systems into living, growing, adapting, and changing systems that can survive and perhaps one day, even thrive.

At the present time over 100 human service delivery programs from around the country and internationally are working through the implementation process. A number of programs have become Sanctuary certified. They include adult inpatient psychiatric and substance abuse facilities, domestic violence shelters, residential programs and group homes for children, schools and educational programs, juvenile justice facilities, and a number of large programs that have a wide variety of inpatient, outpatient, partial, and residential programs. We don't know yet if they will all be able to bring about organizational change. Each program we train is its own small social laboratory and these are very difficult times. But we are learning a great deal about change and the challenges of change, and we are doing our best to document what we are learning so that the knowledge can be passed on as our predecessors passed on knowledge to us.

Sanctuary Model: A New Operating System for Organizations

Based on the information from the previous chapters, what conclusions can we draw about what has to change? We know that mental models determine what we think, feel, and act and usually at an unconscious level. So we need a new mental model, a new operating system. What would be the basic premises of such an operating system?

Confronted with the reality that our systems of care are both alive *and* "trauma organized," it is clear that three essential tasks need to be accomplished: *(1)* the development of a model of intervention that can be broadly applied across the population; can be shared between staff, clients, and families; is consistent with established good practice; and allows for the uniqueness of each setting; *(2)* practically integrating the system by developing more trust among organizational members, better communication networks, feedback loops, shared decision making, and conflict resolution practices; and *(3)* using the developed infrastructure to synthesize a variety of treatment approaches and techniques into a progressive map of recovery for each client. What has emerged from our experience to date is the Sanctuary Model, an evidence-supported plan, process, and method for creating trauma-sensitive, democratic, nonviolent cultures that are far better equipped to engage in the innovative treatment planning and implementation that is necessary to adequately respond to the extremely complex and deeply embedded injuries that our clients have sustained. As an organizational culture intervention, it is designed to facilitate the development of structures, processes, and behaviors on the part of staff, clients, and the community as a whole that can counteract the biological, emotional, cognitive, social, and existential wounds suffered by the victims of traumatic experience and by extended exposure to adversity.

"Creating Sanctuary" refers to the shared experience of creating and maintaining physical, psychological, social, and moral safety within a social environment—any social environment—and thus reducing systemic violence. The Sanctuary Commitments are tied directly to trauma-informed treatment goals. The process of "Creating Sanctuary" begins with getting everyone on the same page—surfacing, sharing, arguing about, and finally agreeing on the basic values, beliefs, guiding principles, and philosophical principles that are to guide decisions, decision-making processes, conflict resolution skills, and behavior.

Trauma-informed change requires a change in the basic mental models upon which thought and action are based; without such change, treatment is bound to fall unnecessarily short of full recovery or fail entirely. This change in mental models must occur on the part of the clients, their families, the staff, and the leaders of the organization. Mental models exist at the level of very basic assumptions, far below conscious awareness and everyday function, and yet they guide and determine what we can and cannot think about and act upon [680].

A story that illustrates the shift that staff members must take is illustrated next. It is a story compiled by Siobhan Masterson, the former Sanctuary facilitator at Andrus:

> A teenage boy named Tom was living in a residential cottage. He had come in the year before as aggressive, disheveled, and confused. One of the team members left the agency and was replaced as the cottage director by a man named Harry. Tom and Harry did work together and got along, but Tom was still very upset about the loss. He started to act as he did when he first entered residential care, starting fights, yelling, and so on. One morning he came up behind Harry and hit him. Harry was startled and upset, but he had been on a Sanctuary core team and truly understood what might be going on underneath the surface for this child. He also understood that safety was paramount. So the team got several people together: the Sanctuary coordinator, the psychiatrist, the therapist, another director, the child, and Harry. They sat together with him and told him how much they all cared about him. They shared with him all the ways that he had touched them. Then they said that he was at a crossroads of doing things the old way, the way he used to do them, and a new way, a way he was just learning, and they believed in him to do it the new way. But he would need to work, and it would be a challenge. Tom came around, agreed to a safety plan, and besides apologizing to Harry, he was given the homework of asking at least three staff members how they handle their anger and what they've learned about managing emotions. The boy struggled over the next year, but he continued to demonstrate growth and wisdom, turning a corner to carrying himself with far more pride, gravitating to healthier relationships, and even helping in a group to teach the younger kids how to manage emotions.

If you read that story and notice that it seems like the adults dealt with the child in a kind, compassionate, and commonsense fashion, you are right. If you read the story and believe that this is just common sense, you are right as well—it's just that there seems to be a shortfall currently in that elusive quality.

And if you work in a mental health setting you may be aware that it takes a great deal of unlearning and relearning on the part of the individual staff members and the organization as a whole to arrive at just such simple strategies.

The Sanctuary Model is structured around a philosophy of belief and practice that create a process enabling organizations to shift their mental models. In the next volume, *Restoring Sanctuary: A New Operating System for Human Service Organizations*, we will detail the elements of this process and give examples of how the model is being used and the results of implementing a new methodology. Here we are going to provide an introduction to the ideas and the methodology that we are using.

For a complex organization to function you need just the right number of principles that guide short-term, everyday conduct as well as long-term strategy. Too many rules and a system becomes rigid, inflexible, and even paralyzed. Too few and it becomes purely individualistic and chaotic. The Sanctuary Commitments structure the organizational norms that determine the organizational culture. The seven Sanctuary Commitments represent the guiding principles for implementation of the Sanctuary Model—the basic structural elements of the Sanctuary "operating system"—and each commitment supports trauma recovery goals for clients, staff, and the organization as a whole.

We didn't invent these principles. Other than the newer scientific findings around trauma and attachment, these commitments represent universal principles, ancient wisdom that is as old as human groups. We have simply compiled them, articulated them into a cohesive whole, and developed a methodology to get disparate groups organized around them. And they cannot be "cherry-picked." All seven Sanctuary Commitments are complexly interactive and interdependent. Take away one and the whole structure may fall apart.

- *Commitment to Nonviolence*—to build safety skills, trust, and resilience in the face of stress and inspire a commitment to wider sociopolitical change
- *Commitment to Emotional Intelligence*—to teach emotional management skills, build respect for emotional labor, minimize the paralyzing effects of fear, and expand awareness of problematic cognitive-behavior patterns and how to change them
- *Commitment to Social Learning*—to build cognitive skills, improve learning and decisions, promote healthy dissent, restore memory, unearth the skeletons in the organizational closet and give them proper burial, and ultimately to have the skills to sustain a learning organization
- *Commitment to Open Communication*—to overcome barriers to healthy communication, discuss the "undiscussables," overcome alexithymia, increase transparency, develop conflict management skills, reinforce healthy boundaries

- *Commitment to Democracy*—to develop civic skills of self-control, self-discipline, to learn to exercise healthy authority and leadership, to develop participatory skills, to overcome helplessness, to develop skills for wrestling with complexity, and to honor the "voices" of self and others
- *Commitment to Social Responsibility*—to harness the energy of reciprocity and a yearning for justice by rebuilding restorative social connection skills, establishing healthy and fair attachment relationships, transforming vengeance into social justice, and concern for the common good
- *Commitment to Growth and Change*—to work through loss in the recognition that all change involves loss; to cease repeating irrelevant or destructive past patterns of thought, feeling, and behavior; and to envision, be guided by, skillfully plan, and prepare for a different and better future

Universal Commitment

The Sanctuary Commitments apply to everyone. Organizational leaders must be fully committed to the process of the Sanctuary Model for it to be effective. This includes the Board of Directors, managers at all levels, and every person who works in the organization. If the organizational leaders do not get onboard, it will not work. If the middle managers do not get onboard, it will not work. If the direct care staff or the indirect care staff do not get onboard, it will not work. At first glance, many organizational leaders hear a review of the Sanctuary Commitments and believe that those commitments already constitute their organizational culture. In many cases this is at least partially true. It is only when leaders engage in a different kind of dialogue with other members of their organizational community that they find out how divergent people's views are on what these commitments mean and how to make them real in everyday interactions. Experience has taught that courageous leadership is critical to system change; without it, substantial change is unlikely to occur.

S.E.L.F.: A Nonlinear Organizing Framework

S.E.L.F. is an acronym that represents the four key interdependent aspects of recovery from bad experiences. S.E.L.F. provides a nonlinear, cognitive-behavioral therapeutic approach for facilitating movement—regardless of whether we are talking about individual clients, families, staff problems, or whole organizational dilemmas. S.E.L.F. is a compass that allows us to explore all four key domains of healing: *Safety* (attaining safety in self, relationships, and environment); *Emotional management* (identifying levels of various emotions and modulating emotion in response to memories, persons, events); *Loss* (feeling grief and dealing with personal losses and recognizing that all change involves loss); and *Future* (trying out new roles, ways of relating and behaving as a "survivor" to ensure personal safety, envisioning a different and better future). Using S.E.L.F., the clients, their families, and staff are able to embrace a shared, nontechnical and non-pejorative language that allows them all to see the larger recovery process in perspective. The accessible language demystifies what sometimes is seen as confusing and even insulting clinical or psychological terminology that can confound clients and line staff, while still focusing on the aspects of pathological adjustment that pose the greatest problems for any treatment environment

The Sanctuary Institute

The Sanctuary Institute is a 5-day intensive training experience based at Andrus Children's Center in Yonkers, New York. Teams of five to eight people, from various levels of the organization, come together to learn from our faculty, all of whom are colleagues from other organizations implementing Sanctuary. Together teams begin to create a shared vision of the kind of organization they want to create. These teams will eventually become the Sanctuary Steering Committee for their organization. The training experience usually involves several organizations, and generally these organizations are very different in terms of size, scope, region, and mission. This diversity helps to provide a rich learning experience for the participants.

The Sanctuary Steering Committee is instructed to go back to their organization and create a Core Team, a larger, multidisciplinary team that expands its reach into the entire organization. It is this Core Team that will be the activators of the whole system. The Core Team should have representatives from every level of the organization to insure that every "voice" is represented and heard. It is vital that all key organizational leaders become actively involved in the process of change and participate in this Core Team. The Core Team is armed with a *Sanctuary Direct Care Staff Training Manual*, a *Sanctuary Indirect Staff Training Manual*, a *Sanctuary Implementation Manual*, several psychoeducational curricula, and ongoing consultation and technical assistance from Sanctuary faculty members to guide them through the process of Sanctuary Implementation that extends over 3 years and leads to Sanctuary Certification.

Participants report that the week-long training is a powerful experience; some have said even life changing. It needs to be because they have a big job to go home to. They will need to go back to their respective organizations and begin to change the culture of the organization and change long-standing paradigms and patterns of behavior.

The Sanctuary Network and Sanctuary Certification

Our belief in the power of community led us to develop the Sanctuary Institute. The Sanctuary Institute is the gateway to the Sanctuary Network, a community of organizations committed to the development of trauma-informed services. We are all committed to the belief that we can do better for our clients and our colleagues as well as our society if we can accept that the people we serve are not sick or bad, but injured, and that the services we provide must provide hope, promote growth, and inspire change.

Sanctuary is a registered trademark and the right to use the Sanctuary name is contingent on engagement in a certified training program and an agreement to participate in an ongoing, peer-review certification process. It requires a several-year commitment and research is underway in the hope of moving the Sanctuary Model from an "evidence-supported" to an "evidence-based" approach. In this way we hope to establish a method for guaranteeing an acceptable level of fidelity to the original model upon which the research was based [681–684]. The Sanctuary Institute is based at Andrus Children's Center, Yonkers, New York, and information can be found at http://www.andruschildren.org and at www.sanctuaryweb.com.

We will conclude with two personal narratives, the first from Sandy, the last from Brian.

I recently received a letter from a woman who was treated on our unit in 1992 and describes her hospitalization as a "watershed experience." She continues to struggle with depression and posttraumatic stress disorder, but she is still using the tools she developed during her brief stay in the hospital 16 years ago. But she also shared with me the intergenerational impact of her brief stay: "I remember the first time I asserted to my sister's family (when I saw a niece shoving my sister) that violence was unacceptable in my home, and my sister acknowledging that I had changed. Three of the four of us have refused to follow the family pattern and have broken the chain. People are getting help decades ahead of schedule, including two nieces and another sister. Even my father had his depression treated in his last decade of life. I knew that the way he abused us had stemmed from his own abusive childhood. It took years to forgive the man, but I am grateful that on his passing last year, I could freely grieve and own the good he had done to and for me."

We began on our path in the summer of 2001. We assembled a Core Team made up of our best and brightest. Dr. Bloom insisted the Core Team include representation from all our departments and all levels of the organization. I didn't agree to include any of our indirect care staff so we had to clean that up later. Our Core Team was made up of four senior administrators (residential, education and clinical department heads, and myself), two clinical supervisors, two line clinicians, the dean of students from our on-campus school, four teachers, three school milieu staff, two cottage program managers, and three cottage milieu staff. Once assembled, the plan was for the Core Team to sit in a room two days a month for the next year and hammer out the new vision for how our treatment program would work with traumatized children.

Early on there was a lot of talk about democracy and developing a constitution and other subversive ideas. Andrus has a long history of a very top-down, hierarchical management style. The notion of doing something differently, managing or leading in a more open and participatory fashion, was both exciting and intimidating. As time passed it became increasingly evident that this is the only way to go. My initial frustration with the process was not how tough it is for leadership to give up the reins of power; the hard part was there was so little experience at other levels of the organization on what it required to pick up the slack and take on more responsibility for decisions. No matter what leaders said or how they behaved, Core Team members had enormous difficulty with breaking away from old patterns. As a leader it is very difficult to struggle through this process. While Core Team members complain about the evil and punitive autocracy, they also took little initiative to take on projects and make changes. The difficulty for me early on was to resist the impulse to jump in and over-direct the process or to throttle everyone for their passivity. Doing so would not have advanced the group process but would have only served to confirm their belief that as a leader, I was a controlling and scary guy.

Having good intentions and wanting to do the right thing is certainly a good place to start. If you look at the Sanctuary Commitments and say "that's crazy," then you probably will not get much further. By the same token if you look at the Sanctuary Commitments and say "I believe that is the way to go," it does not mean you are there nor does it mean your path will be an easy one. In fact, I believe I still have a long way to go. When I look back on some of the dopey things I have done since we introduced Sanctuary, you might wonder if I have ever heard of the Sanctuary Commitments. At times I have been autocratic, dysregulated, secretive, stuck, selfish, arrogant, and abusive over the past few years. Mind you, not all the time, but from time to time. I am convinced my setbacks have set back the whole process.

As I reflect on our struggles with Sanctuary, I am quite convinced that our struggles are grounded in what a huge cultural shift this is for our organization. This is an organization with a long history of autocratic rule. For the most part it has been a benevolent autocracy, but it was an autocracy none the less. In some ways, a benevolent autocracy is even harder to part with. The way it used to work around here was that senior leaders took care of all the non-treatment matters. Stuff like budgets, billing, compliance, and crisis management were all handled by the "big cheeses." The line staff would do whatever it was they did with clients, but much of this was directed by management as well. There was always some grousing about money, power, position, but it was pretty clear who did what and who did not. The program was simpler, the funding was simpler—life was simpler.

So when you introduce the Sanctuary Model and start talking about democratic processes and shared decision making, the first reaction is that you are either kidding or you have totally lost your mind. Once people discern you are displaying no other symptoms of madness (like wearing your underwear on the outside or showing up to work dressed as a pirate) they then begin to look for evidence that the organization is not really serious about this change. They look for evidence that contradicts what you are telling them is the new world order. In the early stages of the change it is easy to see the inconsistencies and the gaps and easy to believe that this change is all talk. This change is also new to leadership and we are all prone to sliding back to our familiar ways of operating.

Sanctuary has stood the whole culture on its head, and the old order no longer applies. We are trying to find a new way, but it is difficult and painful and some people are holding onto the old order like grim death. Not because it is best, but because it is what we are used to. It has not been particularly challenging to embrace the notion of shared governance, but it has been challenging to sustain it. Democracy does not just imply that leadership is willing to share, but that everyone is willing to share responsibility, and we are still working on that notion.

As a leader in the organization, I have found that it is essential to engage in endless self-reflection. With great power comes great responsibility and before wading into the organizational change process, it would be worthwhile to spend some time on the personal discovery and change process that comes with being a leader in a Sanctuary organization. The bottom line is a quote attributed to one of our heroes, Mahatma Gandhi: "Be the change you want to see in the world"

To be continued....in **Restoring Sanctuary: A New Operating System for Organizations.**

References

1. Bloom, S. L. (1997). *Creating Sanctuary: Toward the Evolution of Sane Societies.* New York: Routledge.
2. Bloom, S. L. (1994). The Sanctuary Model: Developing Generic Inpatient Programs for the Treatment of Psychological Trauma. In M. B. Williams & J. F. Sommer (Eds.), *Handbook of Post-Traumatic Therapy, A Practical Guide to Intervention, Treatment, and Research* (pp. 474–449). Greenwood Publishing.
3. Hubble, M. A., Duncan, B. L., & Miller, S. D. (Eds.). (1999). *The Heart and Soul of Change: What Works in Therapy.* Washington, D.C.: American Psychological Press.
4. Bloom, S. L. (2000). Our Hearts and Our Hopes are Turned to Peace: Origins of the ISTSS. In A. Shalev, R. Yehuda, & A. S. McFarlane (Eds.), *International Handbook of Human Response Trauma* (pp. 27–50). New York: Plenum Press.
5. Shorto, R. (2008). *Descartes' Bones: A Skeletal History of the Conflict Between Faith and Reason.* New York: Doubleday.
6. de Geus, A. (1997). *The Living Company: Habits for Survival in a Turbulent Business Environment.* Boston: Harvard Business School Press.
7. Von Bertalanffy, L. (1974). General systems theory and psychiatry. In S. Arieti (Ed.), *American Handbook of Psychiatry, Volume One: The Foundations of Psychiatry* (pp. 1095–1117). New York: Basic Books.
8. Napier, R. W., & Gershenfeld, M. K. (2004). *Groups: Theory and Experience, Seventh Edition.* Boston: Houghton Mifflin.
9. Bentovim, A. (1992). *Trauma-Organized Systems: Physical and Sexual Abuse in Families.* London: Karnac Books.
10. Agazarian, Y., & Peters, R. (1981). *The Visible and the Invisible Group.* Boston: Routledge & Kegan Paul.
11. McEwen, B. (2002). *the End of Stress As We Know It.* Washingon, D.C.: Joseph Henry Press.
12. Middlebrooks, J. S., & Audage, M. C. (2008). The Effects of Childhood Stress on Health Across the Lifespan Atlanta, GA: Centers for Disease Control and Prevention, National Center for Injury Prevention and Control.
13. Van der Kolk, B. (1989). The compulsion to repeat the trauma: Reenactment, revictimization, and masochism. *Psychiatric Clinics Of North America, 12,* 389–411.
14. Van der Kolk, B. A., Peclovitz, D., Roth, S., Mandel, F., McFarlane, A., & Herman, J. L. (1996). Dissociation, somatization, and affect dysregulation: The complexity of adaptation to trauma. *American Journal of Psychiatry, 7,* 83–93.
15. Putnam, F. W. (1997). *Dissociation in Children and Adolescents: A Developmental Perspective.* New York: Guilford.

16. van der Hart, O., Nijenhuis, E. R. S., & Steele, K. (2005). Dissociation: An insufficiently recognized major feature of complex posttraumatic stress disorder. *Journal of Traumatic Stress, 18*(5), 413–423.

17. American Psychiatric Association. (2000). *Diagnostic and Statistical Manual of Mental Disorders DSM-IV-TR Fourth Edition (Text Revision)* Washington, D.C.: American Psychiatric Association.

18. Main, M., & Hess, E. (1990). Parents'unresolved traumatic experiences are related to infant disorganized attachment status: is frightened and/or frightening parental behavior the linking mechanism?. In M. T. Greenberg, D. Cicchetti & E. Cummings (Eds.), *Attachment In The Preschool Years: Theory, Research, And Intervention* (pp. 161–182). Chicago: University of Chicago Press.

19. Schore, A. N. (2009). Relational Trauma and the Developing Right Brain. *Annals of the New York Academy of Sciences, 1159* (Self and Systems Explorations in Contemporary Self Psychology), 189–203.

20. Van der Kolk, B. A. (1987). The separation cry and the trauma response: developmental issues in the psychobiology of attachment and separation. In B. A. Van der Kolk (Ed.), *Psychological Trauma* (pp. 31–62). Washington, D.C.: American Psychiatric Press.

21. Zeanah, C. H., & Zeanah, P. D. (1989). Intergenerational transmission of maltreatment: insights from attachment theory and research. *Psychiatry, 52*(2), 177–196.

22. Briere, J., & Spinazzola, J. (2005). Phenomenology and psychological assessment of complex posttraumatic states. *Journal of Traumatic Stress, 18*(5), 401–412.

23. van der Kolk, A. A., Roth, S., Pelcovitz, D., Sunday, S., & Spinazzola, J. (2005). Disorders of extreme stress: The empirical foundation of a complex adaptation to trauma. *Journal of Traumatic Stress, 18*(5), 389–399.

24. Kilpatrick, D. G. (2005). A special section on complex trauma and a few thoughts about the need for more rigorous research on treatment efficacy, effectiveness, and safety. *Journal of Traumatic Stress, 18*(5), 379–384.

25. Bradley, R., Heim, A., & Westen, D. (2005). Personality constellations in patients with a history of childhood sexual abuse. *Journal of Traumatic Stress, 18*(6), 769–780.

26. Morrill, G. P. (1971). *The Multimillionaire Straphanger: A Life of John Emory Andrus.* Middletown, CT: Wesleyan University Press.

27. Senge, P., Cambron-McCabe, N., Lucas, T., Smith, B., Dutton, J., & Kleiner, A. (2000). *Schools That Learn: A Fifth Discipline Fieldbook for Educataors, Parents, and Everyone Who Cares About Education.* New York: Doubleday.

28. Wheatley, M. J. (1994). *Leadership and the New Science.* San Francisco: Berrett Koehler.

29. Ray, M., & Rinzler, A. (Eds.). (1993). *The New Paradigm in Business: Emerging Strategies for Leadership and Organizational Change.* M. Ray and A. Rinzler. New York: G. P. Putnam's Sons.

30. American Medical Association. (2009). Preamble. *Principles of Medical Ethics, Accessed 12/24/09 at* http://www.ama-assn.org/.

31. American Nursing Association. (1998). Code of Ethics for Nurses. Accessed 12/24/09 at http://www.nursingworld.org/MainMenuCategories/EthicsStandards/CodeofEthicsforNurses.aspx.

32. American Psychological Association. (2003). Preamble and General Principles. Ethical Principles of Psychologists and Code of Conduct. Accessed 12/24/09 at http://www.apa.org/ethics/code/index.aspx#.

33. National Association of Social Workers. (2008). Code of Ethics. Accessed 12/24/09 at http://www.socialworkers.org/pubs/code/code.asp.

34. American Counseling Association. (2005). Code of Ethics. Accessed 12/24/09 at http://www.counseling.org/Resources/CodeOfEthics/TP/Home/CT2.aspx.

35. American Mental Health Counselors Association. (2000). Code of Ethics. Accessed 12/24/09 at http://www.amhca.org/about/default.aspx.

36. Alexander, F. G., & Selesnick, S. T. (1966). *The History of Psychiatry: An Evaluation of Psychiatric Thought and Practice From Prehistoric Times to the Present.* New York: Harper and Row.

37. Siegler, M., & Osmond, H. (1974). *Models of Madness, Models of Medicine.* New York: Macmillan.

38. Smith, D. B. (2009). *The Forensic Case Files: Diagnosing and Treating the Pathologies of the American Health System.* Hackensack, NJ: World Scientific Publishing Company.

39. Dogin, J. (2000). *Development of a cost-effective and clinically relevant means of reimbursement for healthcare service delivery, Unpublished manuscript.*

40. Hill, S. (2010). *Europe's Promise: Why the European Way is the Best Hope in an Insecure Age.* Berkeley, CA: University of California Press.

41. Porter, M. E., & Teisberg, E. O. (2006). *Redefining Health Care: Creating Value-Based Competition on Results.* Boston: Harvard Business School Press.

42. Kessler, R. C., Heeringa, S., Lakoma, M., Petukhova, M., Rupp, A., Schoenbaum, M., et al. (2008). Individual and societal effects of mental disorders on earnings in the United States: results from the National Comorbidity Survey Replication. *American Journal of Psychiatry, 165,* 703–711.

43. Insel, T. R. (2008). Assessing the Economic Costs of Serious Mental Illness. *American Journal of Psychiatry, 165,* 663–665.

44. Substance Abuse and Mental Health Services Administration (SAMHSA) Center for Substance Abuse Prevention (CSAP). (2009). Substance Abuse Prevention Dollars and Cents: A Cost-Benefit Analysis (Vol. DHHS Publication No. (SMA) 07-4298). Rockville, MD: U. S. Department of Health and Human Services.

45. Wang, C.-T., & Holton, J. (2007). Total Estimated Cost of Child Abuse and Neglect in the United States, Economic Impact Study, September 2007. Accessed 12/27/09 at http://www.preventchildabuse.org/about_us/media_releases/pcaa_pew_economic_impact_study_final.pdf. Chicago, IL: Prevent Child Abuse America

46. Slevin, P. (2006). U.S. Prison Study Faults System and the Public. Accessed 12/27/09 at http://www.washingtonpost.com/wp-dyn/content/article/2006/06/07/AR2006060702050.html, *Washington Post.*

47. The Pew Center on the States. (2008). One in 100: Behind Bars in America 2008. Accessed 12/27/09 at http://www.pewcenteronthestates.org/uploadedFiles/One%20in%20100.pdf. Washington, D.C.: The Pew Charitable Trusts.

48. Watt, J. W., & Kallmann, G. L. (1998). Managing professional obligations under managed care: A social work perspective. *Family and Community Health, 21*(2), 40.

49. Abramovitz, M. (2005). The Largely Untold Story of Welfare Reform and the Human Services. *Social Work, 50*(2), 175–186.

50. Miller, I. (1998). Eleven Unethical Managed Care Practices Every Patient Should Know About Retrieved September 17, 2005

51. Furman, R. (2003). Frameworks for understanding value discrepancies and ethical dilemmas in managed mental health for social work in the United States. *International Social Work, 46*(1), 37.

52. Alleman, J. R. (2001). Personal, Practical, and Professional Issues in Providing Managed Mental Health Care: A Discussion for New Psychotherapists. *Ethics & Behavior, 11*(4), 413–429.

53. Backlar, P. (1996). Managed mental health care: Conflicts of interest in the provider/ client relationship. *Community Mental Health Journal, 32*(2), 101–106.
54. Wolff, N., & Schlesinger, M. (2002). Clinicians as Advocates: An Exploratory Study of Responses to Managed Care by Mental Health Professionals. *Journal of Behavioral Health Services & Research, 29*(3), 274.
55. Braun, S. A., & Cox, J. A. (2005). Managed Mental Health Care: Intentional Misdiagnosis of Mental Disorders. *Journal of Counseling & Development, 83*(4), 425–433.
56. Merriam-Webster On-line Dictionary. (2009). Capitalism. Accessed 12/26/09 at http://m-w.com/dictionary/capitalism.
57. http://www.answers.com/topic/siege-mentality.
58. Foucault, M. (1965). *Madness and Civilization: A History of Insanity in the Age of Reason.* New York: Vintage.
59. Barber, C. (2008). *Comfortably Numb: How Psychiatry is Medicating a Nation.* New York: Pantheon.
60. Pascale, R. T., Millemann, M., & Gioja, L. (2000). *Surfing the Edge of Chaos: The Laws of Nature and the New Laws of Business.* New York: Crown Business.
61. Hoge, M. A., Morris, J. A., Daniels, A. S., Stuart, G. W., Huey, L. Y., & Adams, N. (2007). An Action Plan on Behavioral Health Workforce Development: A Framework for Discussion, The Annapolis Coalition on the Behavioral Health Workforce.
62. Bloom, S. L. (2005). The System Bites Back: Politics, Parallel Process, and the Notion of Change. *Therapeutic Community: The International Journal for Therapeutic and Supportive Organizations., 26*(4, Silver Jubilee Issue), 337–354.
63. Shatan, C. (1972, May 6). Post-Vietnam Syndrome, *New York Times, May 6.*
64. Niederland, W. G. (1968). Clinical observations on the "survivor syndrome". *International Journal of Psycho-Analysis, 49,* 313–315.
65. Shatan, C. (1974). Through the membrane of reality: "Impacted grief" and perceptual dissonance in Vietnam combat veterans. *Psychiatric Opinion, 11*(6), 6–16.
66. Burgess, A. W., & Holstrom, L. (1974). Rape trauma syndrome. *American Journal of Psychiatry, 131,* 981–986.
67. Walker, L. (1979). *The Battered Woman.* New York: Harper & Row.
68. Gelles, R. J., & Straus, M. A. (1979). Determinants of violence in the family: Toward a theoretical integration. In W. R. Burr, R. Hill & F. I. Nye (Eds.), *Contemporary Theories About the Family* (pp. 549–580). New York: Free Press.
69. Grace, M. C., Green, B. L., Lindy, J. D., & Leonard, A. C. (1993). The Buffalo Creek disaster: a 14 year follow-up. In J. P. Wilson & B. Raphael (Eds.), *International Handbook of Traumatic Stress Syndromes* (pp. 441–459). New York: Plenum Press.
70. Erickson, K. (1976). *Everything in its path: destruction of community in the Buffalo Creek flood.* New York: Simon & Schuster.
71. Young, M. (1988). The crime victim's movement. In F. Ochberg (Ed.), *Post-Traumatic Therapy and Victims of Violence* (pp. 319–329). New York: Brunner/Mazel.
72. Salasin, S. E. (Ed.). (1981). *Evaluating victim services.* Beverly Hills, CA: Sage Publications.
73. Strenz, T. (1982). The Stockholm Syndrome. In F. Ochberg & D. Soskis (Eds.), *Victims of Terrorism* (pp. 149–164). Boulder, CO: Westview.
74. Kempe, C. H., Silverman, F. N., Steele, B. F., Droegemueller, W., & Silver, H. K. (1962). The battered-child syndrome. *American Journal of Medical Science, 181*(1), 17–24.
75. Finkelhor, D. (1979). *Sexually Victimized Children.* New York: Free Press.
76. Sgroi, S. (1975). Sexual molestation of children: The last frontier in child abuse. *Children Today, 44,* 18–21.

77. Herman, J. L. (1981). *Father-Daughter Incest* Cambridge, MA: Harvard University Press.
78. Terr, L. (1979). Children of Chowchilla: A study of psychic trauma. *Psychoanalytic Study of the Child, 34*, 552–623.
79. Ullman, M. (1969). A unifying concept linking therapeutic and community process. In W. Gray, F. J. Duhl & N. D. Rizzo (Eds.), *General Systems Theory and Psychiatry* (pp. 253–265). Boston: Little, Brown.
80. Foucault, M. (1965). *Madness and Civilization: A History of Insanity in the Age of Reason.* New York: Vintage.
81. Jones, M. (1968). *Beyond the Therapeutic Community: Social Learning and Social Psychiatry.* New Haven, CT: Yale University Press.
82. Engel, G. L. (1980). The clinical application of the biopsychosocial model. *American Journal of Psychiatry, 137*, 535–544.
83. Engel, G. L. (1977). The need for a new medical model: A challenge for biomedicine. *Science, 196*, 129–136.
84. United States Public Health Service Office of the Surgeon General. (1999). Mental Health: A Report of the Surgeon General. Rockville, MD: Department of Health and Human Services, U.S. Public Health Service.
85. Cooper, C. L., Dewe, P. J., & O'Driscoll, M. P. (2001). *Organizational Stress: A Review and Critique of Theory, Research and Applications.* Thousand Oaks, CA: Sage Publications.
86. LeRoy, L., Heldring, M., & Desjardins, E. (2006). Foundations' Roles In Transforming The Mental Health Care System. *Health Affairs, 25*, 1168–1171.
87. Brousseau, R. T., Langill, D., & Pechura, C. M. (2003). Are foundations overlooking mental health?. *Health Affairs, 22*, 222–229.
88. Law, B. C. f. M. H. (2005). Moving On Analysis of Federal Programs Funding Services to Assist Transition-Age Youth with Serious Mental Health Conditions. Accessed 1/08/10 at http://www.bazelon.org/publications/movingon/Analysis.pdf.
89. Bazelon Center for Mental Health Law. (2009, June 24). Still Waiting: The Unfulfilled Promise of Olmstead. Accessed August 24, 2009 at http://www.bazelon.org/pdf/Olmstead_Call-to-Action.pdf.
90. Kanapaux, W. (2003). Vision Offered To Overhaul Nation's Mental Health Care System. *Psychiatric Times, XX*(8).
91. Hay Group. (1999). Health Care Plan Design and Cost Trends: 1988 through 1998. http://www.naphs.org/News/hay99/hay99.pdf. Arlington: Virginia.
92. National Association of Psychiatric Health Systems. (2003). Challenges Facing Behavioral Health Care: The Pressures on Essential Behavioral Healthcare Services. Washington, D.C.: National Association of Psychiatric Health Systems.
93. Bassuk, E. L., Buckner, J. C., Perloff, J. N., & Bassuk, S. S. (1998). Prevalence of mental health and substance use disorders among homeless and low-income housed mothers. *Am J Psychiatry, 155*(11), 1561–1564.
94. Goodman, L. A., Dutton, M. A., & Harris, M. (1995). Episodically homeless women with serious mental illness: prevalence of physical and sexual assault. *Am J Orthopsychiatry, 65*(4), 468–478.
95. Goodman, L. A., Rosenberg, S. D., Mueser, K. T., & Drake, R. E. (1997). Physical and sexual assault history in women with serious mental illness: prevalence, correlates, treatment, and future research directions. *Schizophr Bull, 23*(4), 685–696.
96. Torrey, E. F. (1995). Editorial: Jails and Prisons-America's New Mental Hospitals. *American Journal of Public Health, 85*, 1611–1613.
97. Mowbray, C. T., Grazier, K. L., & Holter, M. (2002). Managed Behavioral Health Care in the Public Sector: Will It Become the Third Shame of the States? *Psychiatr Serv, 53*(2), 157–170. doi: 10.1176/appi.ps.53.2.157

98. National Alliance to End Homelessness. Mental and Physical Health. Accessed 12/30/09 at http://www.endhomelessness.org/section/policy/focusareas/health.

99. James, D. J., & Glaze, L. E. (2006). Mental Health Problems of Prison and Jail Inmates *Bureau of Justice Statistics Special Report, September 2006, NCJ213600.* Washington, D.C.: U.S. Department of Justice.

100. Bazelon Center for Mental Health Law. (2001). *Disintegrating Systems: The State of States' Public Mental Health Systems:* Bazelon Center for Mental Health Law.

101. Kaiser Daily Health Policy Report. (2004). 15,000 Children Incarcerated Because of Lack of Mental Health Treatment in 2003, http://www.kaisernetwork.org/daily_reports/rep_index.cfm?dr_id=24606, July 8

102. Mulligan, K. (2003). Recovery Movement Gains Influence In Mental Health Programs. *Psychiatric News, 38*(1), 10.

103. Posner, J., Eilenberg, J., Harkavy Friedman, J., & Fullilove, M. J. (2008). Quality and Use of Trauma Histories Obtained From Psychiatric Outpatients: A Ten-Year Follow-Up. *Psychiatr Serv, 59*(3), 318–321. doi: 10.1176/appi.ps.59.3.318

104. President's New Freedom Commission on Mental Health. (2002). Interim Report Retrieved September 17, 2005

105. Merry, U., & Brown, G. (1987). *The Neurotic Behavior of Organizations.* New York: Gardner Press.

106. Kets de Vries, M., & Miller, D. (1984). *The Neurotic Organization: Diagnosing & Changing Counterproductive Styles of Management.* New York: John Wiley & Sons.

107. Schwartz, H. S. (1990). *Narcissistic Process and Organizational Decay: The Theory of the Organization Ideal.* New York: New York University Press.

108. Schaef, A. W. (1988). *The Addictive Organization.* New York: Harper & Row.

109. Ryan, K., & Oestreich, D. (1998). *Driving Fear out of the Workplace: Creating the High Trust, High Performance Organization.* San Francisco: Jossey Bass.

110. National Mental Health Association. (2003). Can't Make the Grade: NMHA State Mental Health Assessment Project (pp. www.nmha.org). Alexandria, VA: National Mental Health Association.

111. Middebrooks, J. S., & Audage, N. C. (2008) The Effects of Childhood Stress on Health Across the Lifespan. Atlanta, GA: Centers for Disease Control and Prevention, National Center for Injury Prevention and Control.

112. National Scientific Council on the Developing Child. (2007). The Science of Early Childhood Development,. *Accessed March 23, 2009,* http://www.developingchild.net.

113. National Scientific Council on the Developing Child. (2007). A Science-Based Framework for Early Childhood Policy: Using Evidence to Improve Outcomes in Learning, Behavior, and Health for Vulnerable Children. *Accesses March 23, 2009,* http://www.developingchild.harvard.edu.

114. McEwen, B. S., & Gianaros, P. J. (2010). Central role of the brain in stress and adaptation: Links to socioeconomic status, health, and disease *Annals of the New York Academy of Sciences, 1186,* 190–222.

115. Dietz, P. M., Spitz, A. M., Anda, R. F., Williamson, D. F., McMahon, P. M., Santelli, J. S., et al. (1999). Unintended pregnancy among adult women exposed to abuse or household dysfunction during their childhood. *Journal of the American Medical Association, 282*(14), 1359–1364.

116. Dube, S. R., Anda, R. F., Felitti, V. J., Chapman, D. P., Williamson, D. F., & Giles, W. H. (2001). Childhood abuse, household dysfunction, and the risk of attempted suicide throughout the life span: findings from the Adverse Childhood Experiences Study. *Journal of the American Medical Association, 286*(24), 3089–3096.

117. Dube, S. R., Anda, R. F., Felitti, V. J., Croft, J. B., Edwards, V. J., & Giles, W. H. (2001). Growing up with parental alcohol abuse: exposure to childhood abuse, neglect, and household dysfunction. *Child Abuse and Neglect, 25*(12), 1627–1640.

118. Dube, S. R., Anda, R. F., Felitti, V. J., Edwards, V. J., & Williamson, D. F. (2002). Exposure to abuse, neglect, and household dysfunction among adults who witnessed intimate partner violence as children: implications for health and social services. *Violence and Victims, 17*(1), 3–17.

119. Edwards, V. J., Anda, R. F., Felitti, V. J., & Dube, S. R. (2004). Adverse childhood experiences and health-related quality of life as an adult. In K. A. Kendall-Tackett (Ed.), *Health consequences of abuse in the family: a clinical guide for evidence-based practice* (pp. 81–94). Washington: American Psychological Association.

120. Edwards, V. J., Holden, G. W., Felitti, V. J., & Anda, R. F. (2003). Relationship between multiple forms of childhood maltreatment and adult mental health in community respondents: results from the Adverse Childhood Experiences Study. *American Journal of Psychiatry, 160*(8), 1453–1460.

121. Felitti, V. J., Anda, R. F., Nordenberg, D. F., Williamson, D. F., Spitz, A. M., Edwards, V. J., et al. (1998). Relationship of childhood abuse and household dysfunction to many of the leading causes of death in adults: the Adverse Childhood Experiences (ACE) study. *American Journal of Preventive Medicine, 14*(4), 245–258.

122. Felitti, V. J., & Anda, R. F. (2010). The Relationship of Adverse Childhood Experiences to Adult Medical Disease, Psychiatric Disorders, and Sexual Behavior: Implications for Healthcare In R. Lanius & E. Vermetten (Eds.), *The Hidden Epidemic: The Impact of Early Life Trauma on Health and Disease* (pp. 77–87). New York: Cambridge University Press.

123. Felitti, V. J., Anda, R. F., Nordenberg, D., Williamson, D. F., Spitz, A. M., Edwards, V., et al. (1998). Relationship of childhood abuse and household dysfunction to many of the leading causes of death in adults. The Adverse Childhood Experiences (ACE) Study. *Am J Prev Med, 14*(4), 245–258.

124. Groves B, Zuckerman B, Marans S, & DJ., C. (1993). Silent victims: children who witness violence. *JAMA, 269*, 262–264.

125. Bell, C., & Jenkins, E. (1993). Community violence and children on Chicago's southside. *Psychiatry, 56*, 46–54.

126. Richters, J. E., & Martinez, P. (1993). The NIMH Community Violence Project: I. Children as Victims of and Witnesses to Violence. *Psychiatry, 56*, 7–21.

127. Osofsky, J. D., Wewers, S., Hann, D. M., & Fick, A. C. (1993). Chronic Community Violence: What Is Happening to Our Children? *Psychiatry, 56*, 36–45.

128. Groves, B., Zuckerman B., Marans S., & DJ., C. (1993). Silent victims: children who witness violence. *JAMA, 269*, 262–264.

129. Li, X., Howard, D., Stanton, B., Rachuba, L., & Cross, S. (1998). Distress Symptoms among Urban African-American Children and Adolescents: A Psychometric Evaluation of the Checklist of Children's Distress Symptoms. *Archives of Pediatrics and Adolescent Medicine 152*, 569–577.

130. Finkelhor, D., Turner, H., Ormrod, R., Hamby, S., & Kracke, K. (2009). Children's Exposure to Violence: A Comprehensive National Survey. *Juvenile Justice Bulletin, October, Accessed 1/3/10 at* http://www.ncjrs.gov/pdffiles1/ojjdp/227744.pdf.

131. Glaze, L. E., & Maruschak, L. M. (2008). Parents in Prison and Their Minor Children. Bureau of Justice Statistics Special Report, NCJ 222984, Accessed 1/30/09 at http://www.ojp.usdoj.gov/bjs/pub/pdf/pptmc.pdf.

132. Mauer, M., & King, R. S. (2007). Uneven Justice: State Rates of Incarceration By Race and Ethnicity. Washington, D.C.: Sentencing Project. Accessed 12/30/09 at http://www.sentencingproject.org/doc/publications/rd_stateratesofincbyraceandethnicity.pdf.

133. Knudsen, E. I., Heckman, J. J., Cameron, J. L., & Shonkoff, J. P. (2006). Economic, neurobiological, and behavioral perspectives on building America's future workforce. *Proceedings of the National Academy of Science, 103*(27), 10155–10162.

134. Resnick, H. S., Kilpatrick, D. G., Dansky, B., Saunders, B., & Best, C. (1993). Prevalence of civilian trauma and posttraumatic stress disorder in a representative national sample of women. *Journal of Consulting and Clinical Psychology, 61*(6), 984–991.

135. Norris, F. H. (1992). Epidemiology of trauma: frequency and impact of different potentially traumatic events on different demographic groups. *Journal of Consulting and Clinical Psychology, 60*, 409–418.

136. Kessler, R. C., Sonnega, A., Bromet, E., Hughes, M., & Nelson, C. B. (1995). Posttraumatic stress disorder in the National Comorbidity Survey. *Arch Gen Psychiatry, 52*(12), 1048–1060.

137. Courtois, C. A., & Ford, J. D. (Eds.). (2009). *Treating Complex Traumatic Stress Disorders: An Evidence-Based Guide* New York: Guilford.

138. Van der Kolk, B. (2005). Developmental trauma disorder: Toward a rational diagnosis for children with complex trauma histories. *Psychiatric Annals, 35*(5), 401–408.

139. Herman, J. (1992). *Trauma and Recovery*. New York: Basic Books.

140. National Institute for Occupational Safety and Health. (1999). Stress at Work. Cincinnati, OH: DHHS (NIOSH) Publication No. 99-101, http://www.cdc.gov/niosh/stresswk.html.

141. Ferris, G. R., Frink, D. D., Galang, M. C., Zhou, J., & al, e. (1996). Perceptions of organizational politics: Prediction, stress-related implications, and outcomes. *Human Relations, 49*(2), 233.

142. Gray, P. H. (1999). Mental health in the workplace: Tackling the effects of stress. London, UK: Mental Health Foundation, http://www.mentalhealth.org.uk/html/content/mh_workplace.pdf.

143. Tetrick, L. E., & LaRocco, J. M. (1987). Understanding prediction, and control as moderators of the relationships between perceived stress, satisfaction, and psychological well-being. *Journal of Applied Psychology, 72*, 538–543.

144. Gavin, J. F., & Axelrod, W. L. (1977). Managerial stress and strain in a mining organization. *Journal of Vocational Behavior, 11*, 66–74.

145. Gavin, J. F. (1975). Employee perceptions of the work environment and mental health: A suggestive study. *Journal of Vocational Behavior, 6*, 217–234.

146. Erickson, J. M., Pugh, W. M., & Gunderson, E. E. (1972). Status congruency as a predictor of job satisfaction and life stress. Journal of Applied Psychology. *Journal of Applied Psychology, 56*, 523–525.

147. Tosi, H. (1971). Organizational stress as a moderator of the relationship between influence and role response. *Academy of Management Journal, 14*, 7–20.

148. Lance, C. E., & Richardson, D. R. (1988). Correlates of work and non-work stress and satisfaction among American insulated sojourners. *Human Relations, 41*, 725–738.

149. Hollon, C. J., & Chesser, R. J. (1976). The relationship of personal influence dissonance to job tension, satisfaction, and involvement. Academy of Management Journal. *Academy of Management Journal, 19*, 308–314.

150. Wolfe, I. S. (2004). The Truth about Employee Stress: Bleeding at the Bottom Line. *Business 2 Business, October*(http://www.super-solutions.com/Thetruthaboutworkplacestress.asp).

151. Collie, D. (2004, July 7). Workplace Stress: Expensive Stuff, http://www.emax-health.com/38/473.html Retrieved September 19, 2005

152. Connor, D. F., McIntyre, E. K., Miller, K., Brown, C., Bluestone, H., Daunais, D., et al. (2003). Staff Retention and Turnover in a Residential Treatment Center *Residential Treatment for Children & Youth:*, *2*, 43–53.

153. Foderaro, L. W. (2002, February 15, Accessed August 25, 2008, http://query.nytimes.com/gst/fullpage.html?res=9A05E4DF153FF936A25751C0A9649C8B63&sec=&spon=&pagewanted=all). Violence Is a Symptom of Youth Centers' Struggles *New York Times, February 15, Accessed August 25, 2008,* http://query.nytimes.com/gst/fullpage.html?res=9A05E4DF153FF936A25751C0A9649C8B63&sec=&spon=&pagewanted=all.

154. GAO. (2003). *HHS Could Play a Greater Role in Helping Child Welfare Agencies Recruit and Retain Staff, GAO-03-357,* Accessed August 25, 2008 http://www.gao.gov/new.items/d03357.pdf. (03-357).

155. Woltmann, E. M., Whitley, R., McHugo, G. J., Brunette, M., Torrey, W. C., Coots, L., et al. (2008). The Role of Staff Turnover in the Implementation of Evidence-Based Practices in Mental Health Care. *Psychiatr Serv, 59*(7), 732–737. doi: 10.1176/appi.ps.59.7.732

156. Hobbs, T., & Gable, G. (1998). Coping with litigation stress. *Physician's News Digest, January* http://www.physiciansnews.com/law/198.html Retrieved September 21, 2005

157. Jenkins, R., & Elliott, P. (2004). Stressors, burnout and social support: nurses in acute mental health settings. *Journal of Advanced Nursing, 48*(6), 622–631.

158. Social Work Policy Institute. (2010). High Caseloads: How do they Impact Delivery of Health and Human Services? Research to Practice Brief, January. Washington, D.C.: National Association of Social Workers.

159. Bills, L. J., & Bloom, S. L. (1998). From Chaos to Sanctuary: Trauma-Based Treatment for Women in a State Hospital Systems. In B. L. Levin, A. K. Blanch & A. Jennings (Eds.), *Women's Health Services: A Public Health Perspective* (pp. 348–367). Thousand Oaks, CA: Sage Publications.

160. Dane, B. (2000). Child welfare workers: an innovative approach for interacting with secondary trauma. *Journal of Social Work Education 36*(1), 27–38.

161. Larner, M. B., Stevenson, C. S., & Behrman, R. E. (1998). Protecting children from abuse and neglect: Analysis and recommendations. *The Future of Children. The Future of Children, 8*, 4–22.

162. Mills, C., Stephan, S., Moore, E., Weist, M., Daly, B., & Edwards, M. (2006). The President's New Freedom Commission: Capitalizing on Opportunities to Advance School-Based Mental Health Services. *Clinical Child and Family Psychology Review, 9*(3), 149–161.

163. Institute of Medicine. (2002). *Unequal Treatment: Confronting Racial and Ethnic Disparities in Health Care* Washington, D.C.: National Academies Press.

164. McCorkle, D., & Peacock, C. (2005). Trauma and the Isms - A herd of elephants in the room: A training vignette. *Therapeutic Community: The International Journal for Therapeutic and Supportive Organizations, 26*(1), 127–133.

165. Peacock, C., & Gross, C. (2008). My Identity, My SELF: Addressing the Needs of LGBTQ Youth, Version 3 New York: Jewish Board of Family and Children's Services. Accessed 1/4/09 at http://www.jewishboard.org/main/docs/MIMS_curriculum.pdf.

166. President's New Freedom Commission on Mental Health. (2003). *Achieving the Promise: Transforming Mental Health Care in America.* Rockville, MD: New Freedom Commission on Mental Health.

167. Huang, L., Macbeth, G., dodge, J., & Jacobstein, D. (2004). Transforming the workforce in children's mental health *Administration and Policy in Mental Health, 32*(2), 167–187.

168. Hogue, M. A., & Morris, J. (2007). The National Action Plan on Behavioral Health Workforce Development Annapolis, MD: Presentation to The Annapolis Coalition COCE/COSIG Workgroup October 18.

169. Hoge, M., & Morris, J. (2004). Guest Editors' Introduction: Implementing Best Practices in Behavioral Health Workforce Education—Building a Change Agenda. *Administration and Policy in Mental Health and Mental Health Services Research, 32*(2), 85–89.

170. Manderscheid, R. W., Atay, J. E., Hernández-Cartagena, M. d. R., Edmond, P. Y., Male, A., Parker, A. C., et al. (2000). Chapter 14. Highlights of Organized Mental Health Services in 1998 and Major National and State Trends. In R. W. Manderscheid & M. J. Henderson (Eds.), *Mental Health, United States, 2000.* Rockville, MD: U.S. Department of Health and Human Services, Substance Abuse and Mental Health Services Administration, Center for Mental Health Services (pp. http://mental health.samhsa.gov/publications/allpubs/SMA01-3537/chapter14.asp).

171. Women's Law Project. (2002). Responding to the needs of pregnant and parenting women with substance use disorders in Philadelphia (pp. http://www.womens lawproject.org/reports/Pregnant_parenting_PVS.pdf). Philadelphia: Women's Law Project.

172. Hoge, M. A. (2002). The Training Gap: An Acute Crisis in Behavioral Health Education. *Administration and Policy in Mental Health and Mental Health Services Research, 29*(4), 305–317.

173. Koppelman, J. (2004). The Provider System for Children's Mental Health: Workforce Capacity and Effective Treatment. *NHPF Issue Brief, No. 801*(October 26).

174. Styron, T. H., Shaw, M., McDuffie, E., & Hoge, M. A. (2005). Curriculum resources for training Direct care providers in public Sector mental health. *Administration and Policy in Mental Health and Mental Health Services Research, 32*(5), 633–649.

175. Peter, L. J., & Hull, R. (1969). *The Peter Principle: why things always go wrong. New York: William Morrow and Company.* New York: William Morrow and Company.

176. McClure, R. F., Livingston, R. B., Livingston, K. H., & Gage, R. (2005). A Survey of Practicing Psychotherapists. *Journal of Professional Counseling: Practice, Theory & Research, 33*(1), 35–46.

177. Schlesinger, M., Wynia, M., & Cummins, D. (2000). Some Distinctive Features of the Impact of Managed Care on Psychiatry. *Harvard Review of Psychiatry, 8*(5), 216.

178. Smith, H. B. (1999). Managed Care: A Survey of Counselor Educators and Counselor Practitioners. *Journal of Mental Health Counseling, 21*(3), 270.

179. Whitaker, T., Weismiller, T., and Clark, E.J. (2006). Assuring the sufficiency of frontline workforce: A National Study of Licensed social Workers—Special Report: social Work Services in Behavioral Health Care Settings. Washington, D.C.: National Association of Social Workers.

180. Cable, D. M., & Judge, T. A. (1996). Person-organization fit, job choice decisions, and organizational entry", *Organizational Behavior and Human Decision Processes, 67*, 294–311.

181. Judge, T. A., & Ferris, G. R. (1992). The elusive criterion of fit in human resource staffing decisions. *Human Resource Planning, 15*, 47–67.

182. Caldwell, D., & O'Reilly, C. A. (1990). Measuring person-job fit using a profile comparison process. *Journal of Applied Psychology, 75*, 648–756.

183. Ostroff, C., & Rothausen, T. J. (1997). The moderating effect of tenure in person-environment fit: a field study in educational organizations. *Journal of Occupational and Organizational Psychology, 70,* 173–189.

184. Posner, B. Z. (1992). Person-organization values congruence: no support for individual differences as a moderating variable. *Human Relations, 45*(4), 351–361.

185. Maslach, C., & Leiter, M. P. (1997). *The Truth About Burnout: How Organizations Cause Personal Stress and What To Do About It.* San Francisco: Jossey-Bass.

186. Maslach, C., & Leiter, M. P. (1999). Take this job and. love it! *Psychology Today, 32*(5), 50.

187. Siegall, M., & McDonald, D. (2004). Person-organization value congruence, burnout and diversion of resources. *Personnel Review, 3*(3), 291–301.

188. Peterson, D. (2003). The relationship between ethical pressure, relativistic moral beliefs and organizational commitment. *Journal of Managerial Psychology, 18*(6), 557–572.

189. Gibelman, M., & Mason, S. E. (2002). Treatment choices in a managed care environment: A multi-disciplinary exploration. *Clinical Social Work Journal, 30*(2), 199.

190. Callahan, A. M. (2007). Second Thoughts from the Front Lines. *Social Work, 52*(4), 364.

191. Gabbard, G. O. (1997). In R. K. Schreter, S. S. Sharfstein & C. A. Schreter (Eds.), *Allies and Adversaries: The Impact of Managed Care on Mental Health Services.* Washington, D.C.: American Psychiatric Press.

192. Ware, N. C., Lachicotte, W. S., Kirschner, S. R., Cortes, D. E., & Good, B. J. (2000). Clinician Experiences of Managed Mental Health Care: A Rereading of the Threat. *Medical Anthropology Quarterly, 14*(1), 3–27.

193. Marks, M. L., & Mirvis, P. (1985). Merger syndrome: stress and uncertainty. *Mergers & Acquisitions, Summer,* 50–55.

194. Schein, E. H. (1999). *The Corporate Culture: A Survival Guide. Sense and Nonsense About Culture Change.* San Francisco: Jossey Bass.

195. Nitsun, M. (1996). *The Anti-group: Destructive forces in the group and their creative potential.* London: Routledge.

196. Cheng, Y., Kawachi, I., Coakley, E. H., Schwartz, J., & Colditz, G. (2000). Association between psychosocial work characteristics and health functioning in American women: prospective study. *British Medical Journal, 320*(7247), 1432–1436.

197. Morris, J. A., & Hanley, J. H. (2001). Human Resource Development: A Critical Gap in Child Mental Health Reform. *Administration and Policy in Mental Health and Mental Health Services Research, 28*(3), 219–227.

198. Aarons, G. A., & Sawitzky, A. C. (2006). Organizational Climate Partially Mediates the Effect of Culture on Work Attitudes and Staff Turnover in Mental Health Services. *Administration and Policy in Mental Health and Mental Health Services Research, 33*(3), 289–301.

199. Glisson, C., & Green, P. (2006). The Effects of Organizational Culture and Climate on the Access to Mental Health Care in Child Welfare and Juvenile Justice Systems. *Administration and Policy in Mental Health and Mental Health Services Research, 33*(4), 433–448.

200. Glisson, C. (2002). The Organizational Context of Children's Mental Health Services. *Clinical Child and Family Psychology Review, 5*(4), 233–253.

201. Johnston, K. (1993). *Busting Bureacracy: How To Conquer Your Organization's Worst Enemy.* Tampa, FL: Kaset International.

202. Jennings, A. (2004). The Damaging Consequences of Violence and Trauma Facts, Discussion Points, and Recommendations for the Behavioral Health System (pp. http://www.nasmhpd.org/general_files/publications/ntac_pubs/reports/Trauma %20Services%20doc%20FINAL-04.pdf). Washington, D.C.: National Association of State Mental Health Program Directors.

203. Blanch, A. (2003). Developing trauma-informed behavioral health systems: Report from NTAC's National Experts Meeting on Trauma and Violence. Alexandria, VA: U. S. Department of Health and Human Services, Substance Abuse and Mental Health Services Administration.

204. Huckshorn, K. A. (2005). *Six Core Strategies for Reducing Seclusion and Restraint Use*: http://www.advocacycenter.org/documents/RS_Six_Core_Strategies.pdf.

205. Moskowitz, A., Nadel, L., Watts, P., & Jacobs, W. J. (2008). Delusion atmosphere, the psychotic prodrome, and decontextualized memories. In A. Moskowitz, I. Schäfer & M. J. Dorahy (Eds.), *Psychosis, Trauma and Dissociation: Emerging Perspectives on Severe Psychopathology* (pp. 65–78). New York: John Wiley & Sons.

206. Blackmore, S. (1999). *The Meme Machine*. London: Oxford University Press.

207. Holmes, J. (1993). *John Bowlby and Attachment Theory*. London: Routledge.

208. Rholes, W. S., & Simpson, J. A. (Eds.). (2004). *Adult Attachment: Theory, Research and Clinical Implications*. New York: Guildford.

209. Howe, D., Brandon, M., Hinings, D., & Schofield, G. (1999). *Attachment Theory, Child Maltreatment and Family Support: A Practice and Assessment Model*. London: Macmillan.

210. Bowlby, J. (1980). *Attachment and loss, Volume III: Loss, sadness and depression*. New York: Basic Books.

211. Bowlby, J. (1988). *A Secure Base: Parent-Child Attachment and Healthy Human Development*. New York: Basic Books.

212. Stern, D. (1985). *The interpersonal world of the infant*. New York: Basic Books.

213. Main, M., Kaplan, N., & Cassidy, J. (1985). Security in infancy, childhood, and adulthood: A move to the level of representation. In I. Bretherton & E. Waters (Eds.), *Growing Points of Attachment Theory and Research: Monograph of the Society for Research in Child Development* (Vol. 50, pp. 66–104).

214. Ainsworth, M. D. S., Blehar, M. C., Waters, E., & Wall, S. (1978). *Patterns of Attachment A Psychological Study of the Strange Situation*. Hillsdale, NJ: Erlbaum.

215. Cicchetti, D. P., & Toth, S. L. 1995. A Developmental Psychopathology Perspective on Child Abuse and Neglect. *Journal of the American Academy of Child & Adolescent Psychiatry, 34*(5), 541–565.

216. Eibl-Eibesfeldt, I. (1989). *Human Ethology*. New York: Aldine de Gruyter.

217. Goleman, D. (2006). *Social Intelligence: The New Science of Human Relationships*. New York: Bantam Books.

218. Iacoboni, M. (2008). *Mirroring People: The New Science of How We Connect with Others*. New York: Farrar, Straus and Giroux.

219. National Scientific Council on the Developing Child. (2004). *Young Children Develop in an Environment of Relationships*.

220. Berman, W. H., & Sperling, M. B. (1994). The structure and function of adult attachment. In M. B. Sperling & W. H. Berman (Eds.), *Attachment in Adults: Clinical and Developmental Perspectives* (pp. 1–28). New York: Guilford.

221. Weiss, R. S. (1991). The attachment bond in childhood and adulthood. In C. M. Parkes, J. Stevenson-Hinde & P. Marris (Eds.), *Attachment Across the Life Cycle* (pp. 66–76). London: Routledge.

222. Sroufe, L. A., Carlson, E. A., Levy, A. K., & Egeland, B. (1999). Implications of attachment theory for developmental psychopathology. *Dev Psychopathol, 11*(1), 1–13.

223. Grossman, K. E., & Grossman, K. (1991). Attachment quality as an organizer of emotional and behavioral responses in a longitudinal perspective. In C. M. Parkes, J. Stevenson-Hinde & P. Marris (Eds.), *Attachment Across the Life Cycle.* (pp. 93–114 http://mentalhealth.samhsa.gov/publications/allpubs/SMA01-3537/chapter14. asp). London: Routledge.

224. Bellah, R. N. (1073). Introduction *E. Durkheim, On morality and society: selected writings.* Chicago: The University of Chicago Press.

225. Durkheim, E. (1951). *Suicide: A Study in Sociology.* New York: The Free Press.

226. Bellah, R. N. (1973). Introduction *Emile Durkheim: On Morality and Society: Selected Writings.* Chicago: University of Chicago Press.

227. Caplan, G. (1974). *Support Systems and Community Mental Health.* New York: Behavioral Publications.

228. Mead, G. H. (1934). *Mind, Self and Society.* Chicago: University of Chicago Press.

229. Cooley, C. H. (1962). *Social Organization.* New York: Schocken Books.

230. McDougall, W. (1920). *The Group Mind.* London: Cambridge at the University Press.

231. Campbell, J. (1995). *Understanding John Dewey: Nature and Cooperative Intelligence.* Chicago: Open Court.

232. Douglas, T. (1986). *Group Living.* London: Tavistock Publications.

233. White, W. A. (1919). *Thoughts of a Psychiatrist on the War and After.* New York: Paul Hoeber.

234. Burrow, T. (1984). Trigant Burrow: Toward Social Sanity and Human Survival: Selections From His Writings. In A. Galt (Ed.). New York: Horizon.

235. Burrrow, T. (1926). The laboratory method in psychoanalysis: Its inception and development. *The American Journal of Psychiatry, 5,* 345–355.

236. Burrow, T. (Ed.). (1953). *Science and Man's Behavior: The Contribution of Phylobiology.* New York: Philosophical Library.

237. Frank, L. K. (1936). Society as the patient. *The American Journal of Sociology, 42*(3), 335–344.

238. Szalavitz, M., & Perry, B. (2010). *Born For Love: Why Empathy is Essential and Endangered.* New York: Harper Collins.

239. Brewer, M. B., & Gardner, W. (1996). Who is this "we"? Levels of collective identity and self-representation. *Journal of Personality and Social Psychology, 71,* 83–93.

240. Forsyth, D. R. (1990). *Group Dynamics, Second Edition.* Pacific Grove, CA: Brooks/ Cole.

241. National Scientific Council on the Developing Chilld. (2005). *Excessive Stress Disrupts the Architecture of the Developing Brain.* (2005).

242. Perry, B. D., & Szalavitz, M. (2006). *The Boy Who Was Raised As a Dog: What Traumatized Children Can Teach Us About Loss, Love, and Healing.* New York: Basic Books.

243. Kobak, R., Cassidy, J., & Zir, Y. (2004). Attachment-related trauma and post-traumatic stress disorder: Implications for adult adaptation. In W. S. Rholes & J. A. Simpson (Eds.), *Adult Attachment: Theory, Research and Clinical Implications.* New York: Guilford (pp. 388–407). New York: Guildford.

244. Freyd, J. J. (1996). *Betrayal Trauma: The Logic of Forgetting Childhood Abuse.* Cambridge, MA: Harvard University Press.

245. Pilisuk, M., & Parks, S. H. (1986). *The Healing Web: Social Networks and Human Survival.* Hanover, NH: University Press of New England.

246. Williams, R. B. (1995). Somatic consequences of stress. In M. J. Friedman, D. S. Charney & A. Y. Deutch (Eds.), *Neurobiological and Clinical Consequences of Stress: From Normal Adaptation to PTSD* (pp. 403–412). Philadelphia: Lippincott-Raven.

247. Vaux, A. (1988). *Social Support: Theory, Research, and Intervention.* New York: Praeger.

248. Cassel, J. (1976). The contribution of the social environment to host resistance. *American Journal of Epidemiology, 104,* 107–123.

249. Brewin, C., Andrews, B., & Valentine, J. D. (2000). Meta-analysis of risk factors for posttraumatic stress disorder in trauma-exposed adults. *Journal of Consulting and Clinical psychology, 68*(5), 748–766

250. Flannery, R. B. (1990). Social support and psychological trauma: A methodological review. *Journal of Traumatic Stress, 3*(4), 593–611.

251. Williams, K. D., Forgas, J. P., Von Hippel, W., & Zadro, L. (2005). The social outcast: An overview. In K. D. Williams, J. P. Forgas & W. Von Hippel (Eds.), *The Social Outcast: Ostracism, Social Exclusion, Rejection and Bullying* (pp. 1–16). New York: Taylor Francis.

252. Cacioppa, J. T., & Patrick, W. (2008). *Loneliness: Human Nature and the Need for Social Connection.* New York: W.W. Norton.

253. Festinger, L., Pepitone, A., & Newcomb, T. (1952). Some consequence of deindividuation in a group. *Journal of Abnormal Psychology, 47,* 392–398.

254. Silke, A. (2003). Deindividuation, anonymity, and violence: Findings from Northern Ireland. *The Journal of Social Psychology, 143*(4), 493–499.

255. Horowitz, M. J. (Ed.). (1986). *Stress Response Syndromes (2nd ed.).* Northvale, NJ: Jason Aronson Press.

256. Harber, K. D., & Pennebaker, J. W. (1992). Overcoming traumatic memories. In S. A. Christianson (Ed.), *The Handbook of Emotion and Memory: Research and Theory* (pp. 359–387). Hillsdale, NJ: Lawrence Erlbaum.

257. Marks, I. (1987). *Fears, Phobias and Rituals: Panic, Anxiety and Their Disorders.* New York: Oxford University Press.

258. Bloom, S. L. (2003). *Understanding the Impact of Sexual Assault: The Nature of Traumatic Experience.* Maryland Heights, Missour: GW Medical Publishing, Maryland Heights, Missour.

259. Van der Kolk, B., & Fisler, R. (1995). Dissociation and the fragmentary nature of traumatic memories: Overview and exploratory study. *Journal of Traumatic Stress, 8,* 505–525.

260. Selye, H. (1975). Confusion and controversy in the stress field. *J Human Stress, 1*(2), 37–44.

261. Selye, H. (1973). The evolution of the stress concept. *Am Sci, 61*(6), 692–699.

262. Schumaker, J. F. (1995). *The Corruption of Reality: A Unified Theory of Religion, Hypnosis, and Psychopathology.* Amherst, NY: Prometheus books.

263. St. Pierre, M., Hofinger, G., & Buerschaper, C. (2007). *Crisis Management in Acute Care Settings: Human Factors and Team Psychology in a High Stakes Environment.* New York: Springer-Verlag.

264. Janis, I. L. (1982). Decision making under stress. In L. Goldberger & S. Breznitz (Eds.), *Handbook Of Stress: Theoretical And Clinical Aspects* (pp. 69–87). New York: Free Press.

265. Caine, R. N., & Caine, G. (1994). *Making Connections: Teaching and the Human Brain.* Parsippany, NJ: Dale Seymour Publications.

266. Van der Kolk, B. (1996). Trauma and memory. In B. Van der Kolk, A. McFarlane & L. Weisaeth (Eds.), *Traumatic Stress: The Effects of Overwhelming Experience on Mind, Body and Society* (pp. 279–302). New York: Guilford Press.

267. McEwen, B. S., & Magarinos, A. M. (1997). Stress effects on morphology and function of the hippocampus. In R. Yehuda & A. C. McFarlane (Eds.), *Psychobiology of Posttraumatic Stress Disorder* (Vol. 821, pp. 271–284). New York: New York Academy of Sciences.

268. Roozendaal, B., Quirarte, G. L., & McGaugh, J. L. (1997). Stress-activated hormonal systems and the regulation of memory storage. In: In R. Yehuda & A. C. McFarlane (Eds.), *Psychobiology of Post-traumatic Stress Disorder* (Vol. 821, pp. 247–258). New York: New York Academy of Sciences.

269. Van der Kolk, B. A. (1996). Trauma and memory. In B. A. Van der Kolk, A. C. McFarlane & L. Weisaeth (Eds.), *Traumatic Stress: The Effects of Overwhelming Experience on Mind, Body and Society.* (pp. 279–302). New York: Guilford Press.

270. Taylor, S. E., Klein, L. C., Lewis, B. P., Gruenewald, T. L., Gurung, R. A. R., & Updegraff, J. A. (2000). Biobehavioral responses to stress in females: Tend-and-befriend, not fight-or-flight. *Psychological Review, 107*, 411–429.

271. McLeish, K. (1993). *Key ideas in human thought.* New York: Facts on File.

272. Domhoff, G. W. (2005). *Who Rules America Now? Power, Politics and Social Change, 5th Edition.* New York: McGraw Hill.

273. Korgen, K., & White, J. M. (2007). *The Engaged Sociologist: Connecting the Classroom to the Community.* Thousand Oaks, CA: Pine Forge Press.

274. Van der Kolk, B., Greenberg, M., & Orr, S. (1989). Endogenous opioids, stress induced analgesia, and posttraumatic stress disorder. *Psychopharmacology Bulletin, 25*(417–442).

275. LeDoux, J. (1996). *The Emotional Brain: The Mysterious Underpinnings of Emotional Life.* New York: Simon and Schuster.

276. Van der Kolk, B. A. (2006). Clinical Implications of Neuroscience Research in PTSD. *Annals of the New York Academy of Sciences, 1071* (Psychobiology of Posttraumatic Stress Disorder A Decade of Progress), 277–293.

277. Perry, B. (1994). Neurobiological sequelae of childhood trauma: PTSD in children. In M. Murburg (Ed.), *Catecholamine Function in Posttraumatic Stress Disorders: Emerging Concepts* (pp. 253–276). Washington, D.C.: American Psychiatric Press.

278. Laughlin, C. D., McManus, J., & D'Aquili, E. G. (1979). Introduction. In E. D'Aquili, Laughlin Jr. C.D. & J. McManus (Eds.), *The Spectrum of Ritual: A Biogenetic Structural Analysis.* New York: Columbia University Press.

279. Gazzaniga, M. (1985). *The Social Brain: Discovering the Networks of the Mind.* New York: Basic Books.

280. Janis, I., & Mann, L. (1977). *Decision Making: A Psychological Analysis of Conflict, Choice and Commitment.* New York: Free Press.

281. James, B. (1994). *Handbook for Treatment of Attachment Trauma Problems in Children.* New York: Lexington Books.

282. Freyd, J. J. (1996). *Betrayal Trauma: The Logic of Forgetting Childhood Abuse.* Cambridge MA: Harvard University Press.

283. Rich, J. (2009). *Wrong Place, Wrong Time: Trauma and Violence in the Lives of Young Black Men.* Baltimore: John Hopkins Press.

284. Bremner, J. D. (2002). *Does Stress Damage the Brain?: Understanding Trauma-Related Disorders from a Neurological Perspective.* New York: Norton.

285. Van der Kolk, B. (1996). The body keeps the score: Approaches to the psychobiology of posttraumatic stress disorder. In V. d. K. B., L. Weisaeth & M. A. C. (Eds.), *Traumatic Stress: The Effects of Overwhelming Experience on Mind, Body and Society.* (pp. 214–241). New York: Guilford.

286. Putnam, F. W. (1989). *Diagnosis and Treatment of Multiple Personality Disorder.* New York: Guilford.
287. Perry, B. D. (2009). Examining Child Maltreatment Through a Neurodevelopmental Lens: Clinical Applications of the Neurosequential Model of Therapeutics. *Journal of Loss and Trauma, 14,* 240–255.
288. Rogers, A. G. (2007). *The Unsayable: The Hidden Language of Trauma.* New York: Random House.
289. Krystal, H. (1988). *Integration and self healing: Affect, trauma, alexithymia.* Hillsdale, NJ: Analytic Press.
290. Van der Kolk, B. A., & Perry, J. C. (1991). Childhood origins of self-destructive behavior. *American Journal of Psychiatry, 148*(12), 1665–1671.
291. Briere, J., & Jordan, C. (2009). Childhood Maltreatment, Intervening Variables, and Adult Psychological Difficulties in Women: An Overview. *Trauma Violence Abuse, 10,* 375–388.
292. Pyszczynski, T., Solomon, S., & Greenberg, J. (2003). *In the Wake of 9/11: The Psychology of Terror.* Washington, D.C.: American Psychological Association.
293. van Hiel, A., & De Clercq, B. (2009). Authoritarianism is Good for You: Right-wing Authoritarianism as a Buffering Factor for Mental Distress. *European Journal of Personality, 23,* 33–50.
294. Shay, J. (1994). *Achilles in Vietnam.* New York: Atheneum.
295. Bloom, S. L. (2006). Societal trauma: Democracy in danger. In N. Totten (Ed.), *The Politics of Psychotherapy* (pp. 17–29). New York: Open University Press.
296. Seligman, M. (1992). *Helplessness: On depression, development and death.* New York: W. H. Freeman and Co.
297. Van der Kolk, B. A., Greenberg, M., Boyd, H., & Krystal, J. (1985). Inescapable shock, neurotransmitters, and addiction to trauma: Toward a psychobiology of post traumatic stress. *Biological Psychiatry, 20*(314–325).
298. DeMause. (2002). *The Emotional Life of Nations.* New York: Karnac Books.
299. Schore, A. N. (1994). *Affect Regulation and the Origin of the Self: The Neurobiology of Emotional Development.* Hillsdale, N.J.: Lawrence Erlbaum.
300. Gilligan, J. (1996). *Violence: Our Deadly Epidemic and Its Causes.* New York: G. P. Putnam's Sons.
301. Bloom, S. L. (2001). Commentary: Reflections on the desire for revenge. *Journal of Emotional Abuse, 2*(4), 61–94.
302. Garbarino, J. (1999). *Lost boys: Why our sons turn violent and how we can save them.* New York: The Free Press.
303. Blair, R. J., & Cipolotti, L. (2000). Impaired social response reversal. A case of 'acquired sociopathy'. *Brain, 123*(6), 1122–1141.
304. Bauman, L. J., & Friedman, S. B. (1998). Corporal punishment. *Pediatric Clinics of North America, 45,* 403–414.
305. Gershoff, E. T. (2008). Report on Physical Punishment in the United States: What Research Tells Us About Its Effects on Children. Columbus, OH: Center for Effective Discipline.
306. Afifi, T. O., Brownridge, D. A., Cox, B. J., & Sareen, J. (2006). Physical punishment, childhood abuse and psychiatric disorders. *Child Abuse & Neglect, 30*(10), 1093–1103.
307. Van der Kolk, B., & Greenberg, M. (1987). The psychobiology of the trauma response: Hyperarousal, constriction, and addiction to traumatic reexposure. In B. Van der Kolk (Ed.), *Psychological Trauma* (pp. 63–88). Washington, D.C.: American Psychiatric Press.

308. van der Kolk, B. A., & Ducey, C. P. (1989). The psychological processing of traumatic experience: Rorschach patterns in PTSD. *Journal of Traumatic Stress, 2,* 259–274.
309. Lifton, R. J. (1993). From Hiroshima to the Nazi doctors. In J. P. Wilson & B. Raphael (Eds.), *The International Handbook Of Traumatic Stress Syndromes* (pp. 11–22). New York: Plenum.
310. Karpman, S. B. (1968). Fairy tales and script drama analysis. *Transactional Analysis Bulletin, 7*(26).
311. Karpman, S. B. (1973). 1972 Eric Berne Memorial Scientific Award Lecture. *Transactional Analysis Journal, III,* 73–76.
312. Bloom, S. L. (2007). Beyond the Beveled Mirror: Mourning and Recovery from Childhood Maltreatment. In A. L. Vargas & S. L. Bloom (Eds.), *Loss, Hurt and Hope: The Complex Issues of Bereavement and Trauma in Children* (pp. 4–49). Newcastle, UK: Cambridge Scholars Publishing.
313. Janoff-Bulman, R. (1992). *Shattered assumptions: Towards a new psychology of trauma.* New York: Free Press.
314. Pyszczynski, T. (2004). What Are We So Afraid Of? A Terror Management Theory Perspective on the Politics of Fear. *Social Research, 71*(4), 827.
315. Obholzer, A., & Roberts, V. Z. (1994). The troublesome individual and the troubled institution. In A. Obholzer & V. Z. Roberts (Eds.), *The Uconscious at Work: Individual and Organizational Stress in the Human Services* (pp. 129–138). London: Routledge.
316. Bloom, S. L. (1995). The Germ Theory Of Trauma:The Impossibility of Ethical Neutrality. In B. H. Stamm (Ed.), *Secondary Traumatic Stress: Self Care Issues for Clinicians, Researchers and Educators* (pp. 257–276): Sidran Foundation.
317. Schwartz, M. (1995). Radio interview with Maxim Schwartz, Executive Director, Pasteur Institute, BBC Worldwide Services, National Public Radio, January 24.
318. Yehuda, R., & Bierer, L. M. (2009). The relevance of epigenetics to PTSD: Implications for the DSM-V. *Journal of Traumatic Stress, 22,* 427–434.
319. Becker, E. (1973). *The Denial of Death.* New York: The Free Press.
320. Becker, E. (1975). *Escape from Evil.* New York: The Free Press.
321. Pyszczynski, T., Greenberg, J., Solomon, S., & Maxfield, M. (2006). On the unique psychological import of the human awareness of mortality: Theme and variations. *Psychological Inquiry, 17*(4), 328–356.
322. Rifkin, J. (2009). *The Empathic Civilization.* New York: Jeremy P. Tarcher.
323. Gantt, S. P., & Agazarian, Y. M. (2004). Systems-centered emotional intelligence: Beyond individual systems to organizational systems. *Organizational Analysis, 12*(2), 147–169.
324. Senge, P., Scharmer, C. O., Jaworski, J., & Flowers, B. S. (2004). *Presence: Human Purpose and the Field of the Future.* Cambridge, MA: The Society for Organizational Learning.
325. Ray, M. (1993). What is the New Paradigm in Business? In M. Ray & A. Rinzler (Eds.), *The New Paradigm in Business: Emerging Strategies for Leadership and Organizational Change* (pp. 1–11). New York: G.P. Putnam's Sons.
326. Hewstone, M., Stroebe, W., Codol, J., & Stephenson, G. M. (1989). *Introduction To Social Psychology.* Oxford, England: Basil Blackwell.
327. Gray, W., Duhl, F. J., & Rizzo, N. D. (1969). *General Systems Theory and Psychiatry.* Boston: Little Brown.
328. Gall, J. (2002). *The Systems Bible: The Beginner's Guide to Systems Large and Small, 3rd Edition of Systemantics.* Walker, MN: General Systemantics Press.

329. Ackoff, R. L. (1994). *The Democratic Corporation: A Radical Prescription for Recreating Corporate America and Rediscovering Success*. New York: Oxford University Press.

330. Goldstein, J. (1994). *The Unshackled Organization*. Portland, OR: Productivity Press.

331. Johnson, S. (2001). *Emergence*. New York: Ballantine Books.

332. Holland, J. H. (1998). *Emergence: From Chaos to Order*. Reading, MA: Addison-Wesley.

333. Siegel, D. (1999). *The Developing Mind: Toward a Neurobiology of Interpersonal Experience*. New York: Guilford Press.

334. Goldstone, R. L., Roberts, M. E., & Gureckis, T. M. (2008). Emergent Processes in Group Behavior. *Group Behavior, 17*, 10–15.

335. Lewin, K. (1951). *Field Theory in Social Science: Selected Theoretical Papers*. New York: Harper & Brothers.

336. Bion, W. R. (1961). *Experiences in Groups*. London: Routledge.

337. Kets de Vries, M. (2006). *The Leader on the Cuch: A Clinical Approach to Changing People and Organizations*. San Francisco: Jossey-Bass.

338. Cohen, F. S., Solomon, S., Maxfield, M. G., Pyszczynski, T., & Greenberg, J. (2004). Fatal Attraction:The Effects of Mortality Salience on Evaluations of Charismatic, Task-Oriented, and Relationship-Oriented Leaders. *Psychological Science, 15*(12), 846–851.

339. Axelrod, R. (1984). *The Evolution of Cooperation*. New York: Basic Books.

340. Bloom, S., & Reichert, M. (1998). *Bearing Witness: Violence and Collective Responsibility*. Binghamton NY: Haworth Press.

341. Schimel, J., Simon, L., Greenberg, J., Pyszczynski, T., Solomon, S., Waxmonsky, J., et al. (1999). Stereotypes and terror management: evidence that mortality salience enhances stereotypic thinking and preferences. *J Pers Soc Psychol, 77*(5), 905–926.

342. Volkan, V. (2002). September 11 and Societal Regression. *Group Analysis, 35*(4), 456–483.

343. Janis, I. L. (1983). Groupthink. *Small Groups and Social Interaction, 2*, 39–46.

344. Baumeister, R. F., & Hastings, S. (1997). Distortions of collective memory: How groups flatter and deceive themselves. In J. W. Pennebaker, D. Paez & B. Rimé (Eds.), *Collective Memory of Political Events* (pp. 277–293). Mahwah, NJ: Lawrence Erlbaum.

345. Harber, K. D., & Pennebaker, J. W. (1992). Overcoming traumatic memories. In S. A. Christianson (Ed.), *The Handbook of Emotion and Memory: Research and Theory* (pp. 359–387). Hillsdale, NJ: Lawrence Erlbaum.

346. Pennebaker, J. W., Paez, D., & Rimé, B. (Eds.). (1997). *Collective Memory of Political Events*. Mahwah, NJ: Lawrence Erlbaum.

347. Menzies, I. E. P. (1975). A case study in the functioning of social systems as a defense against anxiety. In A. D. Colman & W. H. Bexton (Eds.), *Group Relations Reader I* (pp. 281–312). Washington, D.C.: A. K. Rice Institute Series.

348. Bloom, S. L. (2004a). Neither liberty nor safety: The impact of fear on individuals, institutions, and societies, Part I. *Psychotherapy and Politics International, 2*(2), 78–98.

349. Bloom, S. L. (2004b). Neither liberty nor safety: The impact of fear on individuals, institutions, and societies, Part II. *Psychotherapy and Politics International, 2*(3), 212–228.

350. Bloom, S. L. (2005a). Neither liberty nor safety: The impact of fear on individuals, institutions, and societies. Part III. *Psychotherapy and Politics International, 3*(2), 96–111.

351. Bloom, S. L. (2005b). Neither liberty nor safety: The impact of fear on individuals, institutions, and societies. Part IV. *Psychotherapy and Politics International, 3*(2), 96–111.

352. Silver, S. (1986). An inpatient program for post-traumatic stress disorder: Context as treatment. In C. Figley (Ed.), *Trauma And Its Wake, Volume II: Post-Traumatic Stress Disorder: Theory, Research And Treatment* (pp. 213–231). New York: Brunner/Mazel.

353. Frueh, B. C., G., K. R., Cusack, K. J., Sauvageot, J. A., Cousins, V. C., Yim, E., et al. (2005). Patients' Reports of Traumatic or Harmful Experiences Within the Psychiatric Setting. *Psychiatric Services, 52*, 1123–1133.

354. Robins, C. S., Sauvageot, J. A., Kusack, K. J., Suffoletta-Maierle, S., & Frueh, B. C. (2005). Consumers' perceptions of negative experiences and "sanctuary harm" in psychiatric settings. *Psychiatric Services, 56*(9), 1134–1138.

355. Erikson, K. (1994). *A new species of trouble: The human experience of modern disasters.* New York: W.W. Norton.

356. Singer, J. (1972). *Boundaries of the Soul: The Practice of Jung's Psychology.* New York: Anchor Books.

357. Hede, A. (2007). The shadow group: Towards an explanation of intepersonal conflict in work groups. *Journal of Managerial Psychology, 22*(1), 25–39.

358. Jacques, E. (1955). The social system as a defense against depressive and persecutory anxiety. In M. Klein, P. Herman & R. Money-Kryle (Eds.), *New Directions in Psycho-analysis* (pp. 478–498). London: Tavistock.

359. Spillius, E. B. (1990). Asylum and Society. In E. Trist & H. Murray (Eds.), *The Social Engagement of Social Science, Volume I: The Socio-Psychological Perspective* (pp. 586–612). London: Free Association Books.

360. Bloom, S. L. (1996). Every Time History Repeats Itself the Price Goes Up: The Social Reenactment of Trauma. *Sexual Addiction and Compulsivity, 3*(3), 161–194.

361. Stokes, J. (1994). The unconscious at work in groups and teams: contributions from the work of W. R. Bion. In A. Oberholzer & V. Roberts (Eds.), *The Unconscious at Work* (pp. 19–27). London: Routledge.

362. Lawrence, W. G. (1995). *The presence of totalitarian states-of-mind in institutions.* Paper presented at the Paper read at the inaugural conference on 'Group Relations', of the Institute of Human Relations, Sofia, Bulgaria, 1995. Accessed November 23, 2006 at http://human-nature.com/free-associations/lawren.html.

363. Catherall, D. R. (1995). Coping with secondary traumatic stress: the importance of the therapist's professional peer group. In B. H. Stamm (Ed.), *Secondary Traumatic Stress: Self-Care Issues for Clinicians, Researchers, & Educators* (pp. 80–92). Lutherville, MD: Sidran Press.

364. Douglas, T. (1995). *Scapegoats: Transferring Blame.* London: Routledge.

365. Catherall, D. R. (1995). Preventing institutional secondary traumatic stress disorder. In C. R. Figley (Ed.), *Compassion Fatigue: Coping with Secondary Traumatic Stress Disorder in Those Who Treat the Traumatized.* New York: Brunner/Mazel.

366. McFarlane, A. C., & van der Kolk, B. A. (1996). Trauma and Its Challenge to Society. In B. Van der Kolk, M. A. C. & L. Weisaeth (Eds.), *Traumatic Stress: The Effects of Overwhelming Experience on Mind, Body and Society. New York, Guilford Press.* (pp. 24–46). New York: Guilford Press.

367. Hinshelwood, R. D. (2001). *Thinking About Institutions: Milieux and Madness.* London: Jessica Kingsley.

368. Szegedy-Maszak, M. (2002, June 3). Consuming passion: The mentally ill are taking charge of their own recovery. But they disagree on what that means. *U.S. News and World Report.*

369. Egan, G. (1994). *Working the Shadow Side: A Guide to Positive Behind-the-Scenes Management*. San Francisco: Jossey-Bass.

370. Bloom, S. L. (2011). Trauma-organized Systems and Parallel Process. In N. Tehrani (Ed.), *Managing Trauma in the Workplace: Supporting Workers and Organizations* (pp. 139–153). London: Routledge.

371. Alderfer, C. P., & Smith, K. K. (1982). Studying Intergroup Relations Embedded in Organizations. *Administrative Science Quarterly, 27*(1), 35.

372. Sullivan, C. C. (2002). Finding the Thou in the I: Countertransference and Parallel Process Analysis in Organizational Research and Consultation. *Journal of Applied Behavioral Science, 38*(3), 375.

373. McNeill, B. W., & Worthen, V. (1989). The Parallel Process in Psychotherapy Supervision. *Professional Psychology: Research and Practice, 20*(5), 329–333.

374. Smith, K. K., & Zane, N. (1999). Organizational reflection: Parallel processes at work in a dual consultation. *The Journal of Applied Behavioral Science, 35*(2), 145–162.

375. Smith, K. K. (1989). The Movement of Conflict in Organizations: The Joint Dynamics of Splitting and Triangulation. *Administrative Science Quarterly, 34*(1), 1.

376. Smith, K. K., Simmons, V. M., & Thames, T. B. (1989). "Fix the Women": An intervention into an organizational conflict based on parallel process thinking. *The Journal of Applied Behavioral Science, 25*(1), 11–29.

377. Stanton, A. H., & Schwartz, M. S. (1954). *The Mental Hospital: A Study of Institutional Participation in Psychiatric Illness and Treatment*. New York: Basic Books.

378. Hassabis, D., HKumaran, D., Vann, S. D., & Maguire, E. A. (2007). Patients with hippocampal amnesia cannot imagine new experiences. *Proceedings of the National Academy of Sciences, PNAS, 104*(5), 1726–1731.

379. Boal, K. B., & Bryson, J. M. (1988). Charismatic leadershp: A Phenomenological and structural approach. In J. G. Hunt, B. R. Baliga, H. P. Dachler & C. A. Schreisheim (Eds.), *Emerging Leadership Vistas* (pp. 5–34). Lexington, MA: Lexington Books.

380. Jick, T. D., & Murray, V. V. (1982). The management of hard times: Budget cutbacks in public sector organizations. *Organization Studies, 3*(2), 141–169.

381. Harvard Business Press. (2008). *Managing Crises: Expert Solutions to Everyday Challenges*. Boston: Harvard Business Press.

382. Mitroff, I. I. (2005). *Why Some Companies Emerge Stronger and Better From a Crisis: 7 Essential Lessons for Surviving disaster*. New York: AMACON.

383. Hatfield, E., Cacioppo, J., & Rapson, R. L. (Eds.). (1994). *Emotional Contagion*. New York: Cambridge University Press.

384. Augustine, N. (2000). Managing the Crisis You Tried to Prevent *Harvard Business Review on Crisis Management* (pp. 1–31). Boston: Harvard Business School Press.

385. NIOSH. (2006). Workplace Violence Prevention, Strategy and Research Needs. Cincinnati, OH: Department of Health and Human Services, Centers for Disease and Control Prevention, National Institute for Occupational Safety and Health, [www.cdc.gov/niosh/conferences/work-violence/].

386. Occupational Safety and Health Administration. (2004). Guidelines for Preventing Workplace Violence for Health Care & Social Service Workers (pp. http://www.osha.gov/Publications/osha3148.pdf). Washington, D.C.: United States Department of Labor.

387. Occupational Safety and Health Administration. (2004). Guidelines for Preventing Workplace Violence for Health Care & Social Service Workers, OSHA 3148-01R 2004. Accessed May 20, 2010 at www.osha.gov. Washington, D.C.: United States Department of Labor.

388. Landau, S. F., & Bendalak, Y. (2008). Personnel exposure to violence in hospital emergency wards: a routine activity approach. *Aggressive Behavior, 34*(1), 88–103.

389. Mayer, B., Smith, F., & King, C. (1999). Factors associated with victimization of personnel in emergency departments. *Journal of Emergency Nursing, 26*, 361–366.

390. Kowalenko, T., Walters, B. L., Khare, R. K., & Compton, S. (2005). Workplace violence: A survey of emergency physicians in the State of Michigan. *Annals of Emergency Medicine, 46*, 142–147.

391. Brady, C., & Dickson, R. (1999). Violence in health care settings. In T. Cox (Ed.), *Work-Related Violence: Assessment and Intervention* (pp. 166–182). London: Routledge.

392. Bureau of Justice. (2001). Violence in the Workplace, 1993-99: Bureau of Justice Statistics Special Report, http://www.ojp.usdoj.gov/bjs/pub/pdf/vw99.pdf. Washington, D.C.: Bureau of Statistics, U.S. Department of Justice.

393. Cunningham, J., Connor, D. F., Miller, K., & Jr., R. H. M. (2003). Staff survey results and characteristics that predict assault and injury to personnel working in mental health facilities. *Aggressive Behavior, 29*(1), 31–40.

394. Carmel H, & M., H. (1989). Staff injuries from in-patient violence. *Hospital and Community Psychiatry, 40*, 41–46.

395. Neuman, J. (2004). Injustice, stress and aggression in organizations. In R. W. Griffin & A. M. O'Leary-Kelly (Eds.), *The Dark Side of Organizational Behavior* (pp. 62–102). San Francisco: Jossey-Bass.

396. Rugulies, R., Christensen, K. B., Borritz, M., Villadsen, E., BÃ¼ltmann, U., & Kristensen, T. S. (2007). The contribution of the psychosocial work environment to sickness absence in human service workers: Results of a 3-year follow-up study. *Work & Stress, 21*(4), 293–311.

397. Spector, P. E., Coulter, M. L., Stockwell, H. G., & Matz, M. W. (2007). Perceived violence climate: A new construct and its relationship to workplace physical violence and verbal aggression, and their potential consequences. *Work and Stress, 21*(2), 21(22): 117130.

398. Björkqvist, K., Österman, K., & Hjelt-Bäck, M. (1994). Aggression among university employees. *Aggressive Behavior, 20*(3), 173–184.

399. Einarsen, S., & Skogstad, A. (1996). Bullying at work: Epidemiological findings in public and private proganizations. *European Journal of Work and Organizational Psychology, 5*, 185–201.

400. Zapf, D., Einarsen, S., Hoel, H., & Vartia, M. (2003). Empirical findings on bullying in the workplace. In S. Einarsen, H. Hoel, D. Zapf & C. L. Cooper (Eds.), *Bullying and Emotional Abuse in the workplace: International Perspectives in Research and Practice.* (pp. 104–126). London: Taylor & Francis.

401. Hoel, H., & Coooper, C. L. (2000). *Destructive Conflict and Bullying at Work.* Manchester, England: Universit of Manchester Institute of Science and Technology.

402. Clements, P. T., DeRanieri, J. T., Clark, K., Manno, M. S., & Kuhn, D. W. (2005). Workplace Violence and Corporate Policy for Health Care Settings *Nursing Economics, 23*(3), 119–124.

403. Bartels, S. J. (1987). The aftermath of suicide on the psychiatric inpatient unit. *General Hospital Psychiatry, 9*(3), 189–197.

404. Bultema, J. (1994). Healing process for the multidisciplinary team: Recovering post-inpatient suicide. *Journal of Psychosocial Nursing & Mental Health Services, 32*(2), 19–24.

405. Alexander, D. A. p. i. m. h., Klein, S. T. r. f., Gray, N. M. r. a., Dewar, I. G. s. r. i. p., & Eagles, J. M. c. p. (2000). Suicide by patients: questionnaire study of its effect on consultant psychiatrists. *British Medical Journal, 320*(7249), 1571–1574.

406. Chemtob, C. M., Hamada, R. S., Bauer, G., Kinney, B., & Torigoe, R. Y. (1988). Patients' Suicides: Frequency and Impact on Psychiatrists. *The American Journal of Psychiatry, 145*(2), 224.

407. Hendin, H., Lipschitz, A., Maltsberger, J. T., Haas, A. P., & Wynecoop, S. (2000). Therapists' reaction to patients' suicides. *The American Journal of Psychiatry, 157*(12), 2022.

408. Ellis, T. E., Dickey, T. O., III, & Jones, E. C. (1998). Patient Suicide in Psychiatry Residency Programs: A National Survey of Training and Postvention Practices. *Acad Psychiatry, 22*(3), 181–189.

409. Brown, H. N. (1987). Patient suicide during residency training: Incidence, implications and program response. *Journal of Psychiatric Education, 11*, 201–206.

410. Jacobson, J. M., Ting, L., Sanders, S., & Harrington, D. (2004). Prevalence of and reactions to fatal and nonfatal client suicidal behavior: A national study of mental health social workers. *Omega, 49*(3), 237–248.

411. Hendin, H., Haas, A. P., Maltsberger, J. T., Szanto, K., & Rabinowicz, H. (2004). Factors Contributing to Therapists' Distress After the Suicide of a Patient. *The American Journal of Psychiatry, 161*(8), 1442.

412. Meyers, T. W., & Cornille, T. A. (2002). The trauma of working with traumatized children. In C. R. Figley (Ed.), *Treating Compassion Fatigue* (pp. 39–56). New York: Brunner-Routledge.

413. Lubrano, A. (2010). Study: To survive, family of four needs nearly $60,000, *Philadelphia Inquirer.*

414. National Child Traumatic Stress Network. (2008). *Child Welfare Trauma Training Toolkit: The Essential Elements, Accessed August 23, 2008,* www.NCTSN.org.

415. Appelbaum, S. H., Gandell, J., Shapiro, B. T., Belisle, P., & Hoeven, E. (2000). Anatomy of a merger: behavior of organizational factors and processes throughout the pre- during and post-stages (part 2). *Management Decision, 38*(10), 674–684.

416. Hirschhorn, L. (1997). *Reworking Authority: Leading and Following in the Post Modern Organization.* Cambridge, Mass: MIT Press.

417. Deci, E. L., & Ryan, R. M. (2000). The "What" and "Why" of Goal Pursuits: Human Needs and the Self-Determination of Behavior. *Psychological Inquiry, 11*(4), 227–268.

418. Lynch, M. F. J., Plant, R. W., & Ryan, R. M. (2005). Psychological Needs and Threat to Safety: Implications for Staff and Patients in a Psychiatric Hospital for Youth. *Professional Psychology: Research and Practice, 36*(4), 415–425.

419. Work & Family Newsbrief. (1999). Fortune's "100 Best" have cultures of trust, pride (February), http://www.workfamily.com/

420. Spector, P. E. (1997). The role of frustration in antisocial behavior at work. In R. A. Giacalone & J. Greenberg (Eds.), *Antisocial Behavior in Organizations* (pp. 1–17). Thousand Oaks, CA: Sage Publications.

421. Elangovan, A. R., & Shapiro, D. L. (1998). Betrayal of trust in organizations. *Academy of Management Review, 23*(3), 547–566.

422. Galford, R., & Drapeau, A. S. (2003). The enemies of trust. *Harvard Business Review, February*, 89–95.

423. Bostock, W. W. (2002). Atrocity, Mundanity and Mental State. *Journal of Mundane Behavior, 3*(3), http://mundanebehavior.org/index2.htm.

424. Walmsley, P. R. (2003). Patient suicide and its effect on staff. *Nursing Management (Harrow), 10*(6), 24–26.

425. Baranowsky, A. B. (2002). The Silencing Response in Clinical Practice: On the road to Dialogue. In C. R. Figley (Ed.), *Treating Compassion Fatigue* (pp. 155–170). New York: Brunner-Routledge.

426. Edmondson, V. C., & Munchus, G. (2007). Managing the unwanted truth: a framework for dissent strategy. *Journal of Organizational Change Management, 20*(6), 747–760.

427. Morrison, E. W., & Milliken, F. J. (2000). Organizational silence: A barrier to change and development in a pluralistic world. *The Academy of Management Review, 25*(4), 706.

428. Joyce, B. & Wallbridge, H. (2003). Effects of suicidal behavior on a psychiatric unit nursing team. *Journal of Psychosocial Nursing & Mental Health Services, 41*(3), 14.

429. Jameton, A. (1984). *Nursing Practice: The Ethical Issues.* Englewood Cliffs, NJ: Prentice-Hall.

430. Austin, W., Rankel, M., Kagan, L., Bergum, V., & Lemermeyer, G. (2005). To stay or to go, to speak or stay silent, to act or not to act: moral distress as experienced by psychologists. *Ethics & Behavior, 15*(3), 197–212.

431. Bell, J., & Breslin, J. M. (2008). Healthcare provider moral distress as a leadership challenge. *JONA'S Healthcare Law, Ethics, and Regulation, 10*(4), 94–97.

432. Satcher, D. (1999). Mental Health: A Report of the Surgeon General. Rockville, MD: U. S. Department of Health and Human Services, Substance Abuse and Mental Health Services Administration, Center for Mental Health Services, National Institutes of Health, National Institute of Mental Health.

433. Mayer, J. D., & Salovey, P. (1997). What is emotional intelligence? In P. Salovey & D. J. Sluyter (Eds.), *Emotional Development and Emotional Intelligence: Educational Implications* (pp. 3–31). New York: Basic Books.

434. Rapisarda, B. A. (2002). The impact of emotional intelligence on work team cohesiveness and performance. *International Journal of Organizational Analysis (1993–2002), 10*(4), 363.

435. Nathanson, D. L. (1992). *Shame and Pride: Affect, Sex, and the Birth of the Self.* New York: W.W. Norton.

436. Hatfield, E., Cacioppa, J. T., & Rapson, R. L. (1994). *Emotional Contagion.* New York: Cambridge University Press.

437. Hochschild, A. R. (1983). *The Managed Heart: Commercialization of Human Feeling.* Berkeley, CA: University of California Press.

438. Heery, E., & Noon, M. (2001). emotional labour *Dictionary of Human Resource Management* (pp. 95–95). New York: Oxford University Press.

439. Othman, A. K., Abdullah, H. S., & Ahmad, J. (2008). Emotional intelligence, emotional labor and work effectiveness in service organizationas: A proposed model *Vision (09722629), 12*(1), 31–42.

440. Miller, K. (2002). The Experience of Emotion in the Workplace: Professing in the Midst of Tragedy. *Management Communication Quarterly, 15*(4), 571.

441. Wilk, S. L., & Moynihan, L. M. (2005). Display Rule "Regulators": The Relationship Between Supervisors and Worker Emotional Exhaustion. *Journal of Applied Psychology, 90*(5), 917–927. doi: 10.1037/0021-9010.90.5.917

442. Glomb, T. M., Kammeyer-Mueller, J. D., & Rotundo, M. (2004). Emotional Labor Demands and Compensating Wage Differentials. *Journal of Applied Psychology, 89*(4), 700–714.

443. Steinberg, R. J. (1999). Emotional labor in job evaluation: Redesigning compensation practices. *Annals of the American Academy of Political and Social Science, 561*, 143–157.

444. Wolf, T. M. (1994). Stress, coping and health: enhancing well-being during medical school. *Medical Education, 28*(1), 6–17; discussion 55–17.

445. Mosley, T. J., Perrin, S., Neral, S., Dubbert, P., Grothues, C., & Pinto, B. (1994). Stress, coping, and well-being among third-year medical students. *Academic Medicine, 69*(9), 765–767.

446. Himmelweit, S. (1999). Caring labor. *Annals of the American Academy of Political and Social Science, 561*, 27–38.

447. George, J. M. (2000). Emotions and leadership: The role of emotional intelligence. *Human Relations, 53*(8), 1027.

448. Brotheridge, C. M., & Lee, R. T. (2008). The emotions of managing: an introduction to the special issue. *Journal of Managerial Psychology, 23*(2), 108–117.

449. Pekrun, R., & Frese, M. (1992). Emotions in work and achievement. *International Review of Industrial and Organizational Psychology, 7*, 153–200.

450. Pfeffer, J. (1998). *The Human Equation: Building Profits by Putting People First.* Boston: Harvard Business School Press.

451. Harvey, M., Novicevic, M. M., Buckley, M. R., & Halbesleben, J. R. B. (2004). The Abilene Paradox After Thirty Years: Global Perspective. *Organizational Dynamics, 33*(2), 215–226.

452. Wright, L. (1996). *Corporate Abuse: How "Lean and Mean" Robs People and Profits.* New York: MacMillan.

453. Collins, R. L. (1975). *Conflict Sociology: Toward an Explanatory Science.* New York: Elsevier Science & Technology Books.

454. Bacal, R. (2004). Organizational Conflict—The Good, the Bad, and the Ugly. *Journal for Quality & Participation, 27*(2), 21–22.

455. Miller, M. R. (1985). Understanding and Resolving Conflict. *Nonprofit World Report, 3*(3), 17–18.

456. Wall, J. A., & Callister, R. R. (1995). Conflict and Its Management *Journal of Management, 21*, 515–558.

457. Berstene, T. (2004). The Inexorable Link Between Conflict and Change. *Journal for Quality & Participation, 27*(2), 4–9.

458. Rahim, M. A. (2002). Toward a theory of managing organizational conflict. *International Journal of Conflict Management, 13*(3), 206.

459. Glasl, F., & Ballreich, R. (2006). Team and Organisational Development as a Means for Conflict Prevention and Resolution (pp. http://www.berghof-handbook.net/documents/publications/ballreich_glasl_handbook.pdf).

460. Bodtker, A. M., & Jameson, J. K. (2001). Emotion in conflict formation and its transformation: Application to organizational conflict management. *The International Journal of Conflict Management, 12*(3), 259–275.

461. Kulik, B. W. (2004). An affective process model of work group diversity, conflict, and performance: a paradigm expansion. *Organizational Analysis, 12*(3), 271–294.

462. Nikolaou, I., & Tsaousis, I. (2002). Emotional Intelligence In The Workplace: Exploring Its Effects On Occupational Stress And Organizational Commitment. *International Journal of Organizational Analysis, 10*(4), 327.

463. Amason, A. C. (1996). Distinguishing the effects of functional and dysfunctional conflict on strategic decision making: Resolving a paradox for top management teams *Academy of Management Journal, 39*, 123–148.

464. Jehn, K. A. (1995). A multimethod examination of the benefits and detriments of intragroup conflict. *Administrative Science Quarterly, 40*(2), 256.

465. Jehn, K. A., Northcraft, G. B., & Neale, M. A. (1999). Why differences make a difference: A field study of diversity, conflict, and performance in workgroups. *Administrative Science Quarterly, 44*(4), 741.

466. Wall, V., & Nolan, L. (1986). Perceptions of inequity, satisfaction, and conflict in task-oriented groups *Human Relations, 39*, 1033–1052.
467. Jehn, K. A. (1997). A qualitative analysis of conflict types and dimensions in organizational groups. *Administrative Science Quarterly, 42*, 530–557.
468. Sunstein, C. R. (2003). *Why Societies Need Dissent.* Cambridge, MA: Harvard University Press.
469. Jehn, K. A., & Mannix, E. A. (2001). The dynamic nature of conflict: A longitudinal study of intragroup conflict and group performance. *Academy of Management Journal, 44*(2), 238.
470. Jehn, K. A. (1997). A qualitative analysis of conflict types and dimensions in organizational groups. *Administrative Science Quarterly, 42*(3), 530.
471. Bourgeois, L. J. (1985). Strategic goals, environmental uncertainty, and economic performance in volatile environments *Academy of Management Journal, 28*, 548–573.
472. Eisenhardt, K. M., & Schoonhoven, C. B. (1990). Organizational Growth: Linking Founding Team, Strategy, Environment, and Growth Among U.S. Semiconductor Ventures, 1978–1988. *Administrative Science Quarterly, 35*, 504–529.
473. Putnam, L. L. (1994). Productive conflict: Negotiation as implicit coordination. *International Journal of Conflict Management, 5*, 285–299.
474. Cosier, R. A., & Rose., G. L. (1977). Cognitive Conflict and Goal Conflict Effects on Task Performance. *Organizational Behavior and Human Performance, 19*, 378–391.
475. Fiol, C. M. (1994). Consensus, diversity and learning organizations. *Organization Science, 5*, 403–420.
476. Schweiger, D., Sandberg, W., & Ragan, J. W. (1986). Group approaches for improving strategic decision making: A comparative analysis of dialectical inquiry, devil's advocacy, and consensus approaches to strategic decison making. *Academy of Management Journal, 29*, 51–71.
477. Moberg, P. J. (2001). Linking conflict strategy to the five-factor model: theoretical and empirical foundations. *International Journal of Conflict Management (1997–2002), 12*(1), 47.
478. Argyris, C. (1990). *Overcoming Organizational Defenses: Facilitating Organizational Learning.* Needham Heights, MA: Allyn & Bacon.
479. Buck, V. (1972). *Working Under Pressure.* London: Staples.
480. McLean, A. (1979). *Work Stress.* New York: Addison-Wesley.
481. LaRocco, J. M., House, J. S., & French, J. R. P., Jr. (1980). Social support, occupational stress, a health. *Journal of Health and Social Behavior, 21*, 202–218.
482. Jex, S. M., & Thomas, J. L. (2003). Relations between stressors and group perceptions: main and mediating effects 1. *Work & Stress, 17*(2), 158.
483. Beer, M., & Spector, B. (1993). Organizational diagnosis: Its role in organizational learning. *Journal of Counseling and Development, 71*, 642–650.
484. Othman, R., & Hashim, N. A. (2004). Typologizing organizational amnesia. *The Learning Organization, 11*(2/3), 273.
485. Kotter, J. P. (2008). *A Sense of Urgency.* Boston: Harvard Business Press.
486. Crossen, M. M., Lane, H. W., & White, R. E. (1999). An organizational learning framework: From intuition to institution. *Academy of Management Review, 24*(3), 522–537.
487. Wells, K. (1991). Long-term residential treatment for Children: Introduction,. *Amer. J. Orthopsychiatry, 61*(3), 324.
488. Lahaie, D. (2005). The impact of corporate memory loss: What happens when a senior executive leaves? *Leadership in Health Services, 18*(3), xxxv–xlvii.

489. Feldman, R. M., & Feldman, S. P. (2006). What links the chain: An essay on organizational remembering as practice. *Organization, 13*(6), 861–887.

490. Conklin, J. E. (2001). Designing organizational memory: Preserving Intellectual Assets in a Knowledge Economy, http://www.touchstone.com/tr/whitepapers.html. Washington, D.C.: Touchstone Consulting.

491. Walsh, J. P., & Ungson, G. R. (1991). Organizational Memory. *Academy of Management. The Academy of Management Review, 16*(1), 57.

492. Scheff, T. J. (Ed.). (1975). *Labeling Madness.* Englewood Cliffs, NJ: Prentice-Hall.

493. Scheff, T. J. (1975). The Labeling Theory of Mental Illness. In T. J. Scheff (Ed.), *Labeling Madness* (pp. 21–33). Englewood Cliffs, NJ: Prentice-Hall.

494. Scheff, T. J. (1984). *Being Mentally Ill: A Sociological Theory, Second Edition.* New York: Aldine.

495. Rosenhan, D. L. (1973). On being sane in insane places. *Science, 179*, 250–256.

496. Rosenhan, D. L. (1975). On being sane in insane places. In T. J. Scheff (Ed.), *Labeling Madness* (pp. 54–74). Englewood Cliffs, NJ: Prentice-Hall.

497. Temerlin, M. K. (1975). Suggestion effects in psychiatric diagnosis. In T. J. Scheff (Ed.), *1975* (pp. 46–53). Englewood Cliffs, NJ: Prentice-Hall.

498. Rosenthal, R. (2002). Covert Communication in Classrooms, Clinic Courtrooms, and Cubicles. *American Psychologist, 57*(11), 839–849.

499. Rosenthal, R. (1995). Critiquing Pygmalion: A 25-year perspective. *Current Directions in Psychological Science, 4*(171–172).

500. Moreno, C., Laje, G., Blanco, C., Jiang, H., Schmidt, A., & Olfson, M. (2007). National trends in the outpatient diagnosis and treatment of bipolar disorder in youth. *Archives of General Psychiatry, 64*(9), 1032–1039.

501. Breslau, N., Davis, G., Andreski, P., & Peterson, P. (1991). Traumatic events and post-traumatic stress disorder in an urban population of young adults. *Archives of General Psychiatry, 48*, 216–222.

502. Kessler, R. C., Davis, C. G., & Kendler, K. S. (1997). Childhood adversity and adult psychiatric disorder in the US National Comorbidity Survey. *Psychol Med, 27*(5), 1101–1119.

503. Argyris, C., & Schon, D. (1996). *Organization Learning II.* Reading, MA: Addison-Wesley.

504. Halbwachs, M. (1992). *On collective memory.* Chicago: University of Chicago Press.

505. Kransdorff, A. (1998). *Corporate Amnesia: Keeping Know-How in the Company.* Woburn, MA: Butterworth-Heineman.

506. NewsBriefs. (2000). More Knowledge; Song strikes chord. *Computing Canada* (May 12).

507. Cole, R. (1993). Learning from learning theory: Implications for quality improvement of turnover, use of contingent workers, and job rotation policies. *Quality Management Journal, 1*, 9–25.

508. Hazell, J. E. (2000). Private sector downsizing: Implications for DOD. *Acquisition Review Quarterly*(March 22).

509. Kransdorff, A. (1997). Fight organizational memory lapse. *Workforce, 76*(9), 34.

510. Frost, P. J. (2003). *Toxic Emotions At Work: How Compassionate Managers Handle Pain and Conflict.* Boston, MA: Harvard Business School.

511. Lievegoed, B. C. J. (1973). *The Developing Organization.* London: Tavistock.

512. Santayana, G. (1998). *The Life of Reason (Great Books in Philosophy)* Amherst, NY: Prometheus Books.

513. Bradford, E. W. (2005). Sued? Calm down! *Medical Economics, 82*(16), 52.

514. Coates, D., Wortman, C. B., & Abben, A. (1979). Reactions to victims. In I. H. Frieze, D. Bar-Tal & J. C. Carroll (Eds.), *New Approaches to Social Problems.* San Francisco: Jossey Bass.

515. Mellers, B. A., Schwartz, A., & Cooke, A. D. J. (1998). Judgment and decision making. *Annual Review of Psychology, 49,* 447.

516. Iannello, K. P. (1992). *Decisions Without Hierarchy: Feminist Interventions in Organization Theory and Practice.* New York: Routledge.

517. Kerr, N. L., & Tindale, R. S. (2004). Group Performance and Decision Making. *Annual Review of Psychology, 55,* 623.

518. Weick, K. E. (2001). *Making Sense of the Organization.* Malden, MA: Blackwell.

519. Kassing, J. W. (1997). Articulating, antagonizing, and displacing: A model of employee dissent. *Communication Studies, 48*(4), 311.

520. Kassing, J. W., & Armstrong, T. A. (2002). Someone's going to hear about this. *Management Communication Quarterly: McQ, 16*(1), 39.

521. Kassing, J. W. (2001). From the looks of things. *Management Communication Quarterly: McQ, 14*(3), 442.

522. Moscovici, S., & Zavalloni, M. (1969). The group as a polarizer of attitudes. *Journal of Personality and Social Psychology, 12,* 125–135.

523. Sunstein, C. R. (2009). *On Rumors: How Falsehoods Spread, Why We Believe Them, What Can Be Done.* New York: Farrar Straua and Giroux.

524. Finet, D. (1994). Sociopolitical consequences of organizational expression. *Journal of Communication, 44*(4), 114.

525. Small, R., Kennedy, K., & Bender, B. (1991). Critical Issues for Practice in Residential Treatment: The View from Within. *American Journal of Orthopsychiatry, 61*(3), 327–337.

526. Wells, K. (1991). Long-term residential treatment for Children: Introduction. *American Journal of Orthopsychiatry, 61*(3), 324.

527. Abramovitz, R., & Bloom, S. L. (2003). Creating Sanctuary in a residential treatment setting for troubled children and adolescents. *Psychiatric Quarterly, 74*(2), 119–135.

528. Bazelon Center for Mental Health Law. (2004). Get It Together: How to Integrate Physical and Mental Health Care for People with Serious Mental Disorders. Washington, D.C.: Bazelon Center for Mental Health Law.

529. Tracy, L. (1994). *Leading the Living Organization: Growth Strategies for Management.* Westport, CT: Quorum Books.

530. Gazzaniga, M. S. (2008). *Human: The Science BEhind What Makes Us Unique.* New York: HarperCollins.

531. Dunbar, R. I. M. (1993). Coevolution of neocortical size, group size and language in humans. Behavioral and Brain Sciences 16(4), 681–735.

532. Gladwell, M. (2002). *The Tipping Point: How Little Things Can Make a Big Difference*: Little, Brown and Company.

533. Kanter, R. M., & Stein, B. A. (1992). *The Challenge of Organizational Change: How Companies Experience It and Leaders Guide It.* New York: The Free Press.

534. Marcus, A. A., & Nichols, M. L. (1999). On the Edge: Heeding the Warnings of Unusual Events. *Organization Science: A Journal of the Institute of Management Sciences, 10*(4), 482.

535. Mandler, G. (1982). Stress and thought processes. In L. Goldberger & S. Breznitz (Eds.), *Handbook of Stress* (pp. 88–104). New York: Free Press.

536. Fulk, J., & Mani, S. (1985). Distortion of communication in hierarchical relationships. In M. McLaughlin (Ed.), *Communication Yearbook 9* (pp. 483–510). Newbury Park, CA: Sage.

537. Stohl, C., & Redding, W. C. (1987). Messages and message exchange processes. In F. M. Jablin, L. L. Putnam, K. H. Roberts & L. W. Porter (Eds.), *Handbook of Organizational Communication* (pp. 451–502). Newbury Park, CA: Sage.

538. Crampton, S. M., Hodge, J. W., & Mishra, J. M. (1998). The informal communication network: Factors influencing grapevine activity. *Public Personnel Management, 27*(4), 569.

539. Rosnow, R. L. (1988). Rumor as Communication: A Contextualist Approach. *Journal of Communication, 38*(1), 10–28.

540. Michelson, G., & Mouly, V. S. (2004). Do loose lips sink ships?: The meaning, antecedents and consequences of rumour and gossip in organisations. *Corporate Communications, 9*(3), 189.

541. Michelson, G., & Mouly, S. (2000). Rumour and gossip in organisations: a conceptual study. *Management Decision, 38*(5), 339.

542. Kurland, N. B., & Pelled, L. H. (2000). Passing the word: Toward a model of gossip and power in the workplace. *Academy of Management. The Academy of Management Review, 25*(2), 428.

543. Baker, J. S., & Jones, M. A. (1996). The poison grapevine: How destructive are gossip and rumor i. *Human Resource Development Quarterly, 7*(1), 75.

544. Morrison, E. W., & Milliken, F. J. (2000). Organizational silence: A barrier to change and development in a pluralistic world. *The Academy of Management Review, 25*(4), 706.

545. Argyris, C. (1993). *Knowledge for Action: A Guide to Overcoming Barriers to Organizational Change*. San Francisco: Jossey-Bass.

546. Hammond, S. A., & Mayfield, A. B. (2004). *The Thin Book of Naming Elephants: How to Surface Undiscussables for Greater Organizational Success*. Bend, OR: Thin Book Publishing Co.

547. Caudill, W. (1958). *The Psychiatric Hospital as a Small Society*. Cambridge, MA: Harvard University Press.

548. Zimbardo, P. (2007). *The Lucifer Effect: Understanding How Good People Turn Evil*. New York: Random House.

549. Kassing, J. W. (1998). Development and validation of the organizational dissent scale. *Management Communication Quarterly: McQ, 12*(2), 183.

550. Michels, R. (1962). *Political parties: A Sociological Study of the Oligarchical Tendencies of Modern Democracy*. New York: Free Press.

551. Ewing, D. (1977). *Freedom Inside the Organization*. New York: Dutton.

552. Sanders, W. (1983). The first amendment and the government workplace: Has the constitution fallen down on the job? *Western Journal of Speech Communication, 47*, 253–276.

553. Scheff, T. J. (1970). Control over policy by attendants in a mental hospital. In H. W. In Polsky, D. S. Claster & C. Goldberg (Eds.), *Social System Perspectives in Residential Institutions* (pp. 240–258). East Lansing, MI: Michigan State University Press.

554. Dalberg-Acton, J. E. E. (1949). *Essays on Freedom and Power*. Boston: Beacon press.

555. DeMause, L. (1974). *The History of Childhood*. New York: Psychohistory Press.

556. Shirtcliff, E. A., Vitacco, M. J., Graf, A. R., Gostisha, A. J., Merz, J. L., & Zahn-Waxler, C. (2009). Neurobiology of empathy and callousness: Implications for the development of antisocial behavior. *Behavioral Sciences & the Law, 27*(2), 137–171.

557. Seabrook, J. (2008). Suffering souls: The Search for the roots of psychopathy. *The New Yorker*, November 10. Retrieved from http://www.newyorker.com/reporting/2008/11/10/081110fa_fact_seabrook

558. Decety, J., Michalska, K. J., Akitsuki, Y., & Lahey, B. B. (2008). Atypical empathic responses in adolescents with aggressive conduct disorder: A functional MRI investigation. *Biological Psychology, In Press, Corrected Proof, Available online 30 September 2008.* Accessed November 13, 2008.

559. Stout, M. (2005). *The Sociopath Next Door.* New York: Broadway Books.

560. Scaer, R. (2005). *The Trauma Spectrum: Hidden Wounds and Human Resiliency.* New York: Norton.

561. Peterson, C., Maier, S. E., & Seligman, M. (1993). *Learned helplessness: A theory for the age of personal control.* New York: Oxford University Press.

562. Amichai-Hamburger, Y., Mikulincer, M., & Zalts, N. (2003). The Effects of Learned Helplessness on the Processing of a Persuasive Message. *Current Psychology, 22*(1), 37.

563. Mikulincer, M. (1989). Coping and learned helplessness: effects of coping strategies on performance following unsolvable problems. *European Journal of Personality, 3*(3), 181–194.

564. Overmier, J. B. (2002). On Learned Helplessness. *Integrative Physiological & Behavioral Science, 37*(1), 4.

565. Campbell, C. R., & Martinko, M. J. (1998). An integrative attributional perspective of empowerment and learned helplessness: A multimethod field study. *Journal of Management, 24*(2), 173–200.

566. McGrath, R. (1994). Organizationally induced helplessness: The antithesis of employment. *Quality Progress*, April, 89–92.

567. Carlson, D. S., & Kacmar, K. M. (1994). Learned helplessness as a predictor of employee outcomes: An applied model. *Human Resource Management Review, 4*(3), 235.

568. Beck, A. J., & Guerino, P. (2010). Sexual Victimization in Juvenile Facilities Reported by Youth, 2008–09 *Bureau of Justice Statistics Special Report*, January 2010, NCJ 228416. Accessed 1/9/10 at http://bjs.ojp.usdoj.gov/content/pub/pdf/svjfry09.pdf. Washington, D.C.: U. S. Department of Justice.

569. UNICEF. (2009). Convention on the Rights of the Child. Accessed 1/9/10 at http://www.unicef.org/crc/.

570. Kankus, R. F., & Cavalier, R. P. (1995). Combating organizationally induced helplessness. *Quality Progress, 28*(12), 89.

571. Martinko, M. J., & Gardner, W. L. (1982). Learned helplessness: An alternative explanation for performance deficits. *Academy of Management. The Academy of Management Review (pre-1986), 7*, 195–204.

572. Schepman, S. B., & Richmond, L. (2003). Employee expectations and motivation: An application from the "learned helplessness" paradigm. *Journal of American Academy of Business, 3*(1/2), 405.

573. Bloom, S. L. (2003). Caring for the Caregiver: Avoiding and Treating Vicarious Trauma. In A. Giardino, E. Datner, J. Asher & Chapter (Eds.), *Sexual Assault, Victimization Across the Lifespan* (pp. 459–470). Maryland Heights, MO: GW Medical Publishing.

574. Young, M. (1998). *Collective Trauma: Insights From a Research Errand,* http://www.aaets.org/article55.htm.

575. Beck, U. (1992). *Risk Society: Towards a New Modernity.* London: Sage.

576. Heyman, B. (Ed.). (1998). *Risk, Health and Health Care—A Qualitative Approach.* London: Arnold Publishers.

577. Skolbekken, J.-A. (1995). The risk epidemic in medical journals. *Social Science & Medicine, 40*(3), 291–305.

578. Giddens, A. (1991). *Modernity and Self-Identity: Self and Society in the Late Modern Age.* Cambridge: Polity Press.

579. Giddens, A. (1998). Risk society: the context of British politics. In J. Franklin (Ed.), *The Politics of Risk Society* (pp. 23–34). Cambridge: Polity Press.

580. McGuire, J. (2004). Minimising harm in violence risk assessment: practical solutions to ethical problems? *Health, Risk & Society, 6*(4), 327–345.

581. Holmes, C. A., & Warelow, P. (1999). Implementing psychiatry as risk management: DSM-IV as a postmodern taxonomy. *Health, Risk & Society, 1*(2), 167.

582. Warner, J., & Gabe, J. (2004). Risk and liminality in mental health social work. *Health, Risk & Society, 6*(4), 387–399.

583. Busfield, J. (2004). Mental health problems, psychotropic drug technologies and risk. *Health, Risk & Society, 6*(4), 361–375.

584. Lipman-Blumen, J. (2004). *Allure of Toxic Leaders: Why We Follow Destructive Bosses and Corrupt Politicians - and How We Can Survive Them.* New York: Oxford University Press.

585. Klein, N. (2007). *The Shock Doctrine: The Rise of Disaster Capitalism.* New York: Metropolitan Books.

586. Murdach, A. D. (1995). Decision-making situations in health care. *Health & Social Work, 20*(3), 187–191.

587. Altemeyer, B. (1996). *The Authoritarian Specter.* Cambridge, Mass.; London: Harvard University Press.

588. Krauss, S. W., Streib, H., Keller, B., & Silver, C. (2006). The Distinction between Authoritarianism and Fundamentalism in Three Cultures: Factor Analysis and Personality Correlates *Psychology of Religion, 28*(1), 341–348.

589. Gladwell, M. (2008). *Outliers: The Story of Success.* New York: Little Brown and Company.

590. Salin, D. (2003). Ways of explaining workplace bullying: A review of enabling, motivating and precipitating structures and processes in the work environment. *Human Relations, 56*(10), 1213.

591. Namie, G., & Namie, R. (2003). *The Bully at Work: What You Can do to Stop the Hurt and Reclaim Your Dignity on the Job.* Naperville, IL: Sourcebooks, Inc.

592. Einarsen, S. (1999). The nature and causes of bullying at work. *International Journal of Manpower, 20*(1/2), 16.

593. Millar, M. (2005). NHS could save millions by tackling workplace bullying, *Personnel Today, 09595848, 9/27/2005.*

594. Brodsky, C. M. (1976). *The Harassed Worker.* Toronto: Lexington Books, D.C. Heath and Company.

595. Leymann, H., & Gustafsson, A. (1996). Mobbing at work and the development of post-traumatic stress disorders. *European Journal of Work and Organizational Psychology, 5,* 251–276.

596. Ashforth, B. (1994). Petty Tyranny in Organizations. *Human Relations, 47*(7), 755–778.

597. McGregor, D. (1960). *The Human Side of Enterprise.* New York: McGraw-Hill.

598. Mansbridge, J. (1973). Time, emotion, and inequality: Three problems of participatory groups. *Journal of Applied Behavioral Science 9,* 351–368.

599. Barker, J. (1993). Tightening the iron cage: Concertive control in the self-managing organization. *Administrative Science Quarterly, 38*, 408–437.

600. Cheney, G. (1995). Democracy in the workplace: Theory and practice from the perspective of communication. *Journal of Applied Communication Research, 23*, 167–200.

601. Argyris, C. (1998). Empowerment: The Emperor's New Clothes. *Harvard Business Review, 76*(3), 98–105.

602. Ciulla, J. B. (Ed.). (2004). *Ethics, the Heart of Leadership, Second Edition.* Westport, CT: Praeger.

603. Wren, T. (1996). The Historical Background of Values in Leadership. 1–11. Retrieved from http://www.academy.umd.edu/Resources/AcademyPublicationsPDF/KLSP/EthicsandLeadership/HistoricalBackground/HistoricalBackground.pdf

604. Stuckless, N., & Goranson, R. (1994). A selected bibliography of literature on revenge. *Psychological Reports 75*, 803–811.

605. Elster, J. (1990). Norms of revenge. *Ethics, 100*, 862–885.

606. Fromm, E. (1973). *The Anatomy of Human Destructiveness.* Greenwich, CT: Fawcett Publications, Inc.

607. Schulman, M., & Mekler, E. (1994). *Bringing Up A Moral Child.* New York: Doubleday.

608. Bloom, P. (2010). The moral life of babies, *New York Times,* pp. 44–49, 56, 62–63, 65.

609. Herzberger, S. D., & Hall, J. A. (1993). Children's evaluations of retaliatory aggression against siblings and friends. *Journal of Interpersonal Violence, 8*(1), 77–93.

610. Staub, E. (1992). Transforming the bystanders: Altruism, caring and social responsibility. In H. Fein (Ed.), *Genocide Watch.* New Haven: Yale Univerity Press.

611. Staub, E. (1989). *The Roots of Evil: The Origins of Genocide and Other Group Violence.* New York: Cambridge University Press.

612. Fogelman, E. (1994). *Conscience & Courage: Rescuers of Jews During the Holocaust.* New York: Anchor Books.

613. Milgram, S. (1974). *Obedience to Authority.* New York: Harper Colophon.

614. Newman, D. M. (2003). *Sociology: Exploring the Architecture of Everyday Life.* Thousand Oaks, CA: Pine Forge Press.

615. Hamilton, V. L., & Sanders, J. (1995). Crimes of obedience and conformity in the workplace: Surveys of Americans, Russians, and Japanese. *Journal of Social Issues, 51*, 67–88.

616. Gamson, W. A., Fireman, B., & Rytina, S. (1982). *Encounters with unjust authority.* Homewood, IL: Dorsey Press.

617. Haney, C., Banks, C., & Zimbardo, P. G. (1973). Interpersonal dynamics in a simulated prison. *International Journal of Criminology and Penology, 1*, 69–97.

618. Kipnis, D., Castell, P. J., Gergen, M., & Mauch, D. (1976). Metamorphic effects of power. *Journal of Applied Psychology, 61*, 127–135.

619. Kelman, H. C., & Hamilton, V. L. (1989). The My Lai Massacre: A Military Crime of Obedience. In H. C. Kelman & V. L. Hamilton (Eds.), *Crimes of Obedience* (pp. 1–20). New Haven: Yale University Press.

620. Figley, C. (1995). *Compassion fatigue: Coping with secondary traumatic stress disorder in those who treat the traumatized.* New York: Brunner/Mazel.

621. Stamm, B. H. (1995). *Secondary Traumatic Stress: Self Care Issues for Clinicians, Researchers and Educators.* Baltimore, MD: Sidran Foundation.

622. Cahn, E. (1949). *The sense of injustice.* New York: New York University Press.

623. Degoey, P. (2000). Contagious justice: Exploring the social construction of justice in organizations. *Research in Organizational Behavior, 22*, 51–102.

624. Ambrose, M. L. (2002). Contemporary justice research: A new look at familiar questions. *Organizational Behavior and Human Decision Processes, 89*(1), 803–812.

625. Cropanzano, R., Bowen, D. E., & Gilliland, S. W. (2007). The Management of Organizational Justice *Academy of Management Perspectives, November*, 34–48.

626. Lind, E. A., Greenberg, J., Scott, K. S., & Welchans, T. D. (2000). The winding road from employee to complainant: Situational and psychological determinants of wrongful termination claims. *Administrative Science Quarterly, 45*, 557–590.

627. Brockner, J. (2006). Why It's So Hard to Be Fair. *Harvard Business Review, Reprint Number R0603H.*

628. Ambrose, M. L., & Schminke, M. (2003). Organization Structure as a Moderator of the Relationship Between Procedural Justice, Interactional Justice, Perceived Organizational Support, and Supervisory Trust. *Journal of Applied Psychology, 88*(2), 295–305.

629. Elovainio, M., Leino-Arjas, P., Vahtera, J., & Kivimäki, M. (2006). Justice at work and cardiovascular mortality: a prospective cohort study. *Journal of Psychosomatic Research, 61*(2), 271–274.

630. Elovainio, M., Kivimäki, M., Steen, N., & Vahtera, J. (2004). Job decision latitude, organizational justice and health: multilevel covariance structure analysis. *Social Science & Medicine, 58*(9), 1659–1669.

631. Elovainio, M., Kivimäki, M., Vahtera, J., Keltikangas-Järvinen, L., & Virtanen, M. (2003). Sleeping Problems and Health Behaviors as Mediators Between Organizational Justice and Health. *Health Psychology, 22*(3), 287–293.

632. Elovainio, M., van den Bos, K., Linna, A., Kivimäki, M., Ala-Mursula, L., Pentti, J., et al. (2005). Combined effects of uncertainty and organizational justice on employee health: Testing the uncertainty management model of fairness judgments among Finnish public sector employees. *Social Science & Medicine, 61*(12), 2501–2512.

633. Spell, C. S., & Arnold, T. J. (2007). A Multi-Level Analysis of Organizational Justice Climate, Structure, and Employee Mental Health. *Journal of Management, 33*(5), 724–751.

634. Tepper, B. J. (2001). Health Consequences of Organizational Injustice: Tests of Main and Interactive Effects. *Organizational Behavior and Human Decision Processes, 86*(2), 197–215.

635. Skarlicki, D. P., & Folger, R. (2004). Broadening our understanding of organizational retaliatory behavior. In R. W. Griffin & A. M. O'Leary-Kelly (Eds.), *The Dark Side of Organizational Behavior* (pp. 373–402). San Francisco: Jossey-Bass.

636. Tripp, T. M., Bies, R. J., & Aquino, K. (2002). Poetic justice or petty jealousy? The aesthetics of revenge. *Organizational Behavior and Human Decision Processes, 89*(1), 966–984.

637. Ambrose, M. L., Seabright, M. A., & Schminke, M. (2002). Sabotage in the workplace: The role of organizational injustice. *Organizational Behavior and Human Decision Processes, 89*(1), 947–965.

638. Huberman, J. (1964). Discipline without punishment. *Harvard Business Review, 42*(4), 62–68.

639. Sims, H. P., Jr. (1980). Further Thoughts on Punishment in Organizations. *Academy of Management. The Academy of Management Review, 5*(1), 133.

640. Butterfield, K. D., Treviño, L. K., Wade, K. J., & Ball, G. A. (2005). Organizational Punishment from the Manager's Perspective: An Exploratory Study. *Journal of Managerial Issues, 17*(3), 363.

641. Arvey, R. D., & Ivancevich, J. M. (1980). Punishment in organizations: A review, propositions, and research suggestions. *The Academy of Management Review, 5*(000001), 123.

642. Hamblin, R. L. (1964). Punitive and non-punitive supervision. *Social Problems, 11*, 345–359.

643. Gross, S. J., & Shapiro, J. P. (2004). Using Multiple Ethical Paradigms and Turbulence Theory in Response to Administrative Dilemmas. *International Studies in Educational Administration, 32*(2), 47–62.

644. Grevin, P. (1990). *Spare the Child: The Religious Roots of Punishment and the Psychological Impact of Physical Abuse.* New York: Vintage.

645. Straus, M. A. (1994). *Beating the Devil Out of Them: Corporal Punishment in American Families.* New York: Lexington Books.

646. Baucus, M. S., & Beck-Dudley, C. L. (2005). Designing Ethical Organizations: Avoiding the Long-Term Negative Effects of Rewards and Punishments. *Journal of Business Ethics, 56*(4), 355–370.

647. Power, F. C., Higgins, A., & Kohlberg, L. (1989). *Lawrence Kohlberg's Approach to Moral Education.* New York: Columbia University Press.

648. Logsdon, J. M., & Yuthas, K. (1997). Corporate social performance, stakeholder orientation and organizational moral development. *Journal of Business Ethics, 16*, 1213–1226.

649. Badaracco, J. L. J., & Webb, A. P. (1995). Business ethics: A view from the trenches. *California Management Review, 37*(2), 8.

650. Trevino, L. K. (1992). Moral Reasoning and Business Ethics: Implications for Research, Education, and Management. *Journal of Business Ethics, 11*(5–6), 445.

651. Bloom, S. L. (2007). Loss in human service organizations. In A. L. Vargas & S. L. Bloom (Eds.), *Loss, Hurt and Hope: The Complex Issues of Bereavement and Trauma in Children* (pp. 142–206). Newcastle, UK: Cambridge Scholars Publishing.

652. Jeffreys, J. S. (2005). *Coping with Workplace Grief: Dealing with Loss, Trauma, and Change, Revised Edition.* Boston, MA: Thomson Course Technology.

653. Rando, T. A. (1993). *Treatment of Complicated Mourning.* Champaign, IL: Research Press.

654. Boss, P. (2006). *Loss. Trauma, and Resilience: Therapeutic Work With Ambiguous Loss.* New York: W.W. Norton.

655. Doka, K., & Davidson, J. (1998). *Living with grief: Who we are, how we grieve.* Washington, D.C.: Brunner/Mazel.

656. Bento, R. F. (1994). When the show must go on: Disenfranchised grief in organizations. *Journal of Managerial Psychology, 9*(6), 35.

657. Gabriel, Y. (1993). Organizational nostalgia - Reflections on 'The Golden Age'. In S. Fineman (Ed.), *Emotion in Organizations* (pp. 118–141). Thousand Oaks, CA: Sage Publications.

658. Hubiak, W. A., & O Donnell, S. J. (1997). Downsizing: A pervasive form of organizational suicide. *National Productivity Review, 16*(2), 31.

659. Buono, A. F., & Bowditch, J. L. (1990). Ethical Considerations in Merger and Acquisition Management: A Human Resource Perspective. *Advanced Management Journal, 55*(4), 18.

660. Carr, A. (2001). Understanding emotion and emotionality in a process of change. *Journal of Organizational Change Management, 14*(5), 421–434.

661. Bloom, S. L. (2003). Bridging the black hole of trauma: The evolutionary necessity of the arts., from www.sanctuaryweb.com

662. Driver, T. F. (1991). *The Magic of Ritual: Our Need for Liberating Rites That Transform Our Lives and Our Communities.* San Francisco: HarperSanFrancisco.

663. Wright, L., & Smye, M. (1996). *Corporate Abuse: How "Lean and Mean" Robs People and Profits.* New York: MacMillan.

664. Ettin, M. R. (1993). Links between group process and social, political, and cultural issues. In H. I. Kaplan & B. J. Sadock (Eds.), *Comprehensive Group Psychotherapy* (pp. 699–715). Baltimore: Williams and Wilkins.

665. Bloom, S. L. (2005). Neither liberty nor safety: The impact of trauma on individuals, institutions, and societies. Part III. *Psychotherapy and Politics International, 3*(2), 96–111.

666. Figley, C. R. (1995). Compassion fatigue as secondary traumatic stress disorder: An overview, in. In C. R. Figley (Ed.), *Compassion fatigue: Coping with secondary traumatic stress disorder in those who treat the traumatized,* (pp. 1–20). New York: Brunner/Mazel.

667. Pearlman, L. (1995). Self Care for Trauma Therapists: Ameliorating Vicarious Traumatization. In B. Stamm (Ed.), *Secondary traumatic stress: Self-care issues for clinicians, researchers, & educators.* (pp. 51–64). Lutherville, MD: Sidran Press.

668. Pines, A. M., & Arenson, E. (1988). *Career Burnout: Causes and Cures.* New York: Free Press.

669. Cordes, C. L., & Dougherty, T. W. (1993). A review and an integration of research on job burnout. *Academy of Management. The Academy of Management Review, 18*(4), 621.

670. Angerer, J. M. (2003). Job burnout. *Journal of Employment Counseling, 40*(3), 98.

671. Golembiewski, R. T., Hilles, R., & Daly, R. (1987). Some Effects of Multiple OD Interventions on Burnout and Work Site Features. *The Journal of Applied Behavioral Science, 23*(3), 295.

672. Weitzel, W., & Jonsson, E. (1989). Decline in Organizations: A Literature Integration and Extension. *Administrative Science Quarterly, 34*(1), 91.

673. Whetten, D. A. (1980). Organizational Decline: A Neglected Topic in Organizational Science. *Academy of Management Review, 5*(4), 577.

674. Menzies, I. E. P. (1975). A case study in the functioning of social systems as a defense against anxiety. In A. D. Coleman & W. H. Bexton (Eds.), *Group Relations Reader I.* Washington, D. C.: Rice Institute Series.

675. Cameron, K. S., Whetten, D. A., & Kim, M. U. (1987). Organizational dysfunctions of decline. *Academy of Management Journal, 30*(1), 126.

676. Mckinley, W. (1993). Organizational decline and adaptation: theoretical controversies. *Organization Science: A Journal of the Institute of Management Sciences, 4*(1), 1.

677. Hager, M., Galaskiewicz, J., Bielefeld, W., & Pins, J. (1999). "Tales from the Grave": Organizations' Accounts of Their Own Demise. In H. K. Anheier (Ed.), *When Things Go Wrong: Organizational Faiilures and Breakdowns* (pp. 51–70). Thousand Oaks, CA: Sage Publications.

678. Seibel, W. (1999). Successful failure: An alternative view of organizational coping. In H. K. Anheier (Ed.), *When Things Go Wrong: Organizational Faiilures and Breakdowns* (pp. 91–104). Thousand Oaks: Sage Publications.

679. Meyer, M., & Zucker, L. (1989). *Permanently Failing Organizations*. Newbury Park, CA: Sage Publications.

680. Senge, P., Kleiner, A., Roberts, C., Ross, R. B., & Smith, B. J. (1994). *The Fifth Discipline Fieldbook: Strategies and Tools for Building a Learning Organization*. New York: Doubleday.

681. Rivard, J. C., Bloom, S. L., Abramovitz, R. A., Pasquale, L., Duncan, M., McCorkle, D., et al. (2003). Assessing the Implementation and Effects of a Trauma-Focused Intervention for Youths in Residential Treatment. *Psychiatric Quarterly, 74*(2), 137–154.

682. Rivard, J. C. (2004). Initial Findings of an Evaluation of a Trauma Recovery Framework in Residential Treatment. *Residential Group Care Quarterly, 5*(1), 3–5.

683. Rivard, J. C., McCorkle, D., Duncan, M. E., Pasquale, L. E., Bloom, S. L., & Abramovitz, R. (2004). Implementing a Trauma Recovery Framework for Youths in Residential Treatment. *Child and Adolescent Social Work Journal, 21*(5), 529–550.

684. Rivard, J. C. (2004). Initial Findings of an Evaluation of a Trauma Recovery Framework in Residential Treatment. *Residential Group Care Quarterly: Child Welfare League of America, 5*(1), 3–5.

Index